The Colonial Life of Pharmaceuticals

Situated at the crossroads between the history of colonialism, of modern Southeast Asia, and of medical pluralism, this history of medicine and health traces the life of pharmaceuticals in Vietnam under French rule. Laurence Monnais examines the globalization of the pharmaceutical industry, looking at both circulation and consumption, considering access to drugs and the existence of multiple therapeutic options in a colonial context. She argues that colonialism was crucial to the world-wide diffusion of modern medicines and speaks to contemporary concerns regarding overreliance on pharmaceuticals, drug toxicity, self-medication, and the accessibility of effective medicines. Retracing the steps by which pharmaceuticals were produced and distributed, readers meet the many players in the process – from colonial doctors to private pharmacists, from consumers to various drug traders and healers. Yet this is not primarily a history of medicines as objects of colonial science, but rather a history of medicines as tools of social change.

Laurence Monnais is Professor of History and Director of the Center for Asian Studies (CETASE) at Université de Montréal, Canada. She specializes in the history of medicine in Southeast Asia, global histories of health, and the history of alternative medicines. A Fellow of the Royal Society of Canada, she is also co-founder and president of HOMSEA (History of Medicine in Southeast Asia).

Global Health Histories

Series editor:

Sanjoy Bhattacharya, University of York

Global Health Histories aims to publish outstanding and innovative scholarship on the history of public health, medicine and science worldwide. By studying the many ways in which the impact of ideas of health and well-being on society were measured and described in different global, international, regional, national and local contexts, books in the series reconceptualize the nature of empire, the nation state, extra-state actors and different forms of globalization. The series showcases new approaches to writing about the connected histories of health and medicine, humanitarianism, and global economic and social development.

The Colonial Life of Pharmaceuticals

Medicines and Modernity in Vietnam

Laurence Monnais

Université de Montréal

Translated by Noémi Tousignant

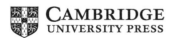
CAMBRIDGE
UNIVERSITY PRESS

CAMBRIDGE
UNIVERSITY PRESS

University Printing House, Cambridge CB2 8BS, United Kingdom

One Liberty Plaza, 20th Floor, New York, NY 10006, USA

477 Williamstown Road, Port Melbourne, VIC 3207, Australia

314-321, 3rd Floor, Plot 3, Splendor Forum, Jasola District Centre, New Delhi - 110025, India

103 Penang Road, #05-06/07, Visioncrest Commercial, Singapore 238467

Cambridge University Press is part of the University of Cambridge.

It furthers the University's mission by disseminating knowledge in the pursuit of education, learning and research at the highest international levels of excellence.

www.cambridge.org
Information on this title: www.cambridge.org/9781108466530
DOI: 10.1017/9781108567152

© Laurence Monnais 2019

This edition is a revised, expanded and updated translation of *Médicaments coloniaux. L'expérience vietnamienne, 1905–1940* (Paris: Les Indes savants, 2014) by Laurence Monnais. It was translated by Noémi Tousignant.

First paperback edition 2022

A catalogue record for this publication is available from the British Library

Library of Congress Cataloging in Publication data
Names: Monnais-Rousselot, Laurence, author. | Tousignant, Noemi, translator.
Title: The colonial life of pharmaceuticals : medicines and modernity in Vietnam / Laurence Monnais ; translated by Noemi Tousignant.
Other titles: Médicaments coloniaux. English | Global health histories (Series)
Description: Cambridge, United Kingdom ; New York, NY : Cambridge University Press, [2019] | Series: Global health histories | "This edition is a revised, expanded and updated translation of Medicaments coloniaux. L'experience Vietnamienne, 1905–1940 (Paris: Les Indes savants, 2014)" | Includes bibliographical references and index.
Identifiers: LCCN 2019008530 | ISBN 9781108474665 (hardback)
Subjects: | MESH: Pharmaceutical Preparations – history | Drug Therapy – history | Colonialism – history | Social Change – history | History, 19th Century | History, 20th Century | Vietnam | France
Classification: LCC RM47.V5 | NLM QV 11 JV6 | DDC 615.109597–dc23
LC record available at https://lccn.loc.gov/2019008530

ISBN 978-1-108-47466-5 Hardback
ISBN 978-1-108-46653-0 Paperback

Contents

Figures

Tables

Acknowledgments

This history of medicines in colonial Vietnam has led many lives. It was born in 2001 out of a research project funded by the Canadian Social Sciences and Humanities Research Council (SSHRC) as I was joining the Université de Montréal as an assistant professor in history and working with a team of wonderful researchers in social sciences and humanities looking at medicines as social objects.

Since then, it has given birth to several articles, in both French and English, and a book, *Médicaments coloniaux. L'expérience vietnamienne, 1905–1940* (Paris: Les Indes savantes) in 2014. It ends now, with this second book. Yet this does not mean that my interest in both the history and anthropology of pharmaceuticals and Vietnamese health practices is going to die.

The Colonial Life of Pharmaceuticals is not merely a translation of *Médicaments coloniaux*. In fact, it is a different book that has grown out of new thoughts, comments, and criticisms that I have received over the past few years; it is a much more mature (and lighter) work.

I do not want to reiterate the thanks I put on paper in 2014. This being said, Noémi Tousignant deserves that I mention her a second time as she has served, once again, as a trustworthy, hardworking, insightful translator, who is never afraid of challenging my ideas and my (very French) pompous style.

I would also like to thank Cambridge University Press and especially senior editor Lucy Rhymer, who happens to commission books in Asian studies, history of Asia, and history of medicine (lucky me!), and the Global Health Histories series editor Sanjoy Bhattacharya. Thank you both for believing in this rebirth and for putting the history of medicine and health in Vietnam on the map.

Abbreviations

Aff po	Fonds des affaires politiques
AFOM	Agence de la France d'outre-mer
AHMC	*Annales d'hygiène et de médecine coloniale*
AIPI	*Archives des Instituts Pasteur d'Indochine*
AMG	Assistance médicale gratuite
AMI	Assistance médicale indigène
Amiraux	Fonds des Amiraux
AMPC	*Annales de médecine et de pharmacie coloniales*
ANOM	Archives nationales d'outre-mer
APPIC	Association professionnelle des pharmaciens de l'Indochine
ARV	antiretroviral drug
BAYB	*Bao an y báo*
BDP	*Báo đông pháp*
BSMI	*Bulletin de la Société médico-chirurgicale de l'Indochine*
BSPE	*Bulletin de la Société de pathologie exotique*
CG	Fonds de la Commission Guernut
DC	Fonds de la Direction du contrôle
DLS	Fonds de la Direction locale de la santé
EFEO	École française d'Extrême-Orient
FEATM	Far Eastern Association for Tropical Medicine
Goucoch	Fonds du Gouvernement de la Cochinchine
Gougal	Fonds du Gouvernement général
Gougal SE	Fonds du Gouvernement général, service économique
IDEO	Imprimerie d'Extrême-Orient
IGHSP	Inspection générale de l'hygiène et de la santé publique
Indo AF	Indochine ancien fonds
Indo NF	Indochine nouveau fonds
PNTV	*Phụ nữ tân van*
OTC	over-the-counter
QE	quinine d'état
RMFEO	*Revue médicale française d'Extrême-Orient*

RSA	Fonds de la Résidence supérieure d'Annam
RST	Fonds de la Résidence supérieure du Tonkin
RST NF	Résidence supérieure du Tonkin nouveau fonds
SDN	Société des nations
STI	sexually-transmitted infection
TC	Troupes coloniales
TKVSCN	*Trung Kỳ vệ sinh chỉ nam*
VNA	Vietnam National Archives
VSB	*Vệ sinh báo*
WHO	World Health Organization

Introduction

Situated at the crossroads between the history of colonialism, of modern Southeast Asia and of medical pluralism, this book traces the "life of pharmaceuticals" in Vietnam under French rule. By focusing on the circulation and consumption of *colonial medicines* from the last third of the nineteenth century to the eve of World War II, it addresses neglected, and sometimes surprising, facets of the medicalization of Vietnamese society.[1] By colonial medicines, I mean not only medicines introduced and distributed by the colonizers, but also, importantly, medicines that were generated within and (re)defined by the process, and experience, of colonization. This book covers a period during which pharmaceuticals as we now know them were being defined, when their characteristics became stabilized and their modalities of distribution were tightened. It illuminates, by placing them side by side, two predominant, apparently contradictory, features of the changing sphere of Vietnamese health care during this period. On the one hand, there were persistent and serious problems of accessibility. On the other hand, a plurality of options was on offer. Constantly under negotiation, these reveal clear manifestations of patient agency. More broadly, I seek to historicize the roles and identities of medicines in the Global South by going back to the early phases of the modern pharmaceutical industry's expansion and globalization, before the advent of antibiotics.[2] Also in these pages, I describe the tricky task of interpreting heterogeneous and fragmented sources, which are full of omissions and of dissonant discourses. I hope this will contribute new ways of investigating and writing (colonial) histories of health.

---

[1] I address medicalization as a historical process that, from the end of the eighteenth century, redefined problems and behaviors as "medical," falling under the purview of medical professionals and institutions, state laws and policies. The process cannot be reduced to social control, even in colonial contexts; rather, it is a negotiated encounter between a "supply" and "demand" that is both variable and complex.

[2] The choice of this chronological endpoint also recognizes World War II as a watershed in the medical history of Vietnam, opening onto thirty-five years of war and instability (beginning with Japanese occupation of Indochina in 1940), associated with major challenges and deficiencies in the provision of health care.

1

Reinterpreting Discrepancies

The government doctors working for the Assistance médicale indigène (AMI; Native Medical Assistance) very rarely wrote about medicines. When medicines were mentioned in the reports that, from 1907, they were required to submit to the Inspection générale d'hygiène et de santé publique (IGHSP; General Inspection of Hygiene and Public Health), this was usually in the budget section.[3] Here, we can sometimes track down a number: an amount allocated to "medicines and materials" – the latter term encompassing surgical instruments, hospital bedding, cleaning and disinfecting products – for the district hospital or clinic under the physician's responsibility. Occasionally, report authors might make some marginal comments on attempts to alleviate the situation (particularly in accounts of local outbreaks of infectious disease) with an emergency pharmaceutical treatment. There were also usually a few lines, often repeated word for word from one report to the next, on the operation of the Service de quinine d'état (State Quinine Service), created in 1909 to distribute quinine in zones of high malaria prevalence. A similar indifference to therapeutics prevailed in medical journals: these published a small number of reports, mostly of hospital-based trials of arsenical or sulfa drugs, the two "wonder drug" classes of the 1910s to 1930s, and of field trials of quinine-based prophylaxis.

Most (of the relatively few) mentions of medicines in colonial sources addressed the problem of inadequate consumption or even outright refusal by "the natives." A common assertion was that, as a general rule, the Vietnamese only deigned to accept the therapeutic options proffered by AMI doctors as "a last resort." For many clinicians, this "last resort recourse" was explained by a shared, indeed a cultural, indifference to disease and its consequences, and a tenacious mistrust of Western medicine.[4] In short, it was a product of collective ignorance paired with

---

[3] The translation of French institutional names, of French colonial categories, and of some pharmaceutical terminology into English poses problems of equivalence in relation to their specific meanings and uses in the context of the French history of colonialism and pharmacy. Original French terms will be given and used wherever appropriate throughout the book, along with a faithful, yet explicit English-language translation, on the basis of the terms used in similar contexts at the time (e.g., the term "native," rather than "indigenous," is the British colonial equivalent of *indigène*).

[4] Contemporary sources referred to the medical system they saw as originating in Europe, and as anchored in scientific validation and discovery, as, alternately, "European," "modern," and "scientific." When I seek to echo actor's emic designations, I also use these terms. In other cases, I use the more neutral term "biomedicine," which refers to the increasingly close relationships between medicine and biological sciences without making claims as to its geographical origins, epistemological universality, or temporal status. In colonial contexts, the use of this term recognizes that "non-Western" medicine can also be "modern," while biomedicine can also be "non-Western."

resistance to change. Its corollary, AMI doctors complained, was that the Vietnamese persisted in trusting "their" medicine. In 1913, the AMI médecin-chef (head doctor) of Ha Giang Province, in Tonkin, the northern part of Vietnam, reported that the sick "would come to [him] only when they have already exhausted the resources of the Chinese pharmacopeia."[5] Eighteen years later, the Directeur local de la santé (local director of health) for the Protectorate of Tonkin wrote, "Clientele – [. . .] We treat one tenth of the population, the chronic, inveterate, the most difficult cases, mostly incurables; nine tenths go to the empirics."[6]

Empirics were practitioners of "Sino-Vietnamese medicine," whose remedies were seen as a major public health risk, either because they were toxic, improperly handled, or therapeutically ineffective.[7] Indeed, the risk of poisoning associated with these "dangerous remedies" was probably the most prevalent theme in colonial discourses on therapeutics. In the very first volume of what would become the colony's main medical journal, the *Bulletin de la Société médico-chirurgicale de l'Indochine* (BSMI; Bulletin of the Medico-Surgical Society of Indochina), established in 1910, Dr. Édouard Sambuc described two cases of fatal poisoning caused by "native medicines" for gonorrhea that happened at the hospital of Haiphong where he worked. In one case, a twenty-five-year-old patient had "suddenly, without any warning sign, chang[ed] expressions, let out a piercing scream and beg[an having] convulsions, los[t] consciousness, making a croaking sound now and then." Sambuc concluded: "We must note [. . .] the rapidity of death, the powerlessness of therapeutics in the face of this poisoning."[8] The sensationalism in the narration of this tragic

[5] "Rapport sanitaire annuel de la province de Ha Giang, 1913," Archives nationales d'outre-mer, Aix-en-Provence, France (hereafter ANOM), Fonds de la Résidence supérieure du Tonkin nouveau fonds (hereafter RST NF) 4014.

[6] "Direction locale de la santé du Tonkin. Rapport annuel de 1931," ANOM, RST NF 3683. Although "empiric" is an often vague designation, in colonial contexts it was usually used to characterize a person or practice as devoid of scientific and rational underpinnings. Many colonial doctors believed that local medical practices, "traditional" practices, were based on trial and error rather than cumulative, validated, and shared knowledge. Although based on an extensive pharmacopeia, Vietnamese medicine could, according to some, hardly claim a scientific status given its lack of "rigorous" knowledge of physiology, anatomy, and symptomatology, of specialization and of diagnostic and therapeutic technologies.

[7] The adjectives "Sino-Vietnamese" and "Sino-Annamese" were used by colonial health authorities to designate the most visible local medical system and to emphasize its Chinese roots. I prefer the term "Vietnamese medicine," which I use to designate dynamic and hybrid traditions that were identified as specific to Vietnam. However, I keep the term "Sino-Vietnamese" to designate the remedies and pharmacopeia used in Vietnamese medicine at the time as well as medical actors who identified themselves as such.

[8] Dr. Édouard Sambuc, "Deux cas mortels d'intoxication par des médicaments indigènes employés contre la blennorragie," BSMI 1 (1910): 502–3, 506.

event was surely meant as counter-propaganda targeting Vietnamese medicine. Yet it also manifested strong colonial anxieties about a wide range of dangerous substances, individuals, and polluted places.[9] These anxieties are more explicit in the following account of an incident that affected a soldier of the Garde indigène (Native Guard) in Nam Dinh, Tonkin, in 1916:

> The unskilled laborer [. . .] Dang-Dinh-Huyen had, in the evening of Tuesday March 14 of this year, during a fit of madness caused by the ingestion of Chinese medicines, ripped apart his clothing, a kaki vest and a kapok jacket, to the point where they are absolutely unusable. Asked about it, Dang-Dinh-Huyen declared the following: having suffered for the last few days from headaches, I decided to go to a seller of Chinese medicines hoping that the medicines that I would get would bring me some relief. I do not know whether the concoction that was sold to me [. . .] did me any good, but what I am sure of, is that it did me lots of harm. Indeed several minutes after absorbing it, I was literally mad, I no longer knew at all what I was doing, thus I had a very unpleasant surprise when, having recovered my sanity, I noted the lamentable state of my belongings.[10]

This type of incident was not uncommon – that is, if we take the health authorities at their word. Apparently, a few young soldiers even died because they had put "too much trust" in their empirics. Such statements clearly reveal AMI doctors' ignorance and contempt of the prevailing models of health and health care among those they sought to convert to the benefits of scientific medicine. They manifest a typical biomedical arrogance toward "the native patient" – viewed as inherently credulous and ignorant, as was indeed also thought of French patients at the time – but also toward any other medical system, considered to be, by definition, irrational, ineffective, even dangerous, and thus de facto made subaltern, if not criminalized outright.[11] Yet according to annual reports of the Bureau d'hygiène (Hygiene Office) of the City of Hanoi, the total number of deaths due to poisoning, both accidental and criminal, caused by toxic substances did not exceed five per one thousand in the period 1923–29. This was comparable to the rate of suicide mortality, but ten times less

---

[9] David Arnold, *Toxic Histories. Poison and Pollution in Modern India* (Cambridge: Cambridge University Press, 2016).

[10] "Décès survenus parmi les volontaires de l'Annam, 1916," ANOM, RST NF 896.

[11] I define "medical system" as a medical culture – that is, a set of shared conceptual foundations and practices, upheld within one or more social groups: Steven Feierman and John M. Janzen, *The Social Basis of Health and Illness in Africa* (Berkeley: University of California Press, 1992), 163–64. On subaltern therapeutics, see: Projit Mukharji and David Hardiman, ed., *Medical Marginality in South Asia: Situating Subaltern Therapeutics* (Abingdon: Routledge, 2012).

than deaths caused by gastroenteritis and forty times less than deaths caused by bronchial pneumonia.[12]

Such oft-repeated remarks do, however, also indicate that even if the Vietnamese consulted AMI doctors only as "a last resort," they did indeed consult them. They thus hint at practices of medical pluralism – that is, of combining the use of biomedicine with one or more other medical systems. This suggests that seeking and taking pharmaceuticals was one of the ways in which the Vietnamese grew increasingly familiar with biomedicine. Indeed, there were also occasional complaints in AMI reports that some patients saw public hospitals as mere "free pharmaceutical shop[s]" and the clinician as an "automatic medicines distributor."[13] From the interwar period, a few medical professionals also began to note that the Vietnamese seemed to "appreciate more and more," and thus to request "some" Western medicines, such as Antipyrin, santonin, and arsenobenzols. They did not, however, ponder the meaning and underlying reasons of lay practices of therapeutic selection and self-medication, nor did they wonder how these practices were changing as a result of colonization. The consumption of medicines by the colonized was seen as inherently problematic (if only because it often bypassed doctors), and certainly not a topic of serious reflection.

Dr. Nguyễn Văn Luyện had, it seems, a different view.[14] After graduating as a state-qualified doctor of medicine in France in 1928, Nguyễn Văn Luyện worked for the AMI before setting up a private practice in 1931 in Hanoi, the colonial capital. At that time, he began devoting part of his career to educating his compatriots about the benefits of biomedicine. He founded and edited the monthly serial *Bao an y báo. Revue de vulgarisation médicale* (BAYB; Popular Medical Magazine), which was published from July 1934 to January 1938. He invited BAYB readers to write to him directly and, in response, offered personalized health advice. This "letters to the editor" rubric took up several pages in each issue. On average, about half of the questions asked in these letters were about medicines used in the past, ongoing courses of treatment, or medicines for potential future use. These included, according to a list I compiled, references to nearly 650 different medicines – including 250 (nearly 40 percent) by name. About 350 (over half) of these medicines were *spécialités pharmaceutiques* (pharmaceutical specialties), trademarked

[12] Gouvernement général de l'Indochine, *Annuaire statistique de l'Indochine, 1923–1929* (Hanoi: Imprimerie d'Extrême-Orient [IDEO], 1931), 111, 126.

[13] Dr. Paucot, "Discussion sur l'emploi du Salvarsan aux colonies," *Bulletin de la Société de pathologie exotique* (BSPE) 6 (1913): 240.

[14] I have respected Vietnamese diacritics whenever possible – that is, when they were specified in my sources.

products manufactured by the pharmaceutical industry.[15] Some of these were toxic but highly effective drugs, such as "914," an arsenobenzol compound used to treat syphilis. Marketed under several brand names, this drug was mentioned fifty-seven times by readers, which averages out to more than once per issue. BAYB readers also evoked cutting-edge products that, in some cases, had arrived in Vietnam only a few months earlier. For example, Folliculine, a synthetic ovarian hormone launched by the French firm Roussel in 1932, was mentioned in early 1934.

The published correspondence between Nguyễn Văn Luyện and his virtual patients contradicts the dominant discourse among AMI doctors. Were I to write a colonial history of medicines based exclusively on an analysis of the letters-to-the-editor section of the BAYB, I would conclude that the Vietnamese consumed medicines profusely, and that pharmaceuticals were widely available, well-trusted, and familiar commodities, and one of the main objectives of therapy-seeking. Letter writers did not, however, consume medicines indiscriminately. They often wondered about a specific product's toxicity and side effects, or another's lack of efficacy, seeking out information for selecting the most effective medicines, with the fewest possible risks. This paints a picture that is very far from the figure of the ignorant, resistant patient or of the occasional yet exasperating consumer, as depicted by medical periodicals and AMI reports.

Toward a Colonial and Vietnamese History of Modern Medicines

One way of reconciling these conflicting discourses would be to point out that Vietnam changed between the first years of the AMI (created in 1905) and the time when the BAYB was published. There is value in this statement. Vietnam garnered the lion's share of attention and resources among the territories that formed the Union indochinoise (Indochinese Union) or French Indochina from 1887 to 1947, placed under the authority of a Gouverneur général (governor general) who represented the French Republic.[16] Here, colonial policies of

---

[15] Translator's note: the specificity of national pharmaceutical markets and industries in the nineteenth and early twentieth centuries generated distinctive terminologies. Thus, there is no commonly-used equivalent term in English for *spécialité pharmaceutique* (sometimes approximated as "proprietary drug"). I have opted to use the literal translation throughout this book.

[16] L'Union indochinoise or Indochine française was created as an administrative umbrella for five distinct territories (*pays*): a colony (Cochinchina), administered by a governor, and four protectorates (Tonkin, Annam, Laos, and Cambodia), administered by Résidents supérieurs (superior residents). I generally use the term "colony" more broadly

centralization, economic exploitation and *mise en valeur* – a policy for "improving" the economic potential of colonies developed and popularized by the Minister of Colonies and former Governor General Albert Sarraut in the early 1920s – were applied with the greatest vigor.[17] Some have characterized this colonization of Vietnam as "total": a "model" totality that joined both colonial enterprises – to exploit and to civilize – at the intersection of which was the project of taking the health of "the natives" in hand.

The drawn-out French conquest and pacification of Indochina in the second half of the nineteenth century was well timed to enlist medicine as a "tool of empire."[18] This was a time when the cultural authority of biomedicine as modern, expert, and scientific was growing. It became a realm of professionals, to be accredited and protected by the state. As the links between the clinic and the laboratory grew stronger, significant progress was made in the scientific understanding and control of tropical diseases. Bacteriology, usually seen as the paragon of this "new" medicine, was, in the French world, dominated by Pasteur and his acolytes (the "Pastorians"). The synchronicity between the "bacteriological revolution" and the stabilization of colonial rule in Indochina created an opening for the Pastorians to quickly export their science and institutions overseas. Indeed, the Pastorian ambition to master tropical pathological environments was welcomed by a colonial government grappling with high rates of mortality and morbidity. It is no coincidence that the first Institut Pasteur d'outre-mer (Overseas Pasteur Institute) was established in Saigon in 1891, only three years after the Parisian headquarters opened its doors. By the late 1930s, there were four Instituts Pasteur in Indochina and three affiliated laboratories. This dense network of research facilities was unparalleled in other colonial territories.[19]

---

to refer to the three Vietnamese territories, or to Indochina as a whole. I use the term "Vietnamese" to designate the ethnic majority of Vietnam (of Việt or Kinh origin), which made up 85 percent of its population at the time. Contemporary sources also used this designation interchangeably with that of "Annamese" (*Annamite*), referring to the population of the precolonial kingdom of Annam.

[17] The best overview of the history of French Indochina is Pierre Brocheux and Daniel Hémery, *Indochine. La colonisation ambiguë, 1858–1954* (La Découverte, 2001 [1994]). On mise en valeur, see Albert Sarraut, *La mise en valeur des colonies* (Paris: Payot, 1923), and Alice Conklin, *A Mission to Civilize: The Republican Idea of Empire in France and West Africa, 1895–1930* (Stanford: Stanford University Press, 1997).

[18] Daniel Headrick, *Tools of Empire. Technology and European Imperialism in the Nineteenth Century* (New York and Oxford: Oxford University Press, 1981).

[19] On the history of the AMI and the role of the Institut Pasteur in Indochina, see Laurence Monnais-Rousselot, *Médecine et colonisation. L'aventure indochinoise, 1860–1939* (Paris: CNRS Editions, 1999).

From 1905, the AMI, a public health care system, was the theatre of an ambiguous – to echo the insightful adjective used by Pierre Brocheux and Daniel Hémery to characterize Indochina's colonization – project to exploit and to modernize, through biomedicine, its agents and techniques. This endeavor was predominantly focused on the collective prevention of infectious diseases, especially those responsible for the greatest burden of morbidity and mortality in the territory. Yet the system also sought to educate the population about the benefits of Western medicine, both directly, through classes and pamphlets on the principles of hygiene, and indirectly, through the provision of free care. As AMI authorities began to take stock of the system's achievements just after World War I, a process of nativization of the health care system was initiated.[20] A growing number of indigenous health care workers were hired by the AMI, including Vietnamese doctors trained at the Hanoi Medical School, which had opened in 1902. During the same period, greater attention was given to mothers and children, as well as to conditions associated with poverty such as tuberculosis and trachoma, and efforts were made to ruralize the provision of medical care. Some statistics, such as the linear rise in the number of outpatient consultations, or the sharp drop in cases of maternal and neonatal tetanus, were encouraging. The interwar period was thus marked by a clear drive to expand both the nature and reach of colonial medicalization, creating new potential points of contact with Vietnamese health practices. By the 1930s, however, the administration was facing a series of crises ranging from the aftermath of the 1929 stock market crash to the radicalization of nationalist movements, as well as demographic pressures in zones of high population density and bitterness arising from the failure of colonial reformism and the abandonment of the policy of *collaboration franco-annamite* (Franco-Vietnamese collaboration).[21] This placed serious constraints on the expansion – dampening optimism about the achievements – of colonial health programs.

---

[20] Laurence Monnais, "'Modern Medicine' in French Colonial Vietnam. From the Importation of a Model to its Nativisation," in *Development of Modern Medicine in Non-European Countries: Historical Perspectives*, ed. Hormoz Ebrahimnejad (London and New York: Routledge, 2008), 127–59.

[21] Official name given to colonial policy on indigenous political participation from 1911, collaboration franco-annamite sought to grant representation to the local population through consultative assemblies elected through suffrage by census (i.e., of taxpayers only). However, the policy did not lead to any consistent reforms on the political status of Indochina and lost the support of local elites from the late 1920s: Agathe Larcher, "La voie étroite des réformes coloniales et la collaboration franco-annamite, 1917–1928," *Revue française d'histoire d'outre-mer* 82, 309 (1995): 397–420.

Given these ongoing constraints, "the passing of time" cannot entirely and convincingly account for the discursive discrepancies concerning the consumption of medicines, as noted previously. It is true that the interwar period was, in Vietnam, one of rapid social change that manifested in a flourishing press, the emergence of new socio-professional categories, dynamic local economies, and even the birth of the first feminist movements.[22] However, these changes were almost exclusively limited to urban areas, mainly to the Union's two largest cities: Hanoi, the colonial capital in the North, and Saigon, the economic capital in the South. This is also where cutting-edge hospitals, scientific laboratories, and retail pharmacies were concentrated. What role might biomedicine, and its medicines, have played in the small provincial cities of Annam,[23] or even in the remote outposts that accounted for the majority of health care facilities that filled the reports submitted to the IGHSP in Hanoi? To what extent did colonization provide access to drugs and to curative, individual, care? There is little indication that AMI doctors dispensed a greater volume of medicines in 1940 than they did in 1905, and it seems unlikely their perspectives changed much. That there is no sub-series on the subject of "medicines" or "pharmaceuticals" in the colonial archives seems, in itself, to reveal the absence of any effective pharmaceutical policy in the colony. These discrepancies must be given a voice rather than muffled. But *how*, using what historiographical, theoretical, or methodological tools, and on the basis of which alternative sources – other than the BAYB, which I discovered by accident when I came upon a (not yet consulted) copy at the National Library of France in Paris?

The first obstacle I encountered as I set out on this long research journey was the lack of historiography on medicines prior to the antibiotic era – that is, before World War II, particularly in settings other than Europe and North America. This is surprising, given that several studies pointed out, long ago, the importance of the years between the 1870s and the 1940s as a period of long "therapeutic transition" if not of "therapeutic revolution."[24] It has also been known that medicines

---

[22] Van Nguyen-Marshall, Lisa Drummond Welch, and Danièle Bélanger, ed., *The Reinvention of Tradition. Modernity and the Middle Class in Urban Vietnam* (Singapore: Asian Research Institute, 2012).

[23] Annam was much less a target of colonial investment than Tonkin, which was seen as having a greater economic potential. The paucity in health archives for the protectorate, relative to Tonkin, is in itself a sign of this disparity. In addition, it should be noted that the archival reference in this book to the Fonds de la Résidence supérieure d'Annam at the Vietnam National Archives (hereafter VNA) is no longer valid. Although it was accurate at the time I consulted this archival collection, it has since been moved to Hué.

[24] On the concept of therapeutic transition, see Harry Marks, *The Progress of Experiment: Science and Therapeutic Reform in the United States, 1900–1990* (Cambridge: Cambridge University Press, 1997), and John Harley Warner, *The Therapeutic Perspective: Medical*

played a key role, from the turn of the twentieth century, in the transformation and globalization of industrial and commercial practices, and in the emergence of health consumerism.[25] A spate of recent work on postwar pharmaceuticals renders obsolete Charles Rosenberg's 1992 observation that historians were ignoring medicines because they saw them as "strange objects."[26] Despite this, medicines rarely occupy a central position in current reflections on the coproduction of imperialism and health.

Guillaume Lachenal's book on Lomidine, a contested wonder drug used in sleeping sickness prophylaxis in 1950s sub-Saharan Africa, is a notable exception.[27] At most, medicines appear in the margins of studies of imperialism, as a modern technology among others (as is the case for quinine), as part of an array of modern consumer goods that may even be seen as "emancipatory," or as evidence of dynamic practices of medical pluralism and of the reinvention of traditional medicines.[28] Therapeutic substances are sometimes evoked to highlight colonial oppression, subjugating the colonized through addiction

Practice, Knowledge and Identity in America, 1820–1885 (Cambridge: Cambridge University Press, 1986). On the idea of a post–World War II therapeutic revolution and its narratives, see Jeremy A. Greene, Flurin Condrau, and Elizabeth Siegel Watkins, ed. *Therapeutic Revolution. Pharmaceutical and Social Change in the Twentieth Century* (Chicago: Chicago University Press, 2016).

[25] Nancy Tomes, "Merchants of Health: Medicine and Consumer Culture in the United States, 1900–1940," *The Journal of American History* 88, 2 (2001): 531–38.

[26] Charles Rosenberg, *Explaining Epidemics and Other Studies in the History of Medicine* (Cambridge: Cambridge University Press, 1992), 10.

[27] Guillaume Lachenal, *Le médicament qui devait sauver l'Afrique. Un scandale pharmaceutique aux colonies* (Paris: La Découverte, 2014), translated as *The Lomidine Files. The Untold Story of a Medical Disaster in Colonial Africa* (Baltimore: Johns Hopkins University Press, 2017). See also Nandini Bhattacharya, "Between the Bazaar and the Bench: Making of the Drugs Trade in Colonial India, ca. 1900–1930," *Medical History* 90, 1 (2016): 61–91; Myriam Mertens, "Chemical Compounds in the Congo: Pharmaceuticals and the 'Crossed History' of Public Health in Belgian Africa" (PhD diss., University of Ghent, 2014), and Noémi Tousignant, "Trypanosomes, Toxicity and Resistance: The Politics of Mass Therapy in French Colonial Africa," *Social History of Medicine* 25, 3 (2012): 625–43.

[28] On consumerism and drugs, see Sarah Hodges, *Contraception, Colonialism, and Commerce. Birth Control in South India, 1920–1940* (Aldershot: Ashgate, 2008); and Timothy Burke, Lifebuoy Men, Lux Women. *Commodification, Consumption, and Cleanliness in Modern Zimbabwe* (London: Leicester University Press, 1996). On therapeutic pluralism and traditional medicines, see Karen E. Flint, *Healing Traditions: African Medicine, Cultural Exchange, and Competition in South Africa, 1820–1948* (Athens: Ohio University Press, 2008); Kavita Sivaramakrishnan, *Old Potions, New Bottles. Recasting Indigenous Medicine in Colonial Punjab (1850–1945)* (Hyderabad: Orient Longman, 2006); Anne Digby, "Self-Medication and the Trade in Medicine within a Multi-Ethnic Context: A Case Study of South Africa from the Mid-Nineteenth to Mid-Twentieth Centuries," *Social History of Medicine* 1, 3 (2005): 439–57; Waltraud Ernst, ed., *Plural Medicine, Tradition and Modernity, 1800–2000* (London and New York: Routledge, 2002).

or compulsory ingestion.[29] Other studies take up therapeutic substances to focus on extractive endeavors, as in early instances of bioprospection and experimentation, conducted with impunity far from the metropolitan gaze.[30] Interest in the coercive dimensions of colonial public health has perhaps led to an overrepresentation of vaccines in the study of colonial medicines. However, while biotherapies should indeed be defined as pharmaceutical products, they are set apart not only by their mode of action, but also by their use as tools of collective prevention, whose administration was tightly controlled by the colonial state.[31]

Given these historiographical gaps, I turned to studies of pharmaceuticals from other disciplines in order to formulate the right questions and to identify productive analytical pathways. Indeed, medical anthropologists have, since the 1980s, paid much more attention to medicines than historians have.[32] Their work has, in particular, developed an approach to medicines focusing on their *biography* or *life cycle,* which is articulated around three, sometimes four stages: production (which includes drug innovation, research, and development); circulation (in which one might concentrate, for example, on the role of retail pharmacies or the uses of prescriptions in orienting distribution); consumption; and, in some cases, a drug's "afterlife," its post-ingestion

---

[29] Ved Baruah, "Addicts, Peddlers and Reformers: A Social History of Opium in Assam, 1826–1947" (PhD diss., Cardiff University, 2017); James H. Mills and Patricia Barton, ed., *Drugs and Empires. Essays in Modern Imperialism and Intoxication, c. 1500–c. 1930* (Basingstoke: Palgrave McMillan, 2000); William Jankowiak and Daniel Bradburd, ed., *Drugs, Labor, and Colonial Expansion* (Tucson: University of Arizona Press, 2003).

[30] Laurence Monnais and Noémi Tousignant, "The Values of Versatility: Pharmacists, Plants, and Place in the French (post)Colonial World," *Comparative Studies in Society & History* 58, 2 (2016): 432–62; Abena Osseo-Asare, *Bitter Roots: The Search for Healing Plants in Africa* (Chicago: University of Chicago Press, 2014); Deborah Neill, "Paul Ehrlich's Colonial Connections: Scientific Networks and Sleeping Sickness Drug Therapy Research, 1900–1914," *Social History of Medicine,* 22, 1 (2009): 61–77; Wolfgang Eckart, "The Colony as Laboratory: German Sleeping Sickness Campaigns in German East Africa and in Togo, 1900–1914," *History & Philosophy of Life Sciences* 24 (2002): 69–89.

[31] For these reasons, I chose to exclude vaccines from my study. This exclusion is further justified by the fact that the production of vaccines and serums was then the prerogative, in Indochina as in France, of the Institut Pasteur, and that contractual agreements between Pasteur and the colonial government made it possible to distribute all vaccines for free in Vietnam via specific channels.

[32] See especially Sjaak Van der Geest, Susan Whyte, and Anita Hardon, "The Anthropology of Pharmaceuticals: A Biographical Approach," *American Review of Anthropology* 25 (1996): 153–78; Sjaak Van der Geest and Susan Whyte, *The Context of Medicines in Developing Countries. Studies in Pharmaceutical Anthropology* (Dordrecht and Boston: Kluwer Academic Publishers, 1988); Charles E. Cunningham, "Thai 'Injection Doctors': Antibiotic Mediators," *Social Science & Medicine* 4 (1970): 1–24.

manifestations.[33] By attending to the meanings invested in medicines across space and over time, this approach is particularly valuable for identifying the multiple determinants of the accessibility of health care. Indeed, it illuminates its many dimensions, which are not only economic and geographical (i.e., how much care costs and where it can be obtained), but as also shaped by other practical and conceptual, even cultural, issues, ranging from forms of interaction with health care professionals to the representations of drug effects. Furthermore, following medicines through these different stages – which also represent sets of relationships and interactions, in which value and meaning are negotiated and transformed – helps highlight the roles played as much by "dominant" pharmaceutical actors (the industry, pharmacists, doctors) as by consumers. It helped, and pushed, me to foreground those who ingest, or who refuse, medicines as playing an active part in their own health care – in other words, to privilege a "bottom-up" construction of the history of health.

Anthropologists of medicines do not begin with a priori judgments of drug consumption as problematic, risky, or irrational. The meanings of observed therapeutic practices become clear only after their specific factors – logics, values, practical obstacles, and advantages – have been identified. This perspective is shared by some sociologists who are committed to studying medicines as *social objects*,[34] and to thereby grasp the full complexity of processes of medicalization. Here, I deploy this capacity to illuminate the flip side of official narratives and practices of colonial medicalization, and therefore to better scrutinize and capture this process as a whole, with its multiple, sometimes conflicting, more and less visible dimensions; its imposed, accepted, refused, and sought-after elements. Pharmaceuticals have highly malleable social meanings, more so than doctors, for example.[35] Furthermore, medicines have a life of their own, a potential for material and therapeutic autonomy. Indeed, despite the proliferation of institutional and legal measures to impose biomedical gatekeepers, namely the doctor and the pharmacist, on access to medicines since the nineteenth century, medicines embody expertise in a way that often makes it possible to bypass the experts.[36] As modern, volatile,

---

[33] Nina Etkin, "'Side Effects': Cultural Constructions and Reinterpretations of Western Pharmaceuticals," *Medical Anthropology Quarterly* 6 (1994): 99–113.

[34] Johanne Collin, Marcelo Otero, and Laurence Monnais, ed., *Le médicament au cœur de la socialité contemporaine. Regards croisés sur un objet complexe* (Sainte Foy: Presses de l'Université du Québec, 2006), 1–15.

[35] Sokhieng Au, *Mixed Medicines. Health and Culture in French Colonial Cambodia* (Chicago: Chicago University Press, 2011), 80.

[36] Sjaak Van der Geest and Susan Whyte, "The Charm of Medicines: Metaphors and Metonyms," *Medical Anthropology Quarterly* 3, 4 (1989): 357–60.

autonomous medical technologies, and as commodities in the making, medicines are also historical objects that can shed light on the social dynamics at work in (colonial) ways of relating to health and to well-being.

Historicizing the "Inappropriate" Consumption of Medicines

Pharmaceuticals are in urgent need of historicization, going beyond the specific context of Vietnam under French rule. We are now in an era, some say, of out-of-control *pharmaceuticalization*.[37] The "pharmaceuticalization of daily life" is epitomized by a rampant, global consumption of drugs such as Lipitor, Plavix, Prozac, and Viagra, paralleled by a race to unleash nature's pharmacological potential and the growing scale of mass production of "neo-traditional" medicines.[38] Pharmaceuticals are at the heart of the quest for health; indeed, medicines have shaped how we define health and disease since at least the late nineteenth century. While relying heavily on pharmaceuticals, health care and public health professionals, policy makers, and managers continue to raise concerns about the role they play in care. These concerns include ever-more complex and potentially risky patterns of consumption, as well as exorbitant costs to national economies. According to the global information and technology services company IMS Health, the global use of medicines will reach 4.5 trillion doses by 2020, costing US$1.4 trillion.[39] Frantic pharmaceutical consumption appears to be rooted in another major problem: the "misuse" (i.e., inappropriate or irrational use, with reference to biomedical standards) of medicines, which is blamed, for example, as the cause of widespread antibiotic resistance. While some drugs are defined as essential[40] or as miraculous, there is still a persisting tendency to judge

---

[37] The term "pharmaceuticalization," in its most neutral historical definition, points to the role played by pharmaceuticals (produced, distributed, consumed), and their many actors, in modern processes of medicalization. However, its use in the fields of anthropology, sociology, or public health often implies a harmful process of "pharmaceutical invasion": Adriana Petryna, Andrew Lakoff, and Arthur Kleinman, ed., *Global Pharmaceuticals. Ethics, Markets, Practices* (Durham and London: Duke University Press, 2006).

[38] Nick J. Fox and Kathie J. Ward, "Pharma in the Bedroom . . . and the Kitchen . . . The Pharmaceuticalisation of Daily Life," *Sociology of Health & Illness* 30, 6 (2008): 856–68.

[39] imshealth.com/en/thought-leadership/ims-institute/reports/global-medicines-use-in-2020.

[40] Jeremy A. Greene, "Making Medicines Essential: The Emergent Centrality of Pharmaceuticals in Global Health," *BioSocieties* 6 (2011): 10–33.

the generalized attraction to pills of all sorts as blind and lazy: as sidestepping healthy lifestyles and the collective prevention of "real" health problems.

The issues arising from the consumption of medicines in the Global South appear to be different from those plaguing high-income countries and, it seems, more "problematic." Often mentioned is the ease and frequency with which prescription-only drugs are obtained without due consultation of a qualified health care professional. This tendency is then linked to high levels of nonadherence to officially recommended uses (dosage, therapeutic indications, course of treatment, etc.) and a profuse circulation of counterfeit products: the World Health Organization (WHO) estimates that 25 percent of the drug market in the Global South is composed of counterfeit medicines, compared to 7 to 15 percent in other countries – although internet purchasing may be narrowing this gap.[41] Pluralistic medical practices are viewed as especially likely to result in harmful drug interactions or, at the very least, to make patients less adherent to biomedical therapeutic principles. The "rediscovery" of so-called traditional medicines and their inclusion within integrative health care systems obtained the WHO's stamp of approval in 1978; its Declaration of Alma-Ata affirms the benefits of promoting medical traditions that are rooted in the values and practices of local communities.[42] Yet this has positioned traditional medicine as an *alternative* to biomedicine, to be fostered in order to meet the goal of providing primary health care "for all" in the face of the obvious impossibility (both material and human) of universal and equitable access to biomedical care.

While it is easy to blame irrational individuals, negligent states, and dysfunctional health care systems for problems of pharmaceutical consumption and accessibility, there is, of course, another important player. In the 1970s and 1980s, a greedy, devious, and far-reaching pharmaceutical industry was accused of launching a global "pharmaceutical invasion." Through aggressive marketing and product distribution, the industry was said to expose vulnerable populations to risky forms and norms of pharmaceutical consumption.[43] The economist Michael Kremer suggests that the distinctive traits of drug consumption in the

---

[41] gphf.org/images/downloads/library/who_factsheet275.pdf.

[42] WHO, Declaration of Alma-Ata International Conference on Primary Health Care, Alma-Ata Kazakhstan, USSR, September 6–12, 1978 (http://who.int/publications/almaa ta_declaration_en.pdf).

[43] On the pharmaceutical invasion of the Global South, see Milton Silverman, Mia Lydecker, and Philip Randolph Lee, *Bad Medicine: The Prescription Drug Industry in the Third World* (Stanford: Stanford University Press, 1992); Diana Melrose, *Bitter Pills: Medicines and the Third World Poor* (Oxford: Oxfam, 1982).

Global South can also be linked to the fact that pharmaceutical products are, compared with the Global North, responsible for a higher share of twentieth-century population-level health gains relative to other medical interventions and technologies.[44] This assertion merits consideration. Indeed, it is worth investigating the process of pharmaceuticalization from the vantage point of multiple genealogies. Although we might catch a whiff of colonial discourses in some interpretations of the current situation, it is surely not enough to denounce as neo-imperialist the pressures and accusations weighing on the consumption of pharmaceuticals in Asia or Africa. We have to go back further, before the years of the pharmaceutical invasion, before Alma-Ata, even before antibiotics, to really understand the meanings and determinants of self-medication and therapeutic pluralism, and to document the history of access to health care as well as the genesis (or absence) of pharmaceutical policies.

Vietnam is particularly suited to, and in need of, such a project of excavation. The consumption of medicines became a source of particular anxiety in the wake of the Đổi mới (renovation era), a set of economic reforms initiated in 1986 toward a "socialist market economy," which led to the privatization of the national health care system from 1989. This entailed a deregulation of the sale of medicines and medical services, and the introduction of restrictions on access to free health care, which, until then, had been universal. By the turn of the twenty-first century, thirty-five thousand pharmacies sold about ten thousand medicines, of which four thousand were manufactured abroad (these were usually more expensive but also more sought-after) – a situation that, some pointed out, was ripe for an explosive proliferation of risky practices such as self-medication.[45] Almost twenty years ago already, the World Bank estimated that two-thirds of all acts of health care seeking consisted of direct purchases of medicines, whether from qualified pharmacists or other types of traders, and that 93 percent of these transactions did not involve

[44] Michael Kremer, "Pharmaceuticals and the Developing World," *The Journal of Economic Perspectives* 16, 4 (2002): 72.
[45] See especially Okumura Junko, Wakai Susumu, and Umenai Takusei, "Drug Utilisation and Self-Medication in Rural Communities," *Social Science & Medicine* 54, 12 (2002): 1876–86; Nguyen Thi Kim Chuc and Goran Tomson, "Doi Moi and Private Pharmacies: A Case Study on Dispensing and Financial Issues in Hanoi, Vietnam," *European Journal of Clinical Pharmacology* 55 (1999): 325–32; Duong Dat Van, C. W. Binns, and Truyen Van Le, "Availability of Antibiotics as Over-the-counter Drugs in Pharmacies: A Threat to Public Health in Vietnam," *Tropical Medicine and International Health* 2, 12 (1997): 1133–39; Ivan Wolffers, "The Role of Pharmaceuticals in the Privatization Process in Vietnam's Health Care System," *Social Science & Medicine* 41, 9 (1995): 1325–32.

a medical prescription.[46] The Vietnamese market for counterfeits offered, according to the WHO, a wide variety of products, including different types of antibiotics, analgesics, antimalarial, psychotropic, and combination drugs, as well as (neo)traditional products.[47]

The country is indeed pervaded by a strong medical culture of its own, which has a long and complex history. The use of the term *thuốc ta* (our medicine) is still used with reference to a distinctively national medicine, whose roots are closely intertwined with the anti-colonial emancipation movement of the 1930s and 1940s. Yet this appellation underplays the long-standing, still strong, if sometimes tense, association between *thuốc bắc*, Chinese medicine from the North, and *thuốc nam*, a southern medicine based on a therapeutic arsenal that draws on Vietnam's extraordinary local biodiversity.[48] Interchanges between "north" and "south" have long been fostered by a busy, extensive, and durable network of channels for the circulation of medicinal plants and substances, which crisscrosses the Vietnamese territory and connects it to its neighbors. The prominent social, economic, and therapeutic role played by those who provide remedies (including but not limited to the biomedically qualified pharmacist) also obviously predates the privatization of the Vietnamese health care system. In addition, it should not be surprising to find a tendency toward self-medication in a country whose predominant East Asian Confucian culture emphasizes the value of managing one's own health, a link that can indeed be discerned through a close reading of health magazines, for example.[49] The markers of these patterns of practice – like those of the pharmaceuticalization of the Global South – have yet to be historicized.

A site of total colonization, Vietnam was, from relatively early on, connected to a global economy that included transnational trade in pharmaceuticals. The pharmaceutical industry was taking off in Europe and North America at the same time as the Southeast Asian territory was

---

[46] World Bank, *Vietnam Living Standards Surveys (1997–1998)* (Washington, DC: World Bank, 2001).

[47] WHO, *Counterfeit and Substandard Drugs in Myanmar and Vietnam* (Geneva: WHO, 1999), http://apps.who.int/medicinedocs/pdf/s2276e/s2276e.pdf. Combination drugs are products that contain several medicines or pharmacologically active substances that are usually taken separately. Common examples are APC (aspirin, phenacetin, caffeine) and PPA (phenobarbital, phenacetin, aspirin).

[48] On the identity of Vietnamese medicine, see Laurence Monnais, C. Michele Thompson, and Ayo Wahlberg, ed., *Southern Medicine for Southern People. Vietnamese Medicine in the Making* (Newcastle upon Tyne: Cambridge Scholars Publishing, 2012). *Thuốc* means remedy, medicine, and tobacco.

[49] Judith Farquhar, "For Your Reading Pleasure: Self-Health (Ziwo Baojian) Information in 1990s Beijing," *Positions. East Asia Culture Critique* 9, 1 (2001): 105–30; David Finer, *Pressing Priorities: Consumer Drug Information in the Vietnamese Marketplace* (Stockholm: Karolinska Institutet, Department of Public Health Sciences / Global Health [IHCAR], 1999).

being placed under colonial rule. This synchronicity had a significant impact. French firms sought out overseas market opportunities as soon as they began to expand, if only to secure their position in an industry that was quickly becoming increasingly competitive.[50] These circumstances are difficult to reconcile with colonial doctors' silence on the subject of medicines. Yet they might make a good starting point in responding to historian David G. Marr's 1987 call to unravel the mystery of the popularity of Western drugs in Vietnam.[51] Pointing out that "Western medicines" were absent, or nearly absent, from pharmacy shelves for nearly four decades, from World War II to the Đổi mới, Marr suggests that we need to look back to the time of colonial rule in order to solve this puzzle. I would add weight to this intuition by pointing out that the Democratic Republic of Vietnam (North Vietnam, 1945–76) implemented an integrative health care system as early as 1954, just after the Geneva Agreements provisionally split the country in two. This was a symbolic and highly political decision, but one that was nevertheless necessarily rooted in a preexisting familiarity with biomedicine, its institutions, agents, and, presumably, its medicines.

Tools for Biographical Writing: About Alternative (Colonial) Sources

Once I set out to explore these questions, I had to tackle the problem of locating sources for writing such a colonial genealogy of pharmaceuticals. Unlike anthropologists, historians are often forced to privilege a macroscopic approach when their documentary sources are not sufficiently fine-grained. With its endpoint in 1940, my study could not rely on oral history interviews or ethnographic observation of historical actors. It was particularly challenged by the lack of voice, in the usual sources, given to producers, distributors, and especially to consumers of medicines, most of whom were twice subaltern: as both lay and colonized subjects. It was thus a matter of both finding new sources and reading old ones in new ways. I used multiple search strategies to uncover potential sources, including some that spoke of medicines only marginally or indirectly; forced a juxtaposition of data on official medical positions and practices with information on actors and practices that were beyond the AMI's purview (whether by definition, indifference, or intentional

---

[50] Sophie Chauveau, *L'invention pharmaceutique. La pharmacie française entre l'état et la société au XXe siècle* (Paris: Sanofi Synthélabo, 1999), 77.

[51] David G. Marr, "Vietnamese Attitudes Regarding Illness and Healing," in *Death and Disease in Southeast Asia. Explorations in Social, Medical, and Demographic History*, ed. Norman G. Owen (Singapore: Oxford University Press, 1987), 182–83.

escape); sought to bring private, informal, and even illegal realities to light; and drew together, within the same frame of reality, the silences in sources with their expressions of judgment, value, ignorance, anxiety, and blame. Throughout, I constantly marked out turning points in drugs' trajectories and remained attentive to the distinct regimes of value through which they passed and were redefined.

While the importation (or exportation, if one is standing on the opposite shore) of pharmaceuticals is not a major dimension of my analysis, I still felt it was necessary to trace the outlines of how medicines made their way to Vietnam from the Euro-American, particularly the French, pharmaceutical industry during the colonial period. I once again found an indifference to medicines in the archival series pertaining to the customs services and chambers of commerce. However, a few serial publications on the commerce and economy of Indochina, as well as the *Annuaire statistique de l'Indochine* (Directory of Statistics of Indochina), allowed me to roughly sketch out the flux of products between metropole and colony, but also, interestingly, between Indochina and some of its neighboring countries.[52] Because the Instituts Pasteur were so influential in Indochina, the Pasteur archives housed in Paris, and especially the files of the institution's Laboratoire de chimie thérapeutique (Laboratory of medicinal chemistry), which became involved in the production and experimentation of new pharmaceutical compounds as early as 1911, were highly informative. This compensated, at least in part, for the unavailability of pharmaceutical industry archives documenting their products and activities in Vietnam during this period.

Acts of legislation that regulated the circulation of medicines into and within the colony were published in the serial *Journal officiel de l'Indochine* (Official Journal of Indochina). These reveal an extremely dense and complex legislative framework that seems typical of the well-known French emphasis on centralization and on the regulation, and protectionism of commercial and professional activity. It also, at least on the surface, contradicts the lack of attention to medicines in the texts of AMI protagonists. Obviously, I also consulted the reports of any administrative agency or institution likely to intervene in the circulation of medicines. These of course included the records of the health services, whose top level, initially a Direction de la santé publique (Directorate of Public Health) that became the IGHSP in 1914, centralized (monthly) and synthesized (annually) reports from the districts and facilities under its

---

[52] I also surveyed the metropolitan journal *Chimie & industrie* (Chemistry and Industry) as well as the *Bulletin économique de l'Indochine* (Economic Bulletin of Indochina), *La quinzaine coloniale* (Colonial Fortnightly), and *La revue coloniale* (The Colonial Review).

authority. I identified and retrieved relevant documentation from the Agence des douanes et régies (Customs and State Monopolies Agency), the Service économique du Gouvernement général (Central Government's Economic Service), the Service judiciaire (Judicial Service), and the Sûreté générale, a security and police service created in 1919. I also managed to obtain reports of the Inspection des pharmacies (Pharmacy Inspection Service), a control service created in 1908. These contain a wealth of information on the practices, both legal and illegal, of various types of medicines-traders, as well as evaluations of the "proper" management of "Western-style" pharmacies. These reports also shed light on the highly versatile Vietnamese market for medicines, compensating, to some extent, for the unavailability of prescription ledgers or other sources of information on the day-to-day operation of pharmacies.

Indochinese and colonial medical journals, despite their previously mentioned relative indifference to medicines, did provide some indications as to which medicines were used in AMI hospitals, with what therapeutic methods and results. A much richer source, however, was the Vietnamese popular press. Colonial Vietnam was home to hundreds of periodicals in French, especially in *quốc ngữ*.[53] By 1939, the official count was of 128 dailies and 176 magazines, bulletins, and serials. Unrivalled in the colonial world, this prolific production has, paradoxically, been relatively neglected as a historical source other than for the analysis of its political role.[54] During the interwar years, the pages of these publications were quickly filled up with publicity for an array of medicines. The Vietnamese press often addressed health topics, in ways that echoed, but could also criticize and deviate from, dominant colonial and medical rhetoric. A close reading of a selection of health magazines such as the previously mentioned BAYB gave me a glimpse of dimensions of local therapeutic consumption that are not addressed in other sources. For example, I was able to find out how readers and their kin learned about some of the pharmaceutical products they had discovered in AMI hospitals or through publicity (see Chapter 5).

Together, these sources provide a range of types of information on the medicines that circulated in Vietnam prior to 1940, or at least, on the

[53] Quốc ngữ is a romanized writing system for the Vietnamese language that was imposed by the colonial administration for administrative correspondence in the late nineteenth century and in schools in the early twentieth century; later it became the official national written language.
[54] Philippe M. F. Peycam, *The Birth of Vietnamese Political Journalism: Saigon, 1916–1930* (New York: Columbia University Press, 2012); Shawn F. McHale, *Print and Power. Confucianism, Communism, and Buddhism in the Making of Modern Vietnam* (Honolulu: University of Hawai'i Press, 2004); David G. Marr, *Vietnamese Traditions on Trial, 1925–1945* (Berkeley: University of California Press, 1981).

products considered worth mentioning, for various reasons, by their authors and protagonists. From this information, I compiled a database of 1,121 drugs and traced their colonial lives. I created separate entries for the different brand names of the same active substance. However, I excluded traditional remedies – or remedies identified as such, as opposed to "modern" medicines – and medicinal species. While it would be impossible to ensure or ascertain that the database is complete, and while it provides incomplete biographical information on some of the medicines it lists, it nevertheless contains a wealth of qualitative information. Usefully, the database distinguishes more popular products – which were well known and/or highly sought after, which had long, successful careers, or which drew particular attention – from those with a short-lived or erratic presence in Vietnam.[55]

Overview of the Book

There are several dimensions of the colonial history of pharmaceuticals that are *not* the primary focus of this book. It is not my intention to revisit Euro-American drug production "from the periphery," or to assess the impact of colonial medicalization projects on a therapeutic transition in the metropole. These are worthwhile objectives, but they are beyond the scope of this project. Also, I do not provide a comprehensive overview of (though I do touch upon) colonial drug research, including bioprospection, and therapeutic trials, in Vietnam. Nor do I reconstruct the underlying logics of colonial practitioners' therapeutic practices and experiments. In other words, this is not primarily a history of medicines as objects of colonial science, but rather, as I hope is clear by now, a history of medicines as tools and objects of social change. My main objective is to examine how, and to what extent, modern medicines and the "colonial situation," to use the French sociologist George Balandier's expression,[56] were mutually transformed. How were medicines shaped and incorporated into changing local health practices in the context of colonial rule, and, conversely, how were they redefined by colonial encounters and experiences?

To fully grasp pharmaceutical consumption patterns and especially their determinants in Vietnam, it is, however, essential to first retrace the steps by which they were produced, defined, and brought to potential Vietnamese consumers. I begin, in Chapter 1, by explaining

[55] I also compiled a database of pharmacists and doctors, allowing for an estimation of their number and to reconstruct some of their professional trajectories.
[56] Georges Balandier, "La situation coloniale. Approche théorique," *Cahiers internationaux de sociologie* 12 (1951): 44–79.

what I mean by *modern*, and *colonial*, medicines. In Chapter 2, I sketch out the outlines of the history of pharmaceutical importation to Indochina, and of the main (and knowable) qualitative and quantitative features of the "medicines market" in Vietnam from the last third of the nineteenth century to the Japanese occupation of French Indochina. Chapter 3 describes the circulation and distribution of *public medicines*, thus illuminating their role in colonial health policy and within the framework of the AMI. These first chapters show how large the gap was between discourses reflecting the intentions of colonial medicalization and the realities of health care implementation. While this gap is most evident in the inadequate distribution and accessibility of both medical services and medicines, it was also exacerbated by the slow, rather reluctant acceptance, by colonial authorities and doctors, of medicines as suitable tools of medicalization.

Chapters 4 and 5 focus on some of the key actors involved in the distribution of pharmaceuticals beyond the public health care system. Beginning, in Chapter 4, in the world of Western-style pharmacists and pharmacies, I then move on to the panoply of actors – professional and lay, colonial and colonized, foreign and local, from health specialists to purely commercial actors – who traded in colonial medicines. This chapter highlights the extraordinary fluidity, productivity, and adaptability of pharmaceutical distribution networks. Such flexibility is perhaps most salient in practices that played on, and sometimes transgressed, the limits of legality, which were delineated by a highly detailed and restrictive, but not always enforced (or enforceable), legislative corpus. Focusing on these illicit practices, Chapter 5 shows how innovative pharmaceutical actors could be, creating new possibilities for individual and collective health care.

Chapters 6 through 8 focus on the consumption of medicines, which depended on these diverse, permeable distribution circuits and a versatile, expanding market. My aim here is to gauge the popularity of modern medicines, especially in the interwar period, and indeed to identify the conditions and possible forms under which medicines might have become popular. This brings me, in Chapter 6, to examine the role of pharmaceuticals within broader transformations in Vietnamese health, health care, and day-to-day therapeutic choices, especially in urban settings where social change was at its most striking, if still uneven. I especially seek to analyze the mutual influence between an emerging health consumerism, which considered medicines less as a colonial "gift" and more as a modern commodity, and "quests for therapy." I follow up on this analysis in Chapter 7 by considering whether, and how, demands for medicines were associated with the acceptance of certain biomedical rules (and the refusal of others), and in Chapter 8, by describing the rise of new forms of therapeutic pluralism. These plural practices were fashioned, of course, by the pressures and opportunities of colonization and colonial medicines, but also by shifts in the conceptualization and practice of Vietnamese medicine, as well as by the health care needs of men and women, children and the elderly.[57]

While this book is not a history of encounters between medical cultures and epistemologies, it nevertheless provides a closeup view of the colonial past of medical pluralism. In this, Vietnam, as part of French Indochina, is a fascinating case study that is particularly illuminating in revisiting the past of the globalization (or not) of individual and collective conceptions of health. In particular, it reveals three dimensions of this past: the enterprise of colonial medicalization as it unfolded in a specific colonial situation; the health perspectives and agency of the colonized; and, finally, the potentially transformative impact of medicines on conceptions of health. Though it was certainly violent and normative, modern colonization did not completely crush the liberty of action of the colonized. As producers, distributors, and consumers of medicines, the Vietnamese participated in many significant ways in the process of their own medicalization. There were many medicalizations in Vietnam, and medicines became key mediators in colonial encounters as a site for the expression of a range of expectations, desires, negotiations, and practices. Almost twenty-five years ago already, historian Luise White suggested that medicines (and other medical technologies), because they elicited seemingly conflicting discourses from colonial and colonized actors, could be taken up as a privileged analytical vantage point on the colonial phenomenon and its legacies.[58] *The Colonial Life of Pharmaceuticals* is a response to her call.

---

[57] It is, however, important to note that the colonized perspectives and practices revealed by these multiple sources are primarily those of men who were educated and lived in the city.

[58] Luise White, "They Could Make Their Victims Dull: Genders and Genres, Fantasies and Cures in Colonial Southern Uganda," *The American Historical Review* 100, 5 (1995): 1379–402.

1   Making Medicines Modern, Making Medicines Colonial

As medicines were imported, distributed, marketed, consumed, and even eventually produced in Vietnam, under the conditions created by colonial health policies and regulation, as well as by dynamic private therapeutic markets and changing practices of health consumption and care, they became, in various ways, *colonial* medicines. In other words, by circulating in colonial Vietnam, modern medicines were transformed in terms of their forms, meanings, effects, and identities. This transformation is a core topic of this book. Yet even outside Vietnam, and notably in the French metropole, the very notion of what a medicine was – its form and appearance, how and by whom it should be made and sold, how it should be regulated and advertised, prescribed, and consumed, how it should be owned, and what it should do – changed profoundly, albeit gradually, between the mid-nineteenth and mid-twentieth centuries. In other words, medicines were undergoing a long and uneven process of becoming modern at the same time as they were becoming colonial. This chapter identifies points of contact between these joint processes, describing the main legislative, industrial, commercial, and scientific trends and actors that made medicines dynamic and heterogeneous objects before and as they were imported to the Southeast Asian colony. A series of major shifts shaped, both directly and indirectly, the kinds of medicines that would enter Vietnam and the ways in which their circulation would be regulated. Among these were the transition from artisanal to industrial modes of production, the increasingly central role of chemistry and pharmacology laboratories in conjunction with the rise of a pharmaceutical industry, and the growing role of the state in protecting public health.

1.1   Modernizing Medicines: A Lexicon of Innovation and Coexistence

What is a modern drug? Historians offer no precise or shared definition. Many attempts draw on juridical criteria that are usually anachronistic and ahistorical, and therefore have limited value in describing the process of therapeutic modernization. Several historians take as their chronological starting point the extraction of alkaloids from plants beginning in the early nineteenth century, suggesting, at least implicitly, that modern medicines be defined by their basis in purified active substances.[1] Some go a step further by listing the basic characteristics that came, over time, to qualify medicines as *modern*. It is a material object, with tangible and calculable "thinginess"; its dosage is precise and, ideally, it is physically and chemically stable.[2] It is mass-produced using standardized procedures. Its therapeutic indications are specified and validated on the basis of consensual criteria. It is also a technical and scientific object that embodies one or more forms of expertise. As its material form becomes increasingly precise and miniaturized, it circulates more freely, with growing ease and speed over time.[3]

Modern medicines did not emerge in isolation or as a single category. As in other European and North American countries, the French drug market in the nineteenth century was divided into different segments according to the nature of products (vegetable, mineral, animal), their therapeutic indication (what they were used for), and their legal status. This division would last into the following century. However, with the introduction of pharmaceutical specialties from the 1850s, another differentiation emerged between *spécialités médicales* (medical specialties) and *spécialités commerciales* (commercial specialties). A further distinction was then made between prescription-only and over-the-counter (OTC) products, while therapeutic classes and pharmaceutical forms would provide additional criteria for classifying medicines.[4] The first specialties coexisted with a profusion of *remèdes secrets* (secret remedies), as well as other medicines that were trademarked but produced on a modest scale in retail pharmacies that had been converted into artisanal production facilities.[5]

---

[1] Alkaloids are pharmacologically active organic chemical compounds. They are the active ingredients in many of the first modern medicines, such as quinine, morphine, and cocaine.

[2] Jacques Azema, "La définition juridique du médicament," in *La philosophie du remède*, ed. Jean-Claude Beaune (Paris: Champ-Vallon, 1993), 37–44.

[3] Christian Bonah and Anne Rasmussen, ed., *Histoire et médicament aux XIXe et XXe siècles* (Paris: Glyphe, 2005), 11.

[4] Sophie Chauveau, "Marché et publicité des médicaments," in Bonah and Rasmussen, *Histoire et médicament*, 192–93.

[5] Translator's note: Literal translations of the terms "medical specialty" and "commercial specialty" are used throughout this book to capture their specific meanings in relation to the history of the French pharmaceutical industry, legislation, and modes of distribution. The French terms "officine" and "pharmacie" have been translated as "pharmacy" (when needed, specified as "private" or "retail"), referring to a retail shop that, according to French law, was owned and managed by a qualified pharmacist, which can also be called a drugstore, a chemist's shop, or (earlier) an apothecary shop.

In parallel, a wide range of older forms of medicines remained omnipresent in pharmacists' daily routines and clinical practice up until after World War II.[6] These were of two types: *préparations magistrales* (magistral formulae), which were prepared to order according to a physician's prescription, and *remèdes officinaux* (officinal remedies), which could be made up in advance according to ingredients and compositions dictated by the Codex, the French official pharmacopeia, and kept in stock.[7] Medical historian Olivier Faure has emphasized the heterogeneity of French retail pharmacists' practices up until the 1920s; as the number of magistral preparations dwindled, they tended to "improvise" preparations, some of which they marketed as specialties.[8] Still, the market was clearly marked by a growing industrialization of drug production that began in the mid-nineteenth century.

The French category of spécialité médicale is not the exact equivalent of that of ethical drug in the Anglo-American context. It does, however, share some of its characteristics: these medicines were explicitly qualified as scientific, specifically as the product of innovation obtained by chemical manipulation and pharmacological testing. They could be innovative by virtue of a novel active ingredient, an original combination of ingredients, or the validation of a new therapeutic indication. Their dispensation was generally restricted to a medical prescription, either because they contained toxic ingredients or because manufacturers themselves sought, in this way, to emphasize their products' scientific legitimacy – as medicines requiring expert guidance. In contrast, commercial specialties, a category parallel to that of patent drugs, often had a basis in existing officinal formulae but were either distributed under a new brand name and/or claimed an "improvement" on pharmacopeia instructions. By the late nineteenth century, commercial specialties were heavily advertised; most were defined as nontoxic, could be sold OTC, and were thus widely used in self-medication. The rapid rise of commercial specialties dovetailed the earlier popularity, accessibility, and deft marketing of secret remedies. Yet pharmacists also sought to distinguish the new medicines by the quality of their design and manufacturing, in which they invested

[6] Jacques Neukirch, "Comment le Français moyen utilise les médicaments?," *Hommes & commerce* 23 (1954): 63–67.

[7] Up until 1963, the Codex was a list of formulae for the compounding of officinal preparations for dispensing in pharmacies. It was regularly updated by order of the state by a commission made up of professors in faculties of pharmacy and medicine. Pharmacists were required to use the most recent version.

[8] Faure finds that pharmaceutical specialties were already catching up with other types of medicines by 1914, and were favored because they allowed for more profit with less work: Olivier Faure, "Les officines pharmaceutiques françaises: de la réalité au mythe, fin XIXe-début XXe siècle," *Revue d'histoire moderne et contemporaine* 43 (1996): 676–77.

out of professional and commercial ambition, as well as to showcase their growing scientific expertise.[9] Indeed, the distinction between medical and commercial specialties was blurred by such claims to scientific quality, as well as by similarities in marketing strategies. As we will see, this confusion was also present, even amplified, in the Vietnamese context.

This gradual modernization also resulted in the juxtaposition of old and new material forms of presentation and packaging. Even as pharmacists continued to compound potions, salves, elixirs, balms, and so on, new pharmaceutical presentations were developed to facilitate the mass production and distribution from the mid-nineteenth century. Notable among these were pills, tablets, capsules, gel capsules, granules, ovules, as well as ampoules for injectable preparations. While the hypodermic syringe, first used in medical practice around 1850, emerged from the field of surgery (for anesthesia) rather than the pharmacy sector, its adoption coincided with the introduction of highly active substances. Injection techniques thus came to play an important role in the development of modern therapeutics, helping demonstrate the efficacy of certain products, such as anesthetics, analgesics, and antimicrobial drugs.[10] Standards for shelf life and packaging, as well as for labeling, were introduced alongside the industrialization of drug production. As the art of compounding medicines gradually disappeared, drugs came to be identified with these new material forms.

1.2   Producing Medical Specialties, between Science and Industry

The history of modern drugs is often told as one of pharmacological discovery and of growing alliance between the laboratory and industry. This narrative begins with the extraction of alkaloids. Isolated by the Hanoverian chemist Friedrich Sertüner around 1806, morphine is often identified as one of the first truly active medicines, especially following its intravenous administration from the 1860s to 1870s. From then on, the list of new pharmacologically active substances grew quickly: quinine was isolated from cinchona bark by Joseph Pelletier in 1820, followed by atropine in belladonna and strychnine in Nux vomica, while Albert Niemann extracted cocaine from coca in 1860. New techniques in organic chemistry allowed for a rapid progression: from the isolation and characterization of alkaloids to their synthesis and reproduction,

[9] Chauveau, *L'invention pharmaceutique*, 19–21.
[10] Norman Howard-Jones, "A Critical Study of the Origins and Early Development of Hypodermic Medication," *Journal of the History of Medicine* 2, 2 (1947): 201–49.

and then to the synthesis of novel substances.[11] German chemists first synthesized chloral in 1832 and urea in 1836, followed by other organic compounds.

Another important step was the (serendipitous) discovery of the first synthetic dye, aniline purple, in 1856, which launched a chemical dye industry that would spur the development of pharmaceuticals. The German chemical company Bayer was the first to commercialize a synthetic medicine in 1885: phenacetin or acetophenetidin, a painkiller from which paracetamol/acetaminophen was later derived. Then came acetylsalicylic acid, introduced to the market by Bayer in 1897; it was soon sold around the world under the brand name Aspirin. Another Bayer product, Heroin, the brand name for diacetylmorphine, which was chemically isolated from morphine in London in 1887, was marketed from 1898. In 1903, Bayer commercialized its first sedative, Barbital (Veronal), derived from barbituric acid, which was synthesized in 1864 by future Nobel Prize in Chemistry winner Adolf Von Baeyer.

Through these synthetic drugs, several research laboratories, both private and public, including university labs, came to play a central role in pharmaceutical development and production, along with the chemical industry. By the turn of the twentieth century, the fields of drug research and development (isolation or synthesis of new molecules and the testing of their properties) were being hinged to industrial production through an increasingly dense web of lab-industry connections.[12] In France, this trend is exemplified by the relations cultivated by the firm Établissements Poulenc Frères (later Rhône-Poulenc, incorporated in 1928 after a merger with the Société chimique des usines du Rhône)[13] with the Laboratoire de chimie thérapeutique, a lab created in 1911 as part of the Institut Pasteur in Paris under the direction of pharmacist and former Poulenc chemist Ernest Fourneau. Evidence points to a concrete arrangement between these parties that lasted into the 1930s. Rhône-Poulenc offered material and financial resources, for example by supplying the lab with raw materials and paying some of its researchers' salaries. In return, Fourneau and his collaborators provided the firm with new medicines, including "copies"

[11] However, the standardization of manufacturing processes would take longer, while the means as well as the degree of testing for efficacy and safety would remain highly varied until at least World War II.

[12] Viviane Quirke, *Collaboration in the Pharmaceutical Industry. Changing Relationships in Britain and France 1935–1965* (London: Routledge, 2007).

[13] I use the latter, better-known name of the company to refer to the firm throughout the book. Rhône-Poulenc merged with Hoechst AG to form Aventis in 1999. On the general history of the company, see Pierre Cayez, *Rhône-Poulenc, 1895–1975* (Paris: Armand Colin and Masson, 1988).

of German products recreated with new formulae.[14] In Germany, this type of collusion between the industrial and research sectors was even stronger.[15] Such relations heralded the emergence of a pharmaceutical research and development sector, and its generalization after World War II. The relationship between Poulenc and the Pastorian lab is notable as a precursor of a more widespread trend, but also, as we will see shortly, for its direct consequences on the pharmaceutical market in Vietnam.

These science-industry dynamics, fueled by national and international emulation and competition, stimulated the development of three categories of synthetic antimicrobial therapies in the 1910s to 1930s, which came to play an important role in the treatment of disease worldwide: arsenobenzols, antimalarial drugs, and sulfonamides or sulfa drugs. Arsenical compounds, synthesized from organic by-products of arsenic, led to the first effective synthetic antimicrobial drugs: arsenobenzols. Compound 606 is often identified as the first "magic bullet," and its discoverer, German physician Paul Ehrlich, is commonly celebrated as the founding father of modern chemotherapy.[16] While arsenical compounds were synthesized in France several decades earlier (to be later commercialized as Atoxyl and Tripoxyl), Ehrlich and his team were the first to elucidate their chemical structure and to demonstrate their specific therapeutic action on syphilis and trypanosomiases (sleeping sickness and Chagas disease).

The synthesis of 606 coincided with the discovery of treponema bacteria, the causative agent of syphilis in 1905, followed shortly by the development of the Bordet-Wasserman test for diagnosing and monitoring the disease. The compound was commercialized by several firms, including the German company Hoechst (Salvarsan) and Poulenc (Arsénobenzol Billon). Hoechst, founded as a small dye manufacturer in 1864, had become the first industrial producer of synthetic medicines in 1884 by maintaining close ties with medical researchers such as Ehrlich and the bacteriologist Robert Koch.[17] The distribution of 606 under several brand names was quickly followed by the discovery of Compound 914 (whose brand names included Neosalvarsan, Novarsénobenzol, Uclarsyl, and Rhodarsan Rhône-Poulenc), which

---

[14] Séverine Baverey-Massat-Bourrat, "De la copie au nouveau médicament. Le laboratoire de chimie thérapeutique," *Entreprises & histoire* 36 (2004): 48–63.

[15] Quirke, *Collaboration*, 8, 58.

[16] John Parascandola, "Alkaloids to Arsenicals: Systematic Drug Discovery before the First World War," in *The Inside Story of Medicines: A Symposium*, ed. Elaine Stroud and Gregory Higby (Madison: American Institute for the History of Pharmacy, 1997), 78–79.

[17] Alexandre Blondeau, *Histoire des laboratoires pharmaceutiques en France et de leurs médicaments* (Paris: Le Cherche-midi, 1992, vol. 1), 110–19.

was deemed less toxic and more soluble than 606. New bacteriological knowledge, as well as diagnostic technologies, created the conditions for arsenical compounds to become "revolutionary drugs."[18]

A second strand of research on antimicrobial agents emerged from the accidental observation by a student of Ehrlich's that quinine acted on trypanosomes in experimentally infected mice. The identification of similarities between pathogenic microorganisms opened up new possibilities for the development of antimicrobials. By World War I, a derivative of cupreine, Eucupin, was marketed for external use on wounds, and in 1920, ethacridine (Rivanol) was synthesized, and soon used to treat amoebic dysentery. In parallel, ongoing research on synthetic dyes revealed in 1891 that Plasmodium, the parasite recently discovered by Alphonse Laveran (a Pastorian and military doctor) as the causal agent of malaria, could be stained. Ehrlich thus hypothesized that a change in color might modify the viability of the microorganism, and experimented with methylene blue as a treatment for malaria. Slowed by the lack of animal models of malaria, this line of investigation eventually prompted trials of derivatives of methylene blue in syphilis patients therapeutically infected with malaria – based on the belief that syphilis could be treated by high fever – leading to the first synthetic antimalarial drugs: plasmochine (1926), quinacrine (1932), and chloroquine, synthesized in 1934 and commercialized as Nivaquine after World War II.

Sulfa drugs, the precursors of penicillin and its derivatives (in other words, an early type of antibiotics), were the fruit of a systematic quest for a treatment for internal infections that was driven by the German pharmaceutical firm IG Farben.[19] This quest was entrusted to Gerard Domagk, recruited as director of its Institute of pathology and experimental pathological anatomy in 1927. Using streptococcal infection as an experimental model, Domagk observed the action of phenaxopyridine, a synthetic organic dye. Experiments with similar compounds led the way to sulfonamides. In 1932, sulfamidochrysoidine (Streptozon) was the first drug whose effects were observed to cure an internal infection, and by the end of the year, IG Farben had filed a patent for the molecule under the brand name Protonsil. Domagk only published his results in 1935. By then, Fourneau's lab, in competition with the Germans and in collaboration with Rhône-Poulenc, had already developed antimicrobial medications such as acetarsol, commercialized as Stovarsol. The lab also

[18] J. E. Ross and S. M. Tomkins, "The British Reception of Salvarsan," *Journal of the History of Medicine and Allied Sciences* 52, 4 (1997): 398–423.

[19] John Lesch, "Chemistry and Biomedicine in an Industrial Setting: The Invention of Sulfa Drugs," in *Chemical Sciences in the Modern World*, ed. Seymour H. Mauskopf (Philadelphia: University of Pennsylvania Press, 1993), 158.

reproduced Streptozon to allow for its commercialization in France under the brand name Rubiazol. However, the compound was quickly found to be inactive in vitro, leading to the identification of sulfanilamide, which was not a dye, as its active molecule. This new molecule was then commercialized under several names in France, including Septoplix by the firm Théraplix in 1936.[20] Other derivatives of sulfanilamide were developed, notably Sulfapyridine, by the British firm May & Baker Ltd. Commercialized as Dagénan from 1938, it proved to be particularly active against pneumococcal infections.

These flagship products were not the only ones to make their way to market from the lab. Several other drug categories were also developed during the interwar period, including anesthetics, barbiturates, and products used in opotherapy (or organotherapy, using extracts from animal organs to replace various secretion insufficiencies) and hormone therapy.[21] Thyroxine and insulin were purified from animal organs, and steroids were identified and isolated. By the late 1930s, most vitamins had not only been isolated, but their molecular structure was known and could be synthesized.[22] It should be noted that the rise of vaccine and serum therapies also played a crucial role in the transformation of biotherapies during this period.

1.3   Protecting Innovation . . .

The expanding drug market was fueled not only by these new molecules from the "ethical" drug industry, but also by a proliferation of commercial specialties. From the second half of the nineteenth century, more than seventy thousand medicines were probably available OTC in the French market. A majority of these contained recently discovered alkaloids, and were therefore pharmacologically active. In the 1920s, twenty thousand to thirty thousand substances were associated with about sixty thousand brand names, marketed as both medical and commercial specialties.[23] The identity of commercial specialties was, however, rather nebulous; it raised questions about whether these were really distinct

[20] Daniel Bovet, *Une chimie qui guérit* (Paris: Payot, 1988), 68–69.

[21] Ilana Löwy, "Biotherapies of Chronic Diseases in the Interwar Period: From Witte's Peptone to Penicillium Extract," *Studies in the History and Philosophy of Biological and Biomedical Sciences* 36 (2005): 675–95; Jean-Paul Gaudillière, "Genesis and Development of a Biomedical Object: Styles of Thoughts, Styles of Work and the History of Sex Steroids," *Studies in History and Philosophy of Science* 35, 3 (2004): 525–43.

[22] Miles Weatherhall, *In Search of A Cure: A History of Pharmaceutical Discovery* (Oxford: Oxford University Press, 1990), 140–50.

[23] Chauveau, *L'invention pharmaceutique*, 52–53.

from the older secret remedies, as well as about how to protect both innovation and the public, that is, consumers.

In France, the legality of secret remedies had long been a tricky question. An 1805 decree authorized inventors to continue distributing formulae they had already commercialized. This law also allowed anyone, even non-pharmacists, to submit claims of innovation to the Académie de médecine (Academy of Medicine), which could grant an exclusive right to sell the product for profit, as well as protection from counterfeiting by the "guarantee of the secret of the formula." Such dispositions left loopholes open for a growing range of illegally produced medicines to compete with the legal sector. Although a 1844 law prohibited pharmacists from preparing a large quantity of remedies, other than officinal formulae, "in advance" (i.e., to sell these as ready-made products), they very likely entered the fray by producing their own brands of secret remedies. Increasingly, larger firms also produced secret remedies. Despite the introduction of new laws in 1837, 1842, and 1850, the production of secret remedies was allowed to grow in a climate of tolerance, partly for pragmatic reasons.

In parallel, by the late nineteenth century, producers of commercial specialties were making the most not only of scientific and industrial advances, but also of changes in the nature of the market. The growing diffusion of these specialties, which were generally quite cheap to produce, was both facilitated by, and fed into, a shift in the economic and commercial regulation of pharmaceuticals in France and elsewhere. As a moneymaking business, the drug industry – which was still, at the time, highly fragmented and heterogeneous in size – sought to maximize profits, reduce competition, and protect its branded products. The history of modern drugs is thus also one of changing conditions of ownership and of the protection of innovation. In 1844, the French Assembly of the Constitutional Monarchy had examined the possibility of granting patents to protect therapeutic innovations. This project was supported by some chemists and the nascent industry, but was defeated by opposition from pharmacists and doctors. The latter argued that making remedies the object of intellectual property was wrong. Furthermore, this would create an obstacle to adequate control of quality and efficacy, which only they – not profit-seeking inventors and producers – could ensure. They also won in part because no provisions had been made for a mechanism to authorize the sale of patented medicines.[24]

---

[24] Jean-Paul Gaudillière, "Drugs Trajectories," *Studies in the History of Biological and Biomedical Sciences* 36 (2005): 136.

French resistance to the patenting of medicines did not, however, prevent the proliferation of trademarks. Following the example set by other industrial sectors, an 1857 law allowed for the trademarking of specific procedures (extraction, synthesis, vitamin separation), thus offering protection from counterfeiting.[25] Substances themselves were excluded from intellectual property, and the names of a brand and of a medicinal substance could not be identical. Under this juridical framework, the French firm Dausse, for example, could legally affix its name to products based on plant extracts that had a long history of therapeutic use and figured in the French pharmacopeia, such as valerian (Valériane Dausse), gentian (Gentiane Dausse), and belladonna (Belladone Dausse). What the firm sought to brand was a specific material form and the guarantee of product stability, thus advertising the firm's expertise in handling plant substances.[26] The industrialization and growth of the pharmaceutical sector soon made the 1844 decision irrelevant. Discussions about pharmaceutical patenting reemerged in France after World War I, in response to concerns about German dominance of the European drug and chemical industries, yet a bill proposed in 1927 was then abandoned.[27] From 1916, a tax of 6 percent was levied on the sale of medicines that did not display a list of ingredients on their packaging. Beginning in 1923, foreign pharmaceuticals could only be sold if labeled with the name and dosage of their active substances. Secret remedies were definitively outlawed in 1926. A decree stated that medicines prepared in advance for public distribution (these were now explicitly referred to as spécialités pharmaceutiques and were clearly widely available by this time) would not "be considered secret remedies," provided they were clearly labeled with the name and dosage of each of their active ingredients, as well as the name and address of the producer.

There was no significant legislative reform, however, until a licensing system was established in 1941. The license protected conditions of sale rather than invention per se, but it nevertheless rested on an evaluation of efficacy, safety, as well as originality.[28] Firms that invested in research

---

[25] Maurice Cassier, "Brevets pharmaceutiques et santé publique en France. Opposition et dispositifs spécifiques d'appropriation des médicaments entre 1791 et 2004," *Entreprise & histoire* 36 (2004): 29–46.

[26] Gaudillière, "Drugs Trajectories," 128.

[27] The bill proposed a general system of patents on procedures in chemistry and pharmacy, thus replacing the patent on chemical substances. The idea was to follow the German model, both because it presented greater incentives for invention of new procedures and would prevent German firms from filing patents in France for chemical substances, which offered a broader monopoly than the patent on procedures.

[28] Sophie Chauveau, "Genèse de la 'sécurité sanitaire': les produits pharmaceutiques en France aux XIXe et XXe siècles," *Revue d'histoire moderne et contemporaine* 51, 2 (2004): 98–99.

laboratories could also pursue other forms of protection. From 1900, the Office national de la protection industrielle (National Office of Industrial Protection) determined, on a case-by-case basis, what mechanisms might apply to the invention of synthetic molecules or of other therapeutic substances. Procedures that led to well-defined chemical products could be patented, with minimal negative impact on public health since the product could also be obtained by alternative means. The patent application was denied if the procedure led to a chemically-indeterminate substance or a simple mixture. By the mid-1930s, evaluation criteria were revised to include tests and biological standards in response to growing demand for this type of patent, as well as the introduction of new types of molecules such as hormones. Thus, in 1937–38, Rhône-Poulenc obtained three patents on procedures for the preparation of derivatives of benzenesulfonamide, while several other firms obtained patents for hormone- and organ-based preparations on the basis of specific extraction processes.[29] From the 1920s, drug producers also routinely registered product formulae to protect these against fraud at a university laboratory. Eventually, this laboratory became the National Drug Control Laboratory and was accredited by the French government for the analysis of new pharmaceuticals.

This scramble for patents – which largely bypassed the principle of non-patentability of medicines – is proof of the rapid emergence, over the space of a few decades, of a dynamic and innovative drug market in France that was keen to develop measures of protection against domestic as well as foreign competition. Drug producers from individual pharmacists to industrial firms formed collectives, such as the Union des fabricants (Union of producers), established in 1872, and the Chambre syndicale des fabricants de produits pharmaceutiques (Syndicate of pharmaceutical producers), formed in 1879. These sought to control fraud, set pricing policies, and secure access to conformity testing in advance of legislation on these matters. Alliances even reached across borders. For example, an alliance between Rhône-Poulenc and May & Baker Ltd. was initially formed to give the British firm access to the production of a French arsenical compound during World War I. It led to a progressive merger that would allow the French firm to benefit from the British research lab.[30] Yet given that pharmaceuticals were patentable in several countries such as the United States and Germany, French legislation was felt by many to be overly restrictive. Indeed, as we will

---

[29] Blondeau, *Histoire des laboratoires*, 228–39.
[30] John Lesch, *The First Miracle Drugs. How the Sulfa Drugs Transformed Medicine* (Oxford and New York: Oxford University Press, 2007).

see, French pharmaceutical regulation in general tended, even beyond the issue of intellectual property, to be highly restrictive.

1.4   ... And Protecting the Public

The regulation of secret remedies must also be understood in light of the growing preoccupation of modern states, and of health care professionals, with public protection from dangerous and inefficient drugs. Medicines were made modern by the new forms of production, marketing, and chemical manipulation described previously, but also by legislation that redefined medicines as objects of public health regulation, therapeutic efficacy, expertise, and professional prerogatives (and not just of commercial property). From the beginning of the nineteenth century, the professionalization of medicine and pharmacy in both Europe and North America was buttressed by monopolies over some areas of practice that involved medicines. In parallel, new concerns about the potential toxicity of medicines warranted growing state intervention into pharmaceutical markets in many countries, including France. In the name of public health and safety, the space restricted to pharmacists and doctors expanded, covering an ever-larger number of substances and practices.

Pharmacists' exclusive right to prepare, dispense, and sell drugs "in medicinal quantity" (for retail sale) to the public, as well as their monopoly over filling medical prescriptions, was defined in France by the law of Germinal year XI (April 11, 1803). Pharmacists were qualified as such by holding a diploma from one of the pharmacy schools accredited by the state, and by the purchase of a business license for their pharmacy. They also had to be at least twenty-five years old, and own their pharmacy, but could not own more than one business. This law distinguished between pharmacists, as professionals, and grocers, wholesale druggists, and herbalists.[31] Until 1898, there were two classes of pharmacists: *pharmaciens de première classe* (first-class pharmacists) held full state diplomas, while *pharmaciens de deuxième classe* (second-class pharmacists) graduated from a shorter, more practical-oriented training program. The latter had limited professional prerogatives; in particular, they could not set up shop outside the jurisdiction of the local jury that had recognized their right to practice. By contrast, the training of first-class pharmacists was

---

[31] Herbalists were allowed (until 1941) to continue selling medicinal plants or their parts, fresh or dried, provided they passed an examination by a school of pharmacy or a medical jury. Legislation on toxic substances would, however, significantly restrict both herbalists' and druggists' field of practice. Also, in rural areas, the sale of medicines by non-pharmacists, usually by doctors (a practice called *propharmacie* [propharmacy]), continued to be tolerated.

increasingly rigorous. By the end of the nineteenth century, they could claim to be real scientists, usually chemists.

Parts of the 1803 ruling soon became inapplicable. The law itself was contradictory, in putting forward a restrictive definition of medicines (i.e., magistral and officinal preparations) that, according to article 32, only pharmacists were qualified to prepare. The emerging pharmaceutical industry, especially, quickly made some dimensions of this new monopoly obsolete, or at least problematic. At the same time, many pharmacists, drawing on the possibilities opened by scientific and technological advances, and surely responding to a popular demand, equipped their shops for the serial production and marketing of a range of "house" medicines.[32] New mechanisms were created to control this trend. For instance, a 1905 law on fraud control, which replaced a July 1824 bill on drug alterations that had quickly become irrelevant, included dispositions for the prosecution of pharmacists guilty of practicing sophistication, which referred to the sale of specialties that did not correspond to the formulation on their label.

In parallel, medicines were increasingly limited, at least in theory, to prescription-only sale in France and elsewhere. The isolation and synthesis of active substances brought the question of toxicity to the fore. The intimate link between pharmacology and toxicology was emphasized as early as 1822 by the physiologist François Magendie, who demonstrated, in particular, how pure substances can alter the tissues to which they attach themselves.[33] By the mid-nineteenth century, manufacturers' freedom to choose the level of sales restriction on their products was increasingly overruled by an ever-stricter regulation of substances defined as toxic. In response to a sensational case of domestic poisoning, the Lafarge case (1840), a law was passed in 1845 to define the conditions under which *substances vénéneuses* (poisonous substances) could be dispensed: exclusively by pharmacists and only upon receipt of a doctor's prescription that included a date, signature, and specific dosage. Indeed, dosage was increasingly seen as key to determining whether the action of a pure substance would be therapeutic or harmful, and soon became a crucial consideration in the production and control of medicines more broadly.

The law required pharmacists to record every move of these poisonous substances in a register, and to keep these "in a safe place, under lock and key." The first list of these restricted substances was released in 1846.

---

[32] Anne Rasmussen, "Les enjeux d'une histoire des formes pharmaceutiques: la galénique, l'officine et l'industrie (XIXe-début XXe siècle)," *Entreprises & histoire* 36 (2004): 17–20.

[33] François Magendie, *Formulaire pour la préparation et l'emploi de plusieurs nouveaux médicaments tels la noix vomique, la morphine, etc.* (Paris: Méquignon-Marvis, 1822).

It contained seventy-two items, including opium and its preparations and derivatives (such as morphine, codeine, laudanum). The lists would keep getting longer over the years. In 1895, phosphorus as well as all vaccines and therapeutic serums – with the exception of smallpox vaccine, which was already in use in mass vaccination campaigns – were added, as well as therapeutic substances administered by injection. This expanded the terrain reserved to the doctor-pharmacist couple, contributing to the protection of both their professional and economic interests and to the emergence of a new, modern therapeutic relationship between doctor, pharmacist, and patient. The Inspection des pharmacies, formally established in July of 1908, was meant to enforce these laws on fraud and the sale of toxic substances.

Restrictions were further tightened in response to international pressures on national governments to restrict access to narcotic substances. Older concerns about toxicity were joined by the growing recognition of addiction as a social problem.[34] From China to France, across colonial empires and in North America, concerns were voiced about the dangers of opium and its derivatives, whether consumed for therapeutic or recreational purposes. Many secret remedies and commercial specialties, sold as syrups, bars, and drops, still contained opium and morphine. The French law of 1916 on toxic substances reflects this new preoccupation with narcotics. Unanimously approved by Parliament, the law distinguished between three categories of substances: schedule A (highly toxic), schedule B (narcotics), and schedule C (slightly or moderately toxic and not subject to prescription). It also set a minimal toxic dose that determined whether products were subject to prescription. Substances were to be identified by a color-coded label, and those classified in schedules A and B were to be stored separately. The list of toxic items included about 140 substances and their salts, as well as several pharmacopeia-based preparations, such as Fowler's Solution (containing potassium arsenate), Kendal Black Drops (opium-based), and Sirop Gibert (a syrup combining iodide of mercury and potassium).

The control of toxic substances continued to be tightened during the interwar years as substances were added to or moved between restricted schedules (e.g., the alkaloids of opium and their salts and derivatives were moved to schedule A in the 1920s) and as specific provisions were implemented to further restrict the circulation of narcotics.[35]

---

[34] John Hoffman, "The Historical Shift in the Perception of Opiates: From Medicine to Social Menace," *Journal of Psychoactive Drugs* 22, 1 (1990): 53–62.

[35] The control of schedule B substances would be even more strictly codified by a 1930 decree that restricted their production and circulation to individuals having obtained a nominal authorization to do so.

1.5   Specificity, Popularity, and the Therapeutic Transition

Tightening the control of toxic substances clearly reinforced the power of the prescriber, during a time when the "modern doctor" was professionalizing in France. Six years before the category of second-class pharmacist was abandoned, an 1892 law had likewise eliminated the parallel status of second-class doctor, or *officier de santé* (health officer), who was allowed to work outside the main urban areas. Hereafter, only those holding a state doctorate in medicine were qualified to practice medicine. The right to prescribe was thus restricted to a single class of qualified practitioners.

Yet it seems that many doctors were reluctant to deploy this power to prescribe. Many historians have noted a tendency toward therapeutic skepticism, even *therapeutic nihilism*, among physicians in several industrializing countries in the second half of the nineteenth century. They suggest that this suspicion of therapeutics was associated with a rejection of "heroic medicine." Popular over the previous century, this "heroic trend" favored treatments that produced immediate effects that were powerful and perceptible; it was later criticized as ineffective and risky.[36] In addition, most remedies, up until the late nineteenth century, acted either on symptoms (such as fever or pain) or on a physiological function (digestion, for example). Many thus had a wide range of therapeutic indications (i.e., were seen as panacea) or were used as mere "adjuvant therapies."[37] The goal, for clinicians, had been to formulate magistral preparations that were suited to the specific nature of individual patients' conditions and characteristics.

From the late nineteenth century, the action of medicines was, by contrast, increasingly targeted at a specific pathology: either a causative microorganism (hence the popularity of the image of the magic bullet) or a cellular or physiological disease process. At the same time, diseases were increasingly defined as specific entities that were independent of patients' idiosyncratic constitutions. The clinician's task was no longer to define the specificity of patients, but instead to identify a treatment that was specific to the disease in order to prescribe the "right product," an "antidote."[38] While different medical and therapeutic systems previously had much in common, this paradigm change increasingly made

---

[36] Warner, *The Therapeutic Perspective.*

[37] An adjuvant therapy is given in addition to the primary or initial therapy in order to bolster its effect. At this time, the idea was usually to maintain or strenghten the patient's general condition to better tolerate therapy, resist the disease, or ease recovery and often consisted in a specific diet or tonics.

[38] François Dagognet, *La raison et les remèdes* (Paris: Presses universitaires de France, 1964), 13.

biomedicine incommensurable with other forms of therapy, which, as we will see in Chapters 5 and 7, manifested itself in colonial views of Vietnamese medicine and remedies. This shift, however, only happened slowly.

Indeed, doctors continued, for quite some time, to question the universality and specificity of therapy. They suggested instead that individual and environmental influences affected therapeutic action beyond matters of biological causation and pharmacodynamics.[39] A movement toward rational therapeutics emerged in the early twentieth century to promote the scientific elucidation of mechanisms of drug action prior to the introduction of therapies in clinical practice. A rational drug was defined as one with laboratory-proven effects, and ideally one that acted on the causes rather than the symptoms of disease. Rational therapeutics also referred to clinical judgment in the selection, dosage, and administration of drugs on the basis of knowledge of pharmacological action.[40] Until the efficacy of arsenical drugs was demonstrated on the eve of World War I, many doctors remained skeptical of the benefits of drug-based therapeutic interventions. Even by then, claims for scientific medicine continued to be anchored in the prevention (rather than curative treatment) of disease through sanitation and public health measures and, of course, vaccination. In addition, doctors staunchly refused to endorse secret remedies, even when these offered the only possibility of relief, considering them to be synonymous with (risky) practices of self-medication. Mistrust of both medicines and patients was mutually reinforcing.[41]

Thus some doctors may well have used their power to restrict rather than promote their patients' access to prescription-only drugs. In addition, the therapeutic relationship became more rigid, increasingly subordinating the patient's "lay" knowledge to the expert, as the only "one who knows." This shift not only changed the nature of the therapeutic encounter, but also had an impact on access to treatment, for many doctors continued to conflate pharmaceutical specialties with unorthodox therapies and charlatanism. This wariness seems to have been particularly persistent among French doctors, who continued to decry the demise of the more trustworthy magistral formulations, perhaps as late as the 1940s. Indeed, in 1943, doctor and pharmacist René Hazard, one of the architects of the post–World War II International

---

[39] Recently contested by the development of pharmacogenomics, this issue of specificity and universality of a drug effect remains controversial.

[40] Marks, *The Progress*, 19–33.

[41] Olivier Faure, *Les Français et leur médecine au XIXe siècle* (Paris: Belin, 1993), 221.

Pharmacopeia,[42] essentially accused doctors of prescribing specialties merely out of laziness:

Some of these [specialties] entail modes of preparation that require specially equipped laboratories; their utility is not under question. For the rest, most are either products with standards of purity no greater than those of the Pharmacopeia, or they are mixtures of medicines combined on the basis of therapeutic notions that are sometimes dubious. Many of these could disappear with no loss to the patient [. . .] In truth, the roots of the success of most of these specialties can be found, it must be said, in the failure of many doctors to educate themselves in the art of formulating.[43]

If French doctors long hesitated to promote medicines as an avenue of medical modernization, others – notably, pharmaceutical producers, distributors, and consumers – quickly seized the possibilities offered by pharmaceuticals. Up until at least the 1910s, it seems likely that medicines, primarily commercial specialties, were largely consumed without any medical supervision. The figure of the pharmacist symbolized these tensions and ambiguities of the pharmaceutical market. Increasingly identified as modern health care professionals and as scientists, who were, however, subjected to doctors' prescribing power, pharmacists were also becoming highly competitive businesspersons. They marketed a wide range of pharmaceutical products and, in some cases, engaged in the development and serial production of commercial specialties. According to several historians of medicine, notably Olivier Faure in the French context, chemists and pharmacists played a major role in the transformation of health practices beginning in the second half of the nineteenth century. At this time, the number of medicines on the market and on display in retail pharmacies grew rapidly, in response to popular expectations and still relatively free of legal restrictions. A large number of products still promised symptomatic relief, rather than curative action on a specific disease. As the heirs of secret remedies, commercial specialties were more likely to be marketed as panaceas than as specific remedies. They often had a general tonic effect, and were thus compatible with still vivid and popular humoural representations of disease, as was emphasized in publicity in order to heighten their appeal.[44]

Despite an official prohibition on advertising medicines by the Germinal law of 1803, the text of 1857, which authorized the

[42] Jeremy A. Greene, *Generic. The Unbranding of Modern Medicine* (Baltimore: Johns Hopkins University Press, 2014), 24–25.

[43] Cited by Gaudillière, "Drugs Trajectories," 132.

[44] Roberta Bivins, *Alternative Medicine. A History* (Oxford: Oxford University Press, 2007), 6–11.

trademarking of medicines, indirectly stimulated publicity that focused on brand promotion. By the twentieth century, the majority of direct-to-public advertisements were for commercial specialties, which were numerous and highly diverse. Indeed, Sophie Chauveau suggests that a distinguishing marker of the emergence of the French drug industry was its strong reliance on publicity, directed both to the medical profession and to the public: in the interwar years, 30 percent of the French press media's advertising profits were obtained from the pharmaceutical industry, ahead of department stores (17.5 percent) and the food industry (8.8 percent).[45] A French appetite for medicines is also evident in the large and growing number of retail pharmacies: from just over six thousand in 1875 to about twelve thousand circa 1910.[46] Despite significant gaps in geographical distribution, largely overlapping those in the health care network, these pharmacies offered a large selection of specialties to a growing clientele, which also expanded with the elimination of competing remedy providers. Retail pharmacies became the only suppliers of mutual insurance societies and of the state-provided Assistance médicale gratuite (AMG; Free Medical Assistance), created in 1893 to provide free health care to needy citizens.[47]

Modern medicines had thus clearly become commodities in France as well as in other industrializing economies by the turn of the twentieth century. Their rise was entangled with the emergence of new understandings of health as the cornerstone of success and social integration.[48] Whether modern medicines were perceived as practical, effective, or simply as attractive – due to skillful marketing in the context of an emerging consumer culture – these became privileged tools in quests for care and relief.[49] But how did these medicines-in-the-making, as modern and modernizing substances, travel to a colony-in-the-making, a space placed under the authority of an increasingly structured colonial administration (including by the proliferation of measures to regulate commercial activities and to protect public health)? In other words: How did medicines become colonial as they were becoming modern? The last two sections of this chapter examine the first, most obvious step in this process: the exportation both of

[45] This provoked growing debate in the 1930s, resulting in the adoption of a law in September 1941, which regulated, to some extent, direct-to-consumer drug advertisement, while publicity for treatments against sexually-transmitted infections (STIs) was proscribed (Chauveau, "Marché et publicité,"193–94, 202–3).
[46] Faure, Les Français et leur médecine, 200.
[47] In the 1930s, 11,000 specialties were admissible to AMG coverage (Faure, Les Français et leur médecine, 225–27, 234–37).
[48] Bonah and Rasmussen, Histoire et médicament, 11.
[49] Chauveau, "Marché et publicité," 196.

medicines themselves and of their regulatory framework from the "West," particularly from the French metropole, to Vietnam. Yet while colonial medicines were initially defined by their status as "imported" and "regulated" – that is, by flows of substances and rules from metropole to colony that were under colonial control – we will see in later chapters that this identity would soon expand and branch out as drugs acquired new forms of colonial life.

1.6   Making Medicines Colonial (Part I): Searching for Markets

It is remarkably difficult to obtain data on the quantity and type of medicines that made their way to Vietnam from the last third of the nineteenth century to 1940. The figures provided by colonial sources are neither complete nor systematic enough for a reliable estimate of the total volume of imports. They give an idea of the magnitude of flows at specific moments, but do not specify how volumes fluctuated over time, or differentiate these precisely according to origin. Figures for the import and export of *espèces médicinales* (medicinal species) were consistently published in the section on foreign commerce of the *Annuaire statistique de l'Indochine*. We thus know that Indochina imported from 1,600 to 3,000 tons of these per year in the 1920s, relative to a range of 31,000 to 45,000 tons of food.[50] However, the *Annuaire* did not regularly report data on the importation of *médicaments composés*, or compound medicines, which are made by pharmacists or drug firms from a combination of ingredients.

In 1913, 228 tons of compound medicines entered Indochina, of which 109 tons (52 percent) came directly from France. This figure rose to 306 in 1923, then to 492 in 1929, while the proportion from France increased to 81 percent then 85 percent. A Customs Agency table for 1937–39 suggests a dip in imports in the 1930s. While the numbers increased at the end of the decade (from 291 to 387 tons), they did not reattain the peak levels of the 1920s.[51] Almost all of these imports (98 percent) were pharmaceutical specialties (medical and commercial), which thus accounted for nearly all of the spending on medicines: twelve million francs in 1927 and twenty-six million in 1939. These weight or money values tell us nothing about the number of products that entered Vietnam, or their identity and indications, whether or not they were

---

[50] Gouvernement général de l'Indochine française, *Annuaire statistique*, 226.
[51] "Tarification douanière des produits pharmaceutiques, 1940," ANOM, Fonds du Gouvernement général (hereafter Gougal) Service économique (hereafter SE) 3316.

toxic. Nor do they say much about the channels through which they were moved and by whom they were sold and purchased.

The database I compiled indicates that at least 1,121 medicines, both simple (containing a single ingredient) and compound medicines, and including various kinds of specialties, were in use in Vietnam at some point during the period from the 1880s to 1940. By comparison, 20,000 to 30,000 products circulated in the metropole in the 1920s. Of the total, 671 products, or about 60 percent, were trademarked. This is certainly an underestimate, given that the origin (production, development, and distribution) of many products remains unidentifiable. The repertory also reveals an increasing proportion of specialties at the expense of simples, which pharmacists would have used to compound their own medicines. This shift toward "ready-made" medicines became increasingly visible in the 1920s and accelerated in the 1930s. The same trend can also be seen in the public supply orders for medicines I found in the colonial archives. In 1897–98, an order list for the military health care services contained only three branded products, all from the same firm (Chloroforme Adrian, Ether sulfurique Adrian, and Arrhenal).[52]

By contrast, a 1936–37 order for AMI facilities in Tonkin listed twenty-one pharmaceutical specialties (out of fifty-six items, making up 37.5 percent). Only four items (7 percent) were active ingredients, and the rest were "chemical substances." The following year, a similar regular order was supplemented by a special order for eighteen products; all were specialties.[53] Among these were cutting-edge products, such as hormone therapies (including Gynoestryl Roussel and Parathyroid Byla), several brands of insulin, and barbiturates (Evipan Roche, Ciba's Dial, Gardénal Rhône-Poulenc, etc.). Some had just been launched on the French market, as was the case of Septazine, a sulfonamide marketed by Rhône-Poulenc.[54] Alongside this rising proportion of specialties and rapid transfer of innovations, the material presentations of drugs also mirrored metropolitan trends in the 1920s and 1930s. While these remained varied, the proportion of pills, tablets, and injectable forms grew at the expense of powders, syrups, and elixirs.

My database also confirms the predominance of the French industry in the Vietnamese pharmaceutical market. Of the 260 firms I identified as

---

[52] "Cahier des charges relatif à la fourniture des médicaments nécessaires à différents services du protectorat du Tonkin pendant les années 1897 et 1898," ANOM, RST 6801.

[53] Adding up both order lists, the proportion of specialties grows to 53 percent, which is similar to the trend in metropolitan public hospitals at the time.

[54] "Services sanitaires et Assistance publique. Achat de médicaments et de matériel pour la Pharmacie centrale de l'AMI du Tonkin, 1936–1940," ANOM, Gougal SE 2920.

selling products in the colony, about 90 percent were based in France, the rest in other European countries and in North America. This is a significant proportion, especially given that my total is quite likely an underestimate. The first edition of Louis Vidal's *Dictionnaire des spécialités pharmaceutiques* (a directory of the pharmaceutical specialties that were available on the French market called, then as now, "le Vidal" by French doctors) listed 131 firms advertising drugs in France in 1914. The 1933 edition named 689. The number of firms selling products in Vietnam (but which did not necessarily have a significant commercial presence or influence) thus largely exceeds the earlier figure, and amounts to about 40 percent of the later one.[55] The following firms, listed in decreasing order, were associated with the largest number of products marketed in the colony: Clin, Comar et Cie, Byla, Robin, Hoffman, Laroche et Cie, Roussel, Ciba, Scientia, J. Logeais, A. Lumière, Bailly, Amido, and Choay.[56] But one firm stands out above the others: Rhône-Poulenc and its commercial subsidiaries Specia (or Société d'expansion chimique, created in 1928) and Théraplix (Société générale d'applications thérapeutiques, 1931). These distributed more than fifty medical specialties in Vietnam before 1940, including most of the innovative synthetic drugs – arsenobenzols, antimalarial drugs, and sulfonamides. There are thus clear indications that the commercial strategies of the main French pharmaceutical firms targeted the colonies as significant potential markets.

Despite sparse available documentation of these firms' overseas marketing practices and distribution networks, several channels can be identified. These include formal distribution agreements made directly with private pharmacists doing business in Vietnam, which will be described in more detail in Chapters 2 and 4. Other firms operated through wholesalers or commercial firms that had well-established networks in East and Southeast Asia. A few companies used advertising agencies to promote their products directly to Vietnamese consumers through the local press. For example, the agency Comptoir international de publicité (International Advertising Service) was based in Paris but

---

[55] Not all firms selling in Vietnam were French, but not all those advertising in Vidal's repertory were either, so this comparison is a rough indication of the proportion of metropolitan firms that sold drugs in the colony. Historians generally agree that it is extremely difficult to count the exact number of drug producers at the time, since they were extremely versatile, disappeared, reappeared, merged, changed names, and varied widely in size and importance.

[56] Other prominent firms include Midy, Lematte, Gibert, Houdé, Astier, Mouneyrat, and Dausse. Notable foreign firms include the German Hoechst, IG Farben, Merck and Bayer, as well as the Swiss Sandoz.

specialized in overseas advertising in the 1930s.[57] Other firms distributed documentation (brochures, prospectus, etc.) to medical personnel in Indochina, which was a common practice in France at the time. Firms even made agreements with the governor general for the distribution of specific products in AMI facilities. Rhône-Poulenc, in particular, quickly developed strong links with local colonial and medical authorities. One might also hypothesize that Vietnam's dense Pastorian network further facilitated the circulation of drugs that came out of Fourneau's lab.

Beyond Rhône-Poulenc's apparent influence over the supply decisions of health authorities, there is also evidence of formal agreements with the colonial government for the experimentation of new medicines in public hospitals. This trend seems to have emerged with the commercialization of Compound 606, when Poulenc's Arsénobenzol Billon was used for the first time in Vietnam during an outbreak of relapsing fever in Tonkin in 1912.[58] Other arsenical compounds (Novarsénobenzol Billon, Acétylarsan, Sulfotreparsenan, Eparséno or aminoarsenophenol, Stovarsol) were experimented later, as were several antimicrobials and antiseptics (Gonacrine, Mixiod, Propidon, Rhodiacarbine), the first synthetic antimalarial drugs (Prémaline, Quiniostovarsol), and sulfonamides (Septazine, Septoplix, Dagénan). Arrangements with the firm were acknowledged in reports of trials published in colonial or tropical medical journals. For example, in 1935, the author of a trial of the antimalarial combination therapy Plasmochine-Atabrine thanked Rhône-Poulenc for "kindly providing the samples enabling the continuation of trials at the indigenous hospital."[59] The following year, Dr. Montel thanked Specia for offering Cysteine free of charge, thus helping him in his quest for an adjuvant drug in the treatment of leprosy.[60] Administrative records also contain evidence of such strategies, as when Théraplix offered free supplies of the new antiseptic and diuretic Dycholium for experimentation in public hospitals in the late 1930s.[61]

The governor general's trust in Rhône-Poulenc's products was bolstered by "gifts," but also, as administrative correspondence indicates, by

[57] "Lettre du Service économique de l'Indochine, à M. J. Tribaudini, pharmacien, 11 mai 1935," ANOM, Fonds de l'Agence de la France d'outre-mer (hereafter AFOM), Box 238, Folder 298.

[58] "Rapport sanitaire annuel de la province de Kien An, 1913," ANOM, RST NF 4018.

[59] Dr. J. E. Martial, "La quinacrine dans la tierce maligne," *Annales d'hygiène et de médecine coloniale* (AHMC) 33 (1935): 310.

[60] M. L. R. Montel, Georges Montel, and Nguyễn Ngọc Nhuận, "Essais de traitement de la lèpre par la Phénol-sulfone-phtaléine," BSPE 29 (1936): 1064–67.

[61] "Services sanitaires. Inspection générale de l'hygiène et de la santé publique. Correspondances diverses, 1938–1943," ANOM, Gougal SE 2919.

the firm's efforts to promote itself as one that was invested in research, particularly in tropical medicine, and in the development of new products for the improvement of health in the tropics. The firm also sponsored study trips, for example of researchers from France interested in conducting therapeutic trials in Indochina.[62] Specia even established an office in Saigon in 1936, located in the city's commercial center, on Catinat Street, where the biggest private pharmacies operated (see Chapter 4). In 1939, the director of the branch was Henri Rochard, a French pharmacist whose official task was to promote the firm's products and to supply both the public and private sector.[63] In parallel, Rhône-Poulenc solicited the Ministry of Colonies, which occasionally intervened in decisions to import and test medicines in Indochina. For instance, following the proposition of the Conseil supérieur de la santé métropolitain (Metropolitan High Health Council), the Ministry authorized the introduction of Rhône-Poulenc's Stovarsol for the treatment of dysentery in Indochina in 1924, then the introduction of Dagénan in 1938.[64] Occasionally, the Ministry also formulated requests to the governor general to distribute medicines, several of which were produced by firms other than Rhône-Poulenc, such as Quinimax in 1936, Bailly in 1937, and Pharmacie Houet in 1938.[65]

A preference for French drugs was thus actively stimulated through a variety of marketing strategies, of which Rhône-Poulenc's are but one example. This preference was also favored by a predominantly protectionist juridical framework for the importation of medicines to French colonies. Although French foreign trade policies had shifted toward free trade in 1860, agricultural and industrial interest groups began lobbying, from the 1870s, for the reintroduction of measures against foreign competition. This led to the adoption of the Tarif Méline in 1892. Implemented in Indochina in the late 1890s, this protectionist system introduced preferential treatment for French imports, including therapeutic products. Foreign medicines could only be imported if they figured in an official pharmacopeia recognized in France (the list excluded all Asian, including the Japanese, pharmacopoeias, an exclusion officially

[62] "Service de santé, divers, 1927–1936," VNA, centre no. 1 (Hanoi), RST 48024.

[63] ANOM, Gougal SE 2919; "Copie du cahier des charges relatif à l'adjudication avec indication des prix de base de la fourniture des spécialités courantes nécessaires au dépôt central de médicaments de l'AMI en Cochinchine pendant l'année 1936," ANOM, Gougal SE 2921; "Produits toxiques, Autorisation personnelle et permanente d'importer en Indochine des substances toxiques du tableau B, 1937–1940," ANOM, Gougal SE 217.

[64] "Emploi aux colonies du produit médicamenteux 'Stovarsol,' 1924," ANOM, Fonds de la Résidence supérieure d'Annam (hereafter RSA) S1.

[65] ANOM, Gougal SE 2920.

justified in terms of public health protection).[66] They were taxed at a rate of 15 to 20 percent of their value.

Modified during World War I, these rules were reapplied in 1921 and finally replaced, in 1926, by a total exemption from import duty for French pharmaceuticals. Medicines were nevertheless subject to a domestic sales tax. Initially applied only to some medicines, notably those containing alcohol and opium of which the sale was under state control, this tax was generalized, at a rate of 2 percent ad valorem, to all products regardless of origin. Import restrictions and duties were also tightened on a number of therapeutic products as a result of international pressures for narcotics control. In the 1930s, Indochina's new autonomy in matters of taxation allowed it to introduce preferential rates for countries that offered reciprocal advantages to Indochinese exports.[67] At this time, Governor General Decoux responded to some French pharmacists' demands by proclaiming an exemption of customs duties on some basic products (chemical substances, vaccines and serums, anesthetics and surgical material) and by reducing taxation rates on others by introducing a universal ad valorem rate.[68]

Although it varied, the taxation regime in Indochina was, on the whole, fairly restrictive, clearly to the advantage of metropolitan pharmaceutical imports. The law theoretically offered further protection from fraud and counterfeiting for products from the French pharmaceutical industry, through the implementation in Indochina, starting in 1909, of the 1857 French legislation on trademarks. And yet, French products remained expensive in comparison with medicines made elsewhere: they cost 25 to 40 percent more, according to Sophie Chauveau's estimations. Chauveau explains this to be the result of an overvaluation of the French franc and the high cost of metropolitan labor as well as overseas advertising, to which I would add, for Vietnam, the expense of transportation (relative pricing issues will be examined in more detail in Chapter 2).[69] Thus economic advantages alone cannot account for the apparent preference given to French products in Vietnam. This suggests that this imperial bias

---

[66] However, the legislation did not exclude "Sino-Vietnamese medicines," which were never prohibited from importation, as we will see in Chapter 5.

[67] Products exported from Indochina (outside the metropole) were taxed upon exit from 1899, which locally based French commercial firms found difficult to understand: Kham Vorapheth, *Commerce et colonisation en Indochine, 1860–1945* (Paris: Les Indes savantes, 2004), 213–16, 252, 277–78.

[68] By contrast, medicinal species would fall under a 75 percent rate category, which provoked the ire of many Vietnamese and Chinese merchants (ANOM, Gougal SE 3316; "Régime tarifaire des espèces médicinales de la pharmacopée sino-annamite, 1941," ANOM, Gougal SE 3108).

[69] Chauveau, *L'invention pharmaceutique*, 76–77.

was also influenced by the previously mentioned marketing strategies. There was, however, another factor: the transfer, to the Vietnamese colonial context, of a restrictive metropolitan legislative framework for the distribution of medicines.

1.7   Making Medicines Colonial (Part II): Exporting Control

Colonial sources tell us much more about rules for importing and distributing medicines in Vietnam than they do about the number and nature of products in circulation. This is a meaningful discrepancy, which I will unpack over the next chapters. Here, I begin by outlining the transfer of a legislative framework that accompanied the search for new markets, and which remade the Vietnamese terrain in which medicines could become *colonial* during this time of therapeutic transition.

The legislative framework for regulating the circulation of medicines in French Indochina was explicitly modeled on metropolitan laws. In and beyond health legislation, France had a tendency to export metropolitan regulations to its colonies without much prior reflection on potential adjustments.[70] Yet the system of pharmaceutical regulation introduced to Vietnam was particularly heavy-handed, particularly early on. This was a product of combined political, economic, and scientific logics that played out on local, imperial, and international scales. The French drug industry's quest to open up overseas markets – which it saw not only as a potentially profitable, but also, probably, as imperative to its survival in an increasingly competitive field – was facilitated by the extension of this regulatory infrastructure. Especially after 1914, French firms looked to the colonies to counteract foreign competition. By 1938, France was the world's third exporter of medicinal products, behind Germany and the United States, but it ranked first for pharmaceutical specialties. About a third of the volume, and a quarter of the value, of these exports went to French colonies.[71] This privileged colonial market required protection on a global scale.

Already-restrictive metropolitan laws were not simply transferred to Vietnam. Restrictions were intensified in response to local colonial anxieties, notably about the "charlatanism" of indigenous therapists and druggists, the toxicity of their remedies, and the "cultural taste" for drugs that was supposedly prevalent among the Vietnamese. Colonial authorities' perception of Vietnamese therapeutic practices as a public

---

[70] Monnais-Rousselot, *Médecine et colonisation*, 83–102. By contrast, drug laws were much less restrictive in the British Empire: Bhattacharya, "Between the Bazaar and the Bench."

[71] Chauveau, *L'invention pharmaceutique*, 76–77.

health risk penetrated and shaped the juridical framing of medicines in the region from the outset, long before the establishment of the AMI in 1905. As the first territory to come under colonial rule in 1860, Cochinchina was also the first to adopt legislation on medicines. The principal target of these early laws was the practice of pharmacy. The first French pharmacists who settled in the colony soon demanded legal recognition and protection of their rights. By 1871, a governor's decree applied the Germinal law, thus proposing a metropolitan regulatory model. By this decree, the right to practice pharmacy was reserved to graduates of French state pharmacy schools. Two subsequent texts, in 1875 and 1876, clarified (to some extent) what this exclusive right meant for potential competitors: the first explicitly forbade "Asian" pharmacies, groceries, and drugstores from selling "European-made" medicines; the second, more specifically, stated that these could only be sold in "European retail pharmacies." In 1879, the rules for opening a private pharmacy were loosened slightly, mainly to allow French second-class pharmacists to practice in Cochinchina, provided they had "demonstrated their knowledge" before a local jury. This amendment was clearly a response to a scarcity of fully trained pharmacists in the colony. By 1884, it was extended to the territory of Annam-Tonkin, where the Germinal law had just been promulgated.

Both categories of pharmacists were subject to the same rules for preparing and dispensing medicines, particularly regarding the sale of medicines classified as toxic by prescription only and the prohibition of secret remedies. The 1879 amendment remained in force until the introduction of a 1913 bill (promulgated in 1919), which nevertheless allowed for exceptions to be made for those granted the title of pharmacist by a local jury before 1913. This text insisted on the pharmacist's exclusive right to dispense all toxic substances, upon presentation of a medical prescription, and to sell the following pharmaceutical products: "1. Special products (specialties) sold for curative purposes; 2. Sterilized or medicated bandage products [. . .]; 3. Medicinal mineral waters, notably purgative waters." Last but not least, it prohibited medical doctors from selling medicines, unless their practice was located at least ten kilometers, in any direction, from the nearest pharmacy.

This extension of pharmacists' monopoly in Vietnam elicited protests from representatives of French commercial companies who had previously sold items such as sterilized bandages. It also extended restrictions on "Sino-Vietnamese pharmacists," who were prohibited from the sale of a wider range of preparations, including a long list of toxic substances. The regulation of medicines was soon stepped up with the establishment of a pharmacy inspection system across Indochina in October 1908, just months after a similar system was created in France.[72] This law was a turning point in the regulation of drug distribution in the colony since it stipulated that all sites in which remedies were sold, both "European" and "Sino-Vietnamese," were to be inspected annually by a commission of professionals. Inspectors' primary task was to verify compliance with pharmacy legislation, particularly pertaining to toxic substances. They also controlled the quality of medicines, and were thus empowered to seize samples of any suspicious product, send them for analysis to the fraud control laboratory, and, if needed, to request, after filing a statement of offense with the health authorities, a judicial prosecution. The 1908 text also specified penalties for fraud, ranging from confiscation to fines and jail time.

The 1908 law appears to have been a rapid, drastic, and profoundly political response to a poisoning scandal that had shaken the colonial state. On June 28, 1908, there was an attempt to poison two hundred soldiers in Hanoi with Datura stramonium, commonly called Datura, a powerful hallucinogen that can be fatal in high doses.[73] It might be a stretch to claim that this medicinal substance was seen by authorities as a weapon capable of destabilizing the colonial order. However, the attempted poisoning also coincided with the expression, by colonial officers, of a more general anxiety about dangerous medicines. Of particular concern were substances imported from "foreign," and especially Asian, countries and/or distributed by Asian intermediaries, especially those from Japan. A model of Asian modernity, Japan was already producing cutting-edge pharmaceuticals at the time. These included several arsenobenzols, which Japanese firms tried, with their government's support, to export as widely as possible in the Southeast Asian region (see Chapters 4 and 5).[74] Japan also harbored young Vietnamese intellectuals having participated in early nationalist movements.[75] On July 5 1908, the superior resident of Annam wrote

---

[72] "Arrêté du 28 octobre 1908 constituant dans chacun des pays de l'Union une commission d'inspection des pharmacies," ANOM, Gougal 17165.

[73] Early warning of the poisoning by a confidante of the perpetrator allowed the victims to be treated promptly. The incident was followed by a wave of arrests: Dr. Boyé, "Empoisonnement de la garnison européenne d'Hanoi par le Datura, 28 Juin 1908," AHMC 12 (1909): 656–60.

[74] On the rise of the Japanese pharmaceutical industry, see Hoi-Eun Kim, "Cure for Empire: The 'Conquer-Russia-Pill,' Pharmaceutical Manufacturers, and the Making of Patriotic Japanese, 1904–45," *Medical History* 57 (2013): 249–68; Timothy Yang, "Selling an Imperial Dream: Japanese Pharmaceuticals, National Power, and the Science of Quinine Self-Sufficiency," *EASTS. East Asian Science, Technology and Society. An International Journal* 6, 1 (2012): 101–25.

[75] Diplomatic relations between Japan and the governor general were tense in consequence of this movement known as Đông du, or "exodus towards the East."

to the governor general: "There have been rumours [. . .] for some time in North Annam that the Japanese are distributing or will come to distribute to Europeans' domestic employees, pseudo-medicines that are in reality poisons for their masters."[76] Poisons were not just a target of policies to protect the health of "ignorant natives"; they also threatened Europeans as apparently political weapons, thus demanding a rapid and effective response. The 1908 incident also certainly drew the attention of colonial authorities to the fact that most Vietnamese had ready access to toxic products, with drastic consequences for the practice of Vietnamese medicine. The 1908 law prohibited its practitioners from using many substances that had long occupied a central place in their therapeutic arsenical, thus beginning to redefine the very identity of their medical system. It determined what counted as a modern drug and who could manipulate it in a colonial setting.

The 1919 bill on the practice of pharmacy in Indochina included the text of the 1916 metropolitan law on toxic substances, thus introducing the A-B-C schedules for classifying these substances. It also ratified measures introduced in 1913 regarding the packaging and labeling of these substances, and requiring that their movements be recorded in ad hoc registers, and that their use in chemical production and industry be officially authorized. The 1919 decree was amended several times, partly in order to transfer modifications in metropolitan legislation but also, again, in response to local issues. In 1923, for instance, the governor general was granted the power to add substances to schedules A and B upon formal proposal made by one of the Union's five Directions locales de la santé (Local Directorates of Health). A year later, apparently in response to pressure from a segment of the colonial medical profession, the colonial government passed a law imposing a prescription on the dispensation of all arsenical compounds, injectable products, and proto-iodide of mercury. Special restrictions were also applied to Vietnamese biomedical doctors and pharmacists. Recurring debates about their professional status had a direct impact on their right to prescribe, prepare, and sell drugs. The graduates of the Hanoi Medical School, which opened a pharmacy section in 1914, were seen as inferior in status and qualification to French medical professionals. For many years, *médecins auxiliaires indigènes* (auxiliary native doctors) could prescribe medicines only in quantities that did not exceed the "medicinal dose" for a twenty-four-hour period. By 1920, *pharmaciens auxiliaires indigènes* (auxiliary

---

[76] "Lettre du Directeur général de la santé au Gouverneur général, Hanoi, septembre 1908," ANOM, Gougal 17165.

native pharmacists) were similarly restricted in the quantity of medicines they were allowed to dispense.

The specific issues raised by opium in Indochina, both as a French colony and as part of what was perceived as a "sick," addicted Asia,[77] stimulated several local texts to reinforce local control over narcotics (schedule B) during the interwar period. Over the first decades of the twentieth century, a series of laws, most formulated as in response to international conferences and conventions, specifically regulated the import and sale of a growing list of drugs classified as narcotics. A 1908 decree imposed restrictions on the importation of opium and its wholesale and retail sale to pharmacists. These restrictions were extended, following the conference of the International Opium Commission in Shanghai (1909), to morphine and codeine in 1911. In 1915, control measures were applied to other alkaloids and derivatives of opium, as well as to cocaine, by promulgating a law that, in ratification of a treaty signed at the First International Opium Conference in The Hague in 1912, had been adopted in France only a few months earlier. Only pharmacists were now authorized to handle and dispense substances such as holocaine, Novocain, alypine, stovaine, and Heroin, while importers and wholesalers were required to provide the identity of a legitimate recipient of shipped stocks to customs authorities. The export of controlled substances was banned unless destined to a hospital. Then, in 1917, a governor general–appointed commission studied a project to regulate preparations containing morphine, in response to concerns about popular and widely accessible anti-opium remedies. A 1922 decree prohibited the exit, re-export, transit, and transshipment of opium and derivatives across the French Empire. An amended International Opium Convention that set limits on the production and commerce of an expanded list of substances, including products with a concentration of morphine above 0.2 percent and cocaine above 0.1 percent, was signed in Geneva in 1925, then ratified by France in 1928, and, again, promulgated in Indochina only months later. From 1930, personal authorization (in a specific individual's name) was required for anyone, including pharmacists, to import and distribute any substance defined as a narcotic by law.

---

[77] From the late nineteenth century, the commerce of opium in Indochina was controlled by a lucrative state monopoly: Philippe Le Failler, *Monopole et prohibition de l'opium en Indochine. Le pilori des chimères* (Paris: L'Harmattan, 2001). The addiction epidemic for which it became blamed was thus not only a social problem, but also a very delicate economic and political one. On the history of narcotics in Asia and its meanings during this period, see Frank Dikötter, Lars Laaman, and Zhou Xun, ed., *Narcotic Culture. A History of Drugs in China* (Chicago: Chicago University Press, 2004).

What pressure! Yet this proliferation of laws proved unable, in France as in Vietnam, to effectively regulate the risks and opportunities arising from rapid changes in the production, distribution and consumption of medicines. Legislation constantly lagged behind techno-scientific advances and was limited in its capacity to react effectively to the intro-duction of innovative, increasingly active, and potentially toxic products to the market. For example, the first barbiturates, which reached Vietnam in the 1930s, were initially classified as schedule B substances and thus, for several years, could be sold without a prescription, despite the fact that they had already caused several lethal incidents.[78] Metropolitan categor-izations of pharmaceutical substances and actors proved even more ill-suited to the heterogeneous, dynamic practices and networks of distribution that emerged in Vietnam. These quickly eluded ever-more-determined attempts to control them. Both the density and ineffective-ness of pharmaceutical legislation in Vietnam were, in part, an echo of efforts (and failures) to control and keep up with the emergence of medicines as modern objects of commerce, science, therapy, and exper-tise in France. The qualities of this legislative framework must also, however, be understood as a response to the specific conditions, and attendant concerns, under which medicines became colonial in Vietnam.

After the middle of the nineteenth century, modern medicines in France and the industrialized world were far from a fixed or simple type of entity. By the interwar period, they were part of a market that was already dense and shot through with tensions and contradictions. Medicines were as numerous as they were heterogeneous, as were their perceptions and practices. Some were synthetic, others derived from animal or plant matter, and they had a wide range of indications. Some were specific curatives, others offered panacea-like relief or tonic effects, and yet others had preventive, diagnostic, or regulatory functions, or were used as replacement therapies. The term "pharmaceutical" had an even broader range of meanings: it included all the materials associated with the pharmacy profession (bandages, insecticides, medicinal plants listed in pharmacopeias), as well as hygienic, nutritional, and cosmetic products.[79] This was a pivotal time of change in the quantity and quality of available medicines, but also one of coexistence between old and modern, scientific and empirical, effective and toxic, pragmatic and allur-ing, regulated and free, prescribed and self-medicated. This long period of therapeutic transition would leave its mark on French colonies, an

---

[78] Dr. Charles Massias, "Intoxication volontaire par les barbituriques, en particulier par le Dial. Vaste ulcération sacrée aiguë due au Dial," BSMI 11 (1933): 589–95.
[79] Azema, "La définition juridique," 38.

imprint that is clearly discernible in both the commercial and legislative strategies that orchestrated the overseas export of a growing set of products and, early on, of a complex legislative arsenal. While these export strategies were not alone in delineating the nature of colonial medicines in Vietnam, it must be emphasized that even in France, the establishment of expert pharmacist and medical monopolies over medicines proved ill-adapted. These monopolies were even less suited for wholesale transfer to Vietnam. In fact, some proposed measures were never implemented, or simply not adopted (sometimes after several unsuccessful attempts). The regulation of pharmaceutical exclusivity was extended and adjusted in response to concerns specific to the Vietnamese context. These attempts were further challenged by the complexity and innovations of the *therapeutic transitions* that played out on Vietnamese soil. Yet while the ever-growing list of restrictions on the distribution of medicines was often unenforced or circumvented, it nonetheless exerted pressures that had a clear and significant impact on the accessibility of medicines, both within the public health care system and beyond it.

2   Medicines in Colonial (Public) Health

The interplay between, on the one hand, apparent official and professional indifference toward medicines and, on the other hand, signs of popular therapeutic enthusiasm, is one of the central threads running throughout this book. This chapter provides a general overview of the place (not) given to medicines in colonial health policies, budgets, and discourse, and of the challenges facing their supply to and distribution in the public system. Of this information, I ask: how, and to what extent, did colonial and health authorities consider medicines as tools suited to the twin projects of medicalization and civilization? And how did this shape the geographical and economic accessibility of colonial medicines per se – that is, the medicines supplied and distributed by the colonial government? There were different types of *public* colonial medicines. Some, like the quinine distributed by the State Quinine Service from 1909, and thus called *quinine d'état* (QE; state quinine), were unquestionably public; and yet, their circulation largely bypassed colonial health care facilities and medical personnel. Others, including many pre-scription-only medicines, were largely reserved to public health care facilities and AMI doctors on paper, yet they were inaccessible to the majority of patients and practitioners. This chapter explores the material and ideological conditions of drug inaccessibility within the Assistance, especially with respect to the most effective and expensive drugs, while the following chapter will describe efforts and failures to broaden access to a specific, restricted range of medicines, including preventive quinine and basic nontoxic remedies. Together, they paint a picture of generalized constraints weighing on the provision of public medicines, which, however, played out quite differently depending on place, population, and category of medicines.

2.1   Medicalizing Vietnam or the Primacy of Prevention

Health was one of the cornerstones of the particularly ambitious experiment of French modern imperialism in Indochina.[1] The most obvious,

---

[1] Monnais-Rousselot, *Médecine et colonisation*; Au, *Mixed Medicines*.

and perhaps most prosaic, explanation for this is the imperative to make the colony profitable, at no cost to the metropole. Achieving this would require a cheap but efficient, and therefore healthy, labor force. This prevailing logic did not, however, completely eliminate reluctance to invest in a public health care system that would place a significant financial burden on the colonial administration. The long-term benefits promised by health programs were not only of economic gain, but also of contributing to the French imperial *mission civilisatrice*, the "civilizing" objective of its colonial project. Plans for a health care system based on biomedicine, and above all on the Pastorian paradigm, claimed it would demonstrate the superiority of French civilization and the benefits of its colonial rule. This might bring the colonized to accept and perhaps even, with the next and healthier generation, to adhere to French and biomedical values.

The first, and lasting, priority of public health measures in the peninsula was mass prevention. Smallpox vaccination campaigns were launched as early as the 1860s, soon after Cochinchina became a formal colony (Figure 2.1). There, vaccination was made compulsory in 1871, three decades before France. Another key objective was sanitation, which was targeted by some of the earliest measures taken by local, primarily municipal, administrations. "Vaccinate, register, disinfect" became the motto of a first generation of health care professionals who struggled with little means and inadequate knowledge of local pathological environments. In 1890, the French colonies were given, by decision of the French state secretariat, a Health Council and a colonial military medical corps (Troupes coloniales, or TC), which paved the way for medicalization initiatives at the level of individual colonies. In Indochina, the framework for a public health system was built under the governorship of Paul Doumer (1897–1902). In 1897, Local Directorates of Health were created for each of Indochina's five territories. The same year, a network of *infirmeries-mobiles* (mobile infirmaries), which had, until then, served the troops conquering Tonkin and Annam, were opened up to local civilians. A year later, as Indochina's budget became increasingly autonomous from the metropole, financial responsibility for health was largely shifted to the five local governments.

In 1902, the brand-new Loi de santé publique, the first major French public health law, was almost immediately implemented in Indochina. It introduced, in particular, compulsory notification for some contagious diseases, and enabled the extension of compulsory smallpox vaccination to the whole Union. After several decades of discussions, a medical school was also established in Hanoi that year. Its goal was to train Viêt, Khmer, and Lao auxiliary doctors to assist French medical staff, but also to

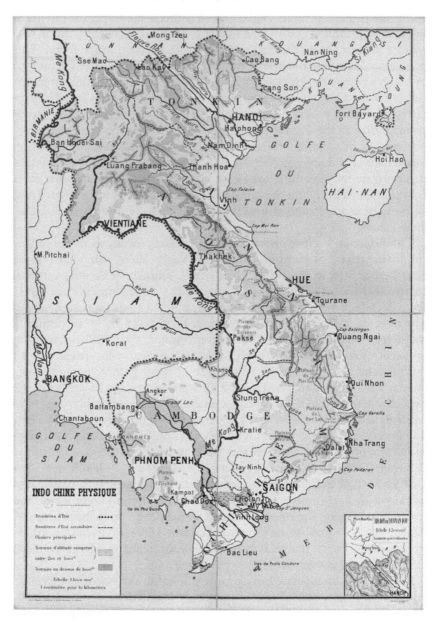

Figure 2.1 Map of French Indochina, 1927 (Service géographique de l'Indochine [Hanoi], 1927, Bibliothèque nationale de France [BNF, Paris], Département Cartes et plans, GE C-5473 (1–4), reproduced with the authorization of the BNF)

counter the influence of "Sino-Vietnamese doctors."[2] In 1905, the creation of a public system for "native health," the AMI, was a major move
toward a coherent health policy on the scale of the Union. This was
primarily a *public health* project rather than a health care initiative. Its
core aim was to prevent and control the transmission and epidemic
resurgence of infectious disease, not to care for individual patients. This
would remain the case for the whole period of colonial rule. The gift AMI
offered was free protection against the deadliest local diseases through
mass immunizations – this "unwavering loyalty" to vaccination, as
Sokhieng Au calls it,[3] was surely marked by the influence of the
Pastorian research network in Indochina – and vertical programs targeting one disease at a time. In return, there was an expectation of good
behavior on the part of the colonized: an acceptance to walk the path of
civilization and medicalization under a benevolent colonial rule.

From the outset, these initiatives faced the challenge of a pathological
environment described by medical officers as a volatile combination of
high morbidity and mortality rates, especially in young children. In the
first decades of the twentieth century, it was estimated that half of
Vietnamese babies died before the age of twelve months. Smallpox,
exacerbated by poor hygiene and nutrition, was a frequent cause of infant
mortality. Neonatal tetanus, a form of tetanus occurring in newborns due
to infection of the umbilical cord cut under unsterilized conditions, which
had become a distant memory in France by that time, is thought to have
killed up to 40 percent of newborns in some areas. Life-threatening
epidemic and endemic diseases were omnipresent, with the greatest
source of anxiety being the mass fatalities caused by outbreaks of smallpox and cholera, and to a lesser extent, of plague. Between 1926 and
1930, for example, 66,179 documented cases of cholera (the real number
is surely higher) were reported as having caused 51,917 deaths in
Indochina, a mortality rate close to 80 percent. Endemic diseases were
also a cause for concern, especially malaria. In 1910, 10,000 patients
were treated for malaria in AMI facilities; ten years later, in 1929, 21,200
were hospitalized for that condition, with a relatively stable mortality rate
hovering around 10 percent. Other common diseases included dysentery
(both bacillary and amoebic), relapsing fever, typhoid fever, diphtheria,
influenza, dengue fever, and beriberi. The impact of tuberculosis, though
difficult to calculate, was likely high: for 1936, the official count was of
11,920 hospitalizations, with a mortality rate of about 11 percent.

---

[2] Laurence Monnais, "La professionnalisation du 'médecin indochinois' au XXe siècle: des
   paradoxes d'une médicalisation coloniale," *Actes de la recherche en sciences sociales* 143
   (2002): 36–43.
[3] Au, *Mixed Medicines*, 33.

Diseases defined as "social" – identified as nurtured or spread by social factors such as poverty, overcrowding, prostitution, regardless of whether they were infectious or not – were also widespread, especially "venereal diseases," as STIs such as syphilis (11,031 hospitalizations reported for 1936) and gonorrhea were called at the time. Leprosy affected an estimated 12,000 to 15,000 individuals around 1900. Many doctors also commented on a pervasive underlying state of polypathology in their patients. As Dr. René Montel, the municipal doctor for Saigon, wrote: "Our patients never present with a single, well-determined and clearly-defined condition; they are [. . .] pluri-infected and carriers of interlocking diseases [. . .] a backdrop of malaria, tuberculosis, syphilis and beriberi [aggravate] co-occurring conditions [. . .] and render the organism vulnerable to all kinds of disease."[4] Such cases were seen as a persistent obstacle to effective medical action throughout the colonial period.

Given these combined obstacles, of polypathology, high rates of infant mortality and the high toll of infectious diseases for which few therapeutic solutions were available at the time, collective preventive action remained the core of health policies. Urban sanitation included pest control and the piping of drinking water. Vaccination campaigns were extended from small-pox to plague, cholera, and, to some extent, tuberculosis. In addition to sanitation and vaccination measures came public education initiatives, held in schools or public conferences to diffuse basic concepts of individual and collective hygiene. At the same time, however, an infrastructure of health care facilities was built up. Urban areas were served by *hôpitaux mixtes* ("mixed" hospitals, open to European and Vietnamese patients) and *hôpitaux indigènes* (native hospitals), while less densely populated areas were scattered with medical outposts, first-aid posts, infirmaries, and maternities. By 1936, there were about 650 AMI facilities in Vietnam; 85 percent of these were small, offering mainly outpatient consultation services.[5]

The doctors who worked in Indochina were, at first, exclusively French military officers of the Marine Corps, and then of the TC created in 1890. With the establishment of the AMI, a civilian medical corps was created that could recruit and retain staff in Indochina, unlike military officers who were rotated across the empire every two or three years. Due to recurrent civilian staff shortages,[6] however, the AMI often "borrowed"

---

[4] "Saigon. Rapport sur l'état sanitaire de la ville de Saigon et sur l'Assistance médicale urbaine, 1908," VNA, centre no. 2 (Ho Chi Minh City), Fonds du Gouvernement de la Cochinchine (hereafter Goucoch) IA.8/077(4).

[5] Monnais-Rousselot, *Médecine et colonisation*, 120.

[6] In contrast with the situation in the British Empire, colonial careers were not compelling to French doctors; overseas salaries were not that attractive, and positions were still available in the metropole.

military doctors from the TC throughout the colonial period. The health care system also relied more and more heavily on doctors trained in Hanoi. From World War I, particular efforts were made to turn out large numbers of auxiliary health workers. Thus, by 1939, the AMI employed more than 4,000 "Indochinese" nurses and midwives alongside approximately 350 doctors. Still, the cost and challenges of staffing, including training and recruitment, and of running this system were formidable; initially, they had been underestimated.

Indochina had two types of budgets: general and local. The general budget covered the costs of running the Union as an autonomous state, including infrastructure that served all of its five territories, such as railways and communication. It was sustained by indirect taxation such as duties imposed on imports, transit, storage, and navigation; the profits generated by state-controlled sales of salt, opium, alcohol, and tobacco, as well as by state-run postal and telecommunications services; and mining dues and estate registration fees. Local budgets, which financed most health-related activities, were generated by the direct taxation of individuals (capitation tax), of property, of economic activity (commerce, river rights), and, from 1938, of income. These budgets thus varied enormously, depending on a region's demographic density, wealth, and economic development. In 1913, Indochina's budget for health was of 1.7 million piasters,[7] and by 1931, it had reached 3 million. Yet it never exceeded 3.8 percent of the Union's general budget. In 1913 as in 1931, roughly 50 percent of this health budget was committed to the construction and maintenance of AMI facilities, 25 percent to hygiene and public health programs (water piping and filtration, sanitation, rat control, etc.), and the rest to health personnel. Although 8 to 12 percent of local budgets were generally committed to health-related costs, these budgets were sometimes, notably in Annam, so small that this added up to a negligible amount. The distribution of funding for health care infrastructure and personnel at the level of provinces was also inequitable, with the ratio of health expenditures per capita spending ranging from one to five.[8]

The system's limitations were soon obvious to colonial authorities, whose responses varied. While Governor General Anthony Klobukoswsi

---

[7] Currency of French Indochina from 1885, the piaster (subdivided into 100 cents) was initially equivalent to the Mexican peso. It remained set by the silver standard until 1920. Due to a rise in the price of silver after World War I, it was pegged to the French franc, thus putting it on a gold exchange standard. Its rate of exchange with the metropolitan currency nevertheless varied widely throughout the colonial period.

[8] "Rapport fait par M. Tupinier, inspecteur des colonies, concernant l'organisation de l'Assistance médicale en Indochine à Hanoi, 4 juin 1937," ANOM, Fonds de la Direction du contrôle (hereafter DC) 703.

(1908–11) proposed to maintain only the bare bones of a system he deemed overly expensive, Albert Sarraut (1911–14, 1916–19) defended the civilizing value of a real medicalization policy. At a time of reaffirmation of Indochina's financial and political autonomy, Sarraut placed the AMI under the direction of the IGHSP. This granted the latter greater power to evaluate, design, and plan its actions (on a five-year basis), according to the needs of local populations and colonial development. Following World War I, increased resources were allocated to health. This was partly a response to the demobilization of French doctors who were returning to the colony, but it also gave recognition to the extraordinary wartime achievements of auxiliary medical staff. Bigger budgets widened the scope for attempts to adapt the system better to local conditions. Large-scale field studies and routine reporting of health staff's observations improved authorities' knowledge of epidemiological patterns. Social diseases (tuberculosis, STIs, trachoma, cancer, malnutrition, and some disabilities) were given greater attention, while new investments in maternal and child health led to the creation of maternities and specialized consultation services as well as Gouttes de lait, centers where new mothers could receive milk as well as other basic supplies and instructions for baby care.

Only a fraction of Indochina's population lived in the major cities; at the time, these were Saigon-Cholon, Hanoi and Haiphong, as well as Hué and Phnom Penh and larger regional capitals such as Nam Dinh City, Ha Dong City, and Thanh Hoa City. The overwhelming majority lived in village communities that were often highly dispersed. Under the aegis of the Assistance rurale (Rural Assistance), created in 1927, a program of mobile medicine was developed to improve rural populations' access to basic health care. The first rural medicines outlets were created in 1920. Alongside intensified efforts to turn out Vietnamese nurses and midwives, a few programs sought to "reeducate" traditional health practitioners such as the bà mụ, the birth attendants who still oversaw most women's deliveries.[9] From at least the mid-1930s, some health authorities, probably prompted by doctors working on the ground, went as far as to suggest measures for integrating Vietnamese medicine into the AMI. However, this integration was to be implemented on the terms, and under the strict

---

[9] On the history of Vietnamese midwives, see Thuy Linh Nguyen, *Childbirth, Maternity and Medical Pluralism in French Colonial Vietnam, 1880–1945* (Rochester, NY: University of Rochester Press, 2016), and Laurence Monnais, "Les premiers pas inédits d'une professionnelle de santé insolite: la sage-femme vietnamienne dans les années 1900–40," in *Le Vietnam au féminin. Viêt Nam: Women's Realities*, ed. Gisèle Bousquet and Nora Taylor (Paris: Les Indes savantes, 2005), 67–106.

control, of the IGHSP. Its aims were minimal and pragmatic: to provide cheap solutions for minor health issues that fell between the gaps of the system's coverage and resources (see Chapter 8).

The impact of these various measures of adaptation, which I call the *nativization* or *indigenization* of the Vietnamese health care system, was variable and constrained by recurring budgetary and staff shortages.[10] Nevertheless, while medicalization is difficult to quantify, colonial health policies did have a perceptible effect on recorded mortality and morbidity rates, especially those attributable to epidemic diseases and to infant mortality. For example, neonatal tetanus vanished from colonial statistics in the 1920s.[11] At the same time, the process of medicalization was clearly two-tiered. The top tier was made up of urban enclaves, in which hospitals, clinics, scientific institutes, and personnel were concentrated. It offered specialized consultation services, cutting-edge technologies, and laboratory analysis. The second covered the rest of the territory, where the majority population often had to make do with rundown facilities, erratic medical tours, and the services of subordinate health care workers. The accessibility of medicines within this public system would be shaped by the following key characteristics: enduring prioritization of preventive health action; persistent urban-rural disparities; and late, and uneven, adaptation to local conditions and demands. Yet the most obvious obstacle to the availability of medicines was the lack of money spent on them, and the challenges of managing their supply and distribution.

2.2 The Many Challenges of Supply

As mentioned previously, budgets for health were highly variable but always tight; this was especially true for spending on medicines, which, despite increases in the 1920s, was never prioritized. The eclectic "materials" heading absorbed only 0.3 percent of the Union's total health budget. Amounts allocated for "materials" appear proportionally higher at the local level, but varied considerably according to the economic vitality of protectorates and provinces, and the choices made by local administrative and medical staff. Large urban hospitals probably

---

[10] Mass prevention was supposed to be more cost-effective. On the other hand, the recurrent shortages in qualified human resources are probably an additional factor explaining the choice to focus in priority on collective prevention and education measures, which required less professional work and supervision, lighter infrastructure, as well as fewer material supplies.

[11] Monnais-Rousselot, *Médecine et colonisation*, 181–82.

got not only the most, but also the "best" (newest, most efficient) medicines.[12]

A snapshot of interprovincial variations in budget size and allocation for medicines can be gleaned from annual health reports for 1912–15. In 1912, the province of Cao Bang in Tonkin spent a high proportion, nearly 25 percent, of its annual health budget on "materials and medicines." At least two factors account for this relatively lavish spending on pharmaceuticals. The province had comparatively light staff costs since, as a military region, many of its doctors were military officers whose salaries were paid directly by the metropole. In addition, the relatively high number of civil servants in this province probably meant that Cao Bang's population was particularly well cared for. By contrast, the nearby Hai Duong Province spent less than 7 percent of its 1915 health budget of 11,294 piasters on medicines (760), while nearly two-thirds (7,300) went to staff costs.[13] Only 600 piasters were spent on medicines in Bac Kan, whose head doctor complained, moreover, that a fifth of this amount went to the cost of transporting medicines to health care facilities and to cover a recent increase in the price of some products.[14] Hung Yen spent 850 piasters on medicines and bandages, yet its head doctor calculated that this averaged out to only 4 cents per patient. As a reference point, a health report for 1913 indicates that a hospitalized patient cost an average of 32 cents a day, of which 7 were for medicines.[15]

Mainly imported from France and subjected to heavy taxation as we have seen, pharmaceuticals remained largely unaffordable for the AMI.[16] On the eve of, and throughout, World War I, budgets for medicines were depleted by general wartime cuts and further strained by a dramatic rise in pharmaceutical prices.[17] In the 1920s, spending on pharmaceuticals increased in both absolute terms and as a proportion of health budgets, reaching 25 percent in some provinces. Yet striking disparities persisted.

---

[12] On the other hand, smaller facilities might have had more flexibility in managing their stocks and distribution. It must be noted that data on budgets for medicines (and, more generally, for health) are difficult to interpret for several reasons, including the fact that they are sometimes given in francs, sometimes in piasters. Because of frequent fluctuation in their exchange rate, this prevents reliable comparisons between budgets and spending proportions.

[13] "Rapport sanitaire annuel de la province de Hai Duong, 1915," ANOM, RST NF 4003.

[14] "Rapport sanitaire annuel de la province de Bac Kan, 1915," ANOM, RST NF 4003.

[15] "Rapport sanitaire annuel de la province de Ha Dong, 1913," ANOM, RST NF 4014.

[16] At the same time, pharmaceuticals were also considered to be expensive in France. There were thus recurring debates about which specialties should be reimbursed through the AMG and French doctors were pressured to favor basic products over specialties and to limit their prescriptions (Faure, *Les Français et leur médecine*, 222–23).

[17] "Importation de produits chimiques et pharmaceutiques en Indochine, 1918," ANOM, Gougal 33693.

Although a significant amount, 273,000 piasters, was allocated to the purchase of materials and medicines in Tonkin in 1931, more than a quarter of this went to the Protectorate's central hospital in Hanoi.[18] In Annam, medicines worth 285,355 piasters were divided up among 20 health care facilities for the period of June 1929 to May 1930. Yet 53 percent of these medicines (in value) made their way to the three main urban centers: Hué (34 percent), Thanh Hoa City (10 percent), and Vinh (9 percent).[19] The upward budgetary trend of the 1920s was then halted by the Great Depression, with significant reductions in health (and drug) spending from 1932. By 1940, the specter of wartime drug shortages once again loomed large. While shortages were due in part to threatened supply routes from the metropole, this obstacle was aggravated by the inadequacy of budgets combined with a surge in the price of medicines that had begun a decade and a half earlier.[20] Medical specialties were becoming particularly expensive. A tube of the sulfa drug Dagénan, for example, cost the AMI 4 to 5 piasters in 1939, including transportation and taxes. This put a full treatment for gonorrhea or meningitis, requiring two to three tubes, out of the reach of most facilities. Rhône-Poulenc's Saigon office helped palliate gaps in the supply of some effective drugs, but at a high price for the health care system.[21]

Wartime shortages provide a striking illustration of the combined effects of budgetary constraints and of the cost and complexity of importing medicines to the colony. Affordability and availability were both recurring problems. While it is difficult to quantify the impact of supply problems on accessibility, or to reconstruct supply circuits in detail, colonial archives do describe many concerns about, and attempts to improve, the efficiency of pharmaceutical supply and distribution within the Vietnamese territory. There were two main routes for supplying medicines to the AMI: a direct route from metropolitan drug firms and commercial distributors and an indirect one that passed through retail pharmacists who had set up shop in the colony. For the latter, a tender system was created in the early years of French presence in Cochinchina to allocate contracts, mainly for the supply of basic medicines intended for the military and the colony's first hospitals. These contracts provided business to a handful of French pharmacists.[22] Bidding rules were

[18] ANOM, RST NF 3683.
[19] "Rapport des services de santé de l'Annam, 1929–1930," ANOM, RSA S1.
[20] ANOM, Gougal 3E 2920.
[21] "Note du contre-amiral secrétaire d'état aux colonies (pour le Ministre, le directeur du service de santé, le Dr Blanchard) au Gouverneur général de l'Indochine, Paris, 30 octobre 1940," ANOM, RST NF 3710.
[22] In localities with too few retail pharmacies for a competitive bidding system, the health authorities could sign contracts directly with individual pharmacists.

formally defined only in 1899 to ensure the fairness of competition, the setting of specifications, and floor prices for each product by the administration and the conformity of deliveries with promised quantities, rates, delivery times, origin, and quality.

The system attracted much criticism, particularly involving accusations directed at private pharmacists for inflating drug prices. Colonial Inspector Le Conte, who evaluated the state of the Indochinese health care system in 1913, concluded that local purchasing put an unnecessary burden on the Union's budget. He gave the example of thymol, a commonly used antiseptic and worm medicine, whose price was more than doubled by local purchasing (36 francs versus a direct import cost of 16.38 francs per kg). Le Conte also noted that Pyramidon tablets, an analgesic and fever-reducing drug derived from phenazone like Antipyrin, cost two and a half times more than the direct import cost when purchased through a local retailer.[23] A 1917 report on the supply of quinine to Cochinchina pointed out that 150 kg of the product were 100 percent more expensive when procured via a Saigon-based pharmacy.[24] Private pharmacists defended these markups as essential to their livelihoods, suggesting that, at the time, public contracts helped their businesses survive. Still, the frugality of public spending on pharmaceuticals meant that some of these contracts were hardly profitable, resulting in very small gains or even losses, as revealed in pharmacists' sometimes heated exchanges with health authorities. For example, in 1936, the bidders for a contract to supply specialties to the AMI in Cochinchina offered rebates of 4 to 18 percent on the floor prices set by the administration.[25]

Pharmacists' ability to ensure regular supplies and keep prices down faced additional constraints. They complained about import regulations and duties, and claimed to be the victims of delays in delivery for which they were wrongfully accused.[26] During the two world wars, in particular, pharmacists put in requests for the relaxation of import regulations. For

---

[23] "Rapport fait par M. Le Conte, inspecteur de 3ᵉ classe des colonies, concernant la vérification du service de M. Clarac, médecin-inspecteur des Troupes coloniales, directeur du service de santé de l'Indochine, Hanoi, 11 février 1913," ANOM, DC 665.

[24] The scarcity of quinine at this time was said not to account for this difference, since it also affected metropolitan suppliers ("Santé. Fourniture de quinine nécessaire au service local de la Cochinchine, 1917," ANOM, Gougal 4447).

[25] ANOM, Gougal SE 2921.

[26] Public tenders and import duties were, more generally, the main points of tension between Indochina's government and private business sector throughout the time of colonial rule: Claire Villemagne-Renard, "Les commerçants et les colons français, acteurs de la vie économique et politique du Tonkin: Les membres des chambres de commerce et des chambres d'agriculture, de leur création aux années Doumer" (paper presented at "Le contact colonial," Université Paris-Sorbonne, France, November 9–10, 2007).

example, in 1915, pharmacists Jean Roux, Louis Blanc, and Edmond Chassagne asked to suspend the prohibition on importing quinine from countries other than France, while Chassagne, in 1918, sought special authorization to obtain commonly used substances and specialties from Japan.[27] Both requests were refused. Pharmacists also protested the colonial administration's growing efforts to bypass them in public pharmaceutical provisioning.[28] In 1935, Pierre Domart went as far as to accuse the AMI of making a profit from the resale of directly imported medicines to other administrative services, at the expense of not only honest businesspeople such as himself but also taxpayers.[29] In Cochinchina, where private pharmacists were more numerous than in other territories, and better able to defend their interests collectively (see Chapter 4), there was also greater use of the tender system.[30] Despite its flaws, the system remained in place until the end of colonial rule.

At the same time, Indochina's health authorities were seeking ways to rationalize, and to control the costs of, pharmaceutical supplying. They lamented that orders had become too complicated for private pharmacists, who were no longer able to fulfill them, and that it was preferable to deal with local branches of pharmaceutical firms such as Rhône-Poulenc's. The creation of three Pharmacies centrales d'approvisionnement (Central Supply Pharmacies) from the mid-1910s was part of this push to streamline public pharmaceutical provisioning and reduce its costs. The first was opened in Hué in 1915 (moving to Tourane in 1930), another was established in Saigon in 1919, and the third opened, a year later, in Hanoi. The supply pharmacies were generally headed either by a TC officer, temporarily "lent" to the AMI for this purpose, or by a privately contracted civilian pharmacist. After a bumpy start, these institutions enabled the AMI to import its medicines directly from the metropole through calls for tenders issued by the Paris-based Agence

---

[27] "Demande d'exonération des droits de douane pour la quinine importée de l'étranger formulée par les pharmaciens de Hanoi et Haiphong, 1915," VNA, centre no. 1, RST 9021; ANOM, Gougal 33693.

[28] "Réclamation de M. Chassagne, pharmacien à Hanoi, contre la décision prise par l'administration de s'approvisionner directement en France pour tous les médicaments nécessaires à l'Assistance médicale du Tonkin, 1919," ANOM, Gougal 17178.

[29] Domart wrote that the Local Directorate of Health in Tonkin benefitted from the reduced cost of direct imports to turn a profit (15 percent commission) from the sale of medicines that could be claimed for reimbursement from different administrative services, rather than to supply its public hospitals ("Au sujet des cessions de médicaments aux divers services locaux par l'Assistance médicale du Tonkin, 1935," VNA, centre no. 1, RST 47980). Indeed, AMI facilities were legally allowed to provide medicines to communes that did not have a pharmacist, at the AMI price increased by 25 percent.

[30] "Rapport annuel d'ensemble sur le fonctionnement de l'inspection, 1928," VNA, centre no. 1, Fonds de l'Inspection générale d'hygiène et de santé publique (hereafter IGHSP) 4.

générale des colonies (General Agency for the Colonies). They thus gave the AMI more direct control over shipping and distribution, and provided it with capacity for onsite conditioning and packaging, thus allowing for some products, including quinine (see Chapter 3), to be imported in bulk.[31] In 1931, the Central Supply Pharmacy of Tonkin had, in addition to a large storeroom for its stocks, a room for compounding officinal preparations. It was equipped with sterilizing apparatus, two presses for making pills and tablets, and two vacuum pumps for filling ampoules. By then, Tonkin purchased nearly 85 percent of its annual quinine requirements directly from France.[32] The pharmacy's staff included one military pharmacist, two auxiliary pharmacists, an accountant, four secretaries, three nurses, and several "coolies." By the mid-1930s, the institution was thriving and making plans to obtain new equipment (boxes, sterilizers, glassware).[33] It also possessed an abundant stock of pharmaceutical products, suggesting that Domart's accusation may have been well founded.

Once they obtained their stocks, the supply pharmacies were in charge of distributing medicines within the AMI. In theory, each health care facility had a retail pharmacy to receive and dispense medicines. In reality, only the largest hospitals had a pharmacy that occupied a distinct room, in which a range of tasks including compounding and packaging were performed. By contrast, many smaller facilities simply allocated a cupboard for medicines and medicinal substances in the corner of a bandage room. Pharmaceutical orders were determined by the head of each facility in compliance with an official nomenclature that set the list of allowable products and quantities. The earliest I found was dated April 1912; it apparently responded to complaints about the patently unfair distribution of medicines among facilities and provinces. All facilities were theoretically entitled to the same medicines, with the allowable quantity calculated on the basis of a rough estimate (by intervals of fifty) of the number of patients seen per day.[34] Deliveries were made every trimester, and then per semester in the 1930s, using a variety of shipment methods. During

[31] "Mission Picanon, rapport sur l'Assistance médicale au Tonkin envoyé au Ministère des colonies, 23 mai 1923," ANOM, DC 670; ANOM, Gougal 17178.

[32] ANOM, RST NF 3683.

[33] "Direction locale de la santé au Tonkin, rapport sanitaire annuel, 1935," ANOM, RST NF 3685.

[34] Special requests could be made for medicines not on this list, but these could not exceed 20 percent of the facility's pharmaceutical budget. By these rules, the largest hospitals were entitled to greater quantities of AMI medicines and a larger range of special requests ("Organisation des services médicaux dans diverses provinces du Tonkin, 1899–1914," VNA, centre no. 1, RST 74506). The nomenclature was only slightly modified over the years, for instance to include more arsenobenzols.

the interwar years, for example, large crates of "commonly used" medicines circulated by sea or rail, while smaller parcels of fragile pharmaceuticals and vaccines, as well as urgent deliveries, were sent by mail or via private shipment companies.[35]

The centralization of supply surely increased its efficiency, but also the weight of its bureaucracy. The system was beset by problems such as delays and unnecessary paperwork. For example, each order from an AMI facility needed to be signed off by the relevant Local Directorate of Health before it was submitted to the Central Supply Pharmacy. Head doctors of provinces occasionally defied the rules in order to purchase medicines directly from private pharmacies, notably during epidemics.[36] During World War II, supply pharmacies also rationed the distribution of medicines to provinces and even requisitioned parts of the stocks held by some hospitals and missionary congregations.[37] Access to regular supplies of medicines was also made more complicated by the intervention of other colonial services: AMI authorities and doctors often complained of excessive zeal on the part of customs officers on the lookout for trafficked narcotics. Crates of medicines might thus be detained for weeks in hot, humid hangars. Not only did this delay their delivery to health care facilities, but it could also impair their chemical stability and bioactivity. Complaints made by AMI doctors do indeed indicate that in the early years especially, there were major problems caused by the deterioration of pharmaceutical quality and efficacy due to heat and humidity, compounded by poor storage conditions, and delays in transportation.[38]

2.3   Free Medicines and Therapeutic Skepticism under Colonial Rule

If and when medicines finally made it to AMI facilities – what then? An additional set of factors determined their accessibility in public health care, whose impact varied from one category of medicines to another, as explored in detail in Chapter 3. Here, I first address two pervasive yet ambiguous issues that deeply affected the accessibility of public

---

[35] ANOM, RSA S1.

[36] "Demandes de médicaments par les services sanitaires et médicaux dans les provinces," VNA, centre no. 1, RST 73636; ANOM, RST NF 4018.

[37] "Perte de quarante caisses de médicaments distribués à l'Assistance de Moncay," ANOM, RST NF 3710; "Tournées d'inspection de M. le Directeur local de la santé et de M. l'Inspecteur général de l'hygiène et de la santé publique, 1942," ANOM, RST NF 630; "Escorte d'une jonque de produits pharmaceutiques sur l'itinéraire Phuly–Ninh Binh–Hanoi, mai 1944," ANOM, RST NF 6722.

[38] "Au sujet des médicaments expédiés au Tonkin par la maison Watson et Cie de Hong Kong, 1911," ANOM, Gougal 18751.

medicines: first, their cost, or rather their provision at no cost as part of free care – the conditions of which were unclear and apparently not very high on the agenda of colonial medical authorities – and second, the prevailing therapeutic skepticism of AMI doctors.

The free provision of health care and medicines was hardly discussed in colonial reports and correspondence. This may, in itself, be a symptom of general indifference to problems of accessibility, but also, perhaps, of a great deal of confusion about the legal conditions of access to free care, or even of a sense of embarrassment about the gulf between the ideals and realities of colonial medicalization. Free medical care for the *"indigents"* (needy) was included in the AMI's foundational text. Yet colonial authorities warned, from the outset, that access to free care did not give the Indochinese population any claim to health care as a right. For example, when the governor of Cochinchina candidly pointed out the legal ambiguity concerning the administration's obligation to provide care, the governor general responded:

The Assistance as it is designed [. . .] is essentially optional. It would be a misinterpretation of the intentions of the chief of the colony to attribute to it a compulsory character [. . .] Besides, a right to obtain treatment entails sanctions, in the hypothetical case that it should be ignored. But as you can see for yourself, nowhere [. . .] is the possibility of recourse [. . .] envisaged. It is intentional that no plans were made for provisions analogous to those of the articles 16, 17 and 18 of the law of 15 July 1893 on Assistance médicale gratuite in France, those which allow any individual to appeal the decision of a communal assistance bureau.[39]

Who, then, might be eligible to obtain medical consultations and treatment for free? How were indigents defined and identified? A card system was set up in Cochinchina to identify eligible individuals. However, it was never extended to Tonkin or Annam, whose populations were deemed "too poor" to implement the system's criteria. Almost everyone in these two protectorates, it seems, was theoretically entitled to free health care, if, of course, they were willing and able to attend an AMI facility.[40] Also eligible for free care were active colonial civil servants and public employees, both French and Vietnamese, including imperial officials (the mandarins who still worked for the Vietnamese court[41]) and their families and, from 1919, war veterans and the disabled.

[39] "Organisation de l'Assistance médicale, pièces de principe, 1904–1909," ANOM, Gougal 6719.
[40] Consultation or hospitalization costs had to be reimbursed by the local budget of the patient's region of origin.
[41] The maintenance of the imperial court by the French authorities was mere form, or almost. It kept only a handful of prerogatives, including the regulation of Vietnamese

Thus free-of-charge care was, in legal terms, applicable to a huge proportion of the colonized population for the whole period of colonial rule. Prior to 1905, public budgets could absorb the limited quantities of medicines that were systematically provided for free in the colony's small network of hospitals and mobile infirmaries. But as both the infrastructural network and the number (and cost) of pharmaceuticals grew, the potential patient pool eligible for free treatment would have quickly outstripped the administration's budgetary resources. Although there is a lack of detailed information on how the system of free medical assistance really worked, it seems quite clear that its goals were unrealistic. It should be mentioned here that in the late 1930s, the population of Indochina has been estimated at twenty-three million inhabitants, of which nineteen million were in Vietnam and nearly fifteen million were in Tonkin and Annam.[42] During the same period, six million people were insured in France and could thus claim reimbursements of 60 percent on the cost of medicines. The reach of the colonial health care system did not come anywhere near these metropolitan figures, even if it was supplemented by some private but nonprofit medical services, such as those run by missionaries, which received supplies from the public system and occasionally donations from private pharmacists.

The high cost of pharmaceuticals may partly explain why the AMI was unable to provide better access. Nevertheless, the low priority of pharmaceuticals in the allocation of meager health budgets is a clear, perhaps the clearest, indication of the marginal role these were given in colonial projects and policies at least until the end of World War I. The persistent orientation of health policies toward prevention tended to minimize the role of curative or palliative drugs. Only substances that could be mass distributed for preventive purposes, such as vaccines and quinine, were seen as apt to further the goals of colonial health policy. Unlike sanitation measures and the principles of hygiene and vaccination, medicines were considered unlikely to foster associations between colonialism, health, civilization, and modernity. Doctors and medical authorities in Vietnam often portrayed drug therapy as either dangerous or ineffective, rendered particularly risky and useless under local conditions. At the turn of the twentieth century, most available medical specialties left them powerless in the face of deadly tropical diseases, while hasty distributions of basic drugs could hardly, as they pointed out, be expected to "impress the natives." The earliest specific, powerful drugs such as

---

medicine. Still, the examination system for entry into mandarinal positions was maintained until 1918.

[42] Brocheux and Hémery, *Indochine*, 248.

arsenical compounds were deemed to be particularly risky in the colonies, because their toxicity might cause accidents given the lack of medical supervision (and tendency to self-medicate) as well as "scare off" potential converts to biomedicine. In other words, the therapeutic skepticism that was still prevalent among the French medical profession gained particular purchase in colonial territories.

In the early years of the twentieth century, several medical officers reported on the failures of therapy in their attempts to control epidemic outbreaks in Vietnam. It seems that they would try any drug they could get their hands on, and often fell back on symptomatic or adjuvant therapies, treating their patients by trial and error and what amounted to a form of therapeutic bricolage. Indeed, some even confessed to having tried out local remedies. Confronted with a cholera epidemic in the Tonkin province of Thai Binh in 1904, Dr. A. Sarrailhé described how, lacking syringes to inject artificial serum, he first let the hospital nuns administer "revulsants, massage, and stimulants" such as caffeine and ether potions. Sarrailhé then took up these methods himself, to which he added hot baths and saline enemas. The result was a 64 percent case fatality rate. He then turned to methodical intravenous injections of 7 percent concentration artificial serum. These apparently caused several deaths, so he decided to "prepare" patients' hearts by injecting ether and caffeine. His fatality rate dropped to 34 percent. Finally, he supplemented this treatment with a "medicated alcohol" from Saigon which, according to several "Vietnamese experts" he knew, had obtained a 75 percent recovery rate. This experiment was disastrous: "three patients, three deaths," he concluded disconsolately.[43]

Other doctors' attempts to treat relapsing fever similarly resulted in repeated failure. Reporting on the epidemics of 1906–7 in Tonkin, Dr. Laurent Gaide listed the medicines his colleagues had tried: quinine, collargol (a colloidal silver preparation, used mainly as an antiseptic), anti-plague serum, several mercury salts, and sodium cacodylate. Only the latter seemed to reduce fever, but required vigorous adjuvant stimulant therapy to "support the heart and strength of the patient" as well as purgatives to alleviate abdominal pain.[44] Two years later, another report listed additional therapeutic experiments with methylene blue, Fowler's or Boudin's syrups, orpiment, Arrhenal, and

---

[43] Dr. A. Sarrailhé, "Rapport sur l'épidémie de choléra de la province de Thai Binh du 20 mars au 23 mai 1904," AHMC, 9 (1906): 54–60.

[44] Dr. Laurent Gaide, "Rapport sur les épidémies de fièvre récurrente au Tonkin," AHMC 11 (1908): 143–45. Relapsing fever, a flea-borne bacterial infection, was endemic in Vietnam at the time, with an average 40 percent fatality rate if untreated. Until 1914, it also regularly emerged as an epidemic.

Atoxyl. None was found to have specific efficacy, and the recommended treatment remained, "by default," to alleviate symptoms and strengthen the patient.[45] In 1910, the first volume of the BSMI included only three articles on curative medicines. Of these, two were reports of adverse effects (the first in relation to a product containing sodium sulphate and the second to an "indigenous medicine"); only one was about the beneficial effects of collargol in the treatment of cholera.[46]

Unsurprisingly then, given the inefficacy of most available medicines in treating tropical pathologies at this time, colonial doctors were skeptical of strategies that would use medicines to reach out to the colonized population. Many were particularly opposed to a 1907 governor general's decree instituting a system of mobile AMI outpatient consultations that entailed free distributions of medicines. Sarrailhé was among them. Not only, he argued, were medicines of little use beyond the relief of a few common symptoms and the treatment of a handful of acute but benign conditions. He also warned that hastily distributed medicines could send the wrong message to the population. He described a hypothetical consultation in some village, crowded with "curious" Vietnamese patients:

The doctor will be very pressed for time, hardly able to examine a complicated case in depth [. . .] Fever will no doubt be the most frequent complaint. But which fever? [. . .] Quinine, administered indiscriminately, will certainly do some measure of good but also lead to many therapeutic failures and deceptions. Cases of bronchitis, pulmonary congestion, pneumonia [. . .] will never be caught early and we cannot hope to treat these in the few days a nomadic doctor will spend in each locality. What about chronic disease [. . .]? What can a single dose of bismuth, tannic syrup, or Brazilian ipecac do? Intestinal diseases call for a rigorous diet as much as medicinal treatment. What can a medicine, even if effective, achieve in a patient incapable of following a special diet? What kind of patients will [. . .] the ambulatory doctor see? Almost always incurables or those whose disease is already very advanced [. . .] It will be very difficult for their simple minds to tolerate the need for a rather long treatment, and for them to lose the illusion of a radical and immediate cure. Can the doctor refuse to treat such uncommitted patients? No, this could go against the objective of mobile consultations. So we will just have to go along with it and tire ourselves out administering eye drops and ointments knowing full well that little good will come of such "fugitive" treatment.[47]

The head doctor of the province of Vinh Yen (Tonkin) reported in 1913 that he had abandoned mobile consultations, declaring these "not

[45] Dr Imbert, "Épidémie de fièvre récurrente," AHMC 13 (1910): 195–98.
[46] Dr. J. Casaux, "Deux cas d'amaurose bilatérale transitoire à la suite d'ingestion de sulfate de soude," BSMI 1 (1910): 257–59; Dr. Georges Barbezieux, "Le Collargol dans le traitement du choléra," BSMI 1 (1910): 362–68; Sambuc, "Deux cas mortels."
[47] Dr. A. Sarrailhé, "Extraits du rapport annuel pour 1910 sur le fonctionnement de l'AMI dans la province de Bien Hoa," AHMC 15 (1912): 304–10.

only a poor investment of resources [. . .] but also at risk of damaging perceptions of the efficacy of Western medicine."[48] His colleague from Bac Giang even opined that the system was a "concession to the native mentality."[49] A year later, a Vietnamese medical officer called mobile consultations "transit camp medicine," likening these to a charlatan distributing his wares at a country fair, not only cheapening the doctor's image, but also threatening the efficacy of his therapeutics. "It saddens me," he added, "to often hear my countrymen say 'not only did the European remedy fail to improve my condition but it even made it worse!'"[50] Vietnamese auxiliary doctors were, at the time, as mistrustful of medicines as their European colleagues.

Responses to the mobile consultation system are a particularly good illustration of doctors' doubts about medicines as tools of medicalization. Given the paucity of effective drugs, how could medicines successfully demonstrate the superiority of European medicine and the benefits of colonial rule? Medicines were to be mistrusted not only because they carried the wrong message about biomedicine, but also, perhaps, because of the ease with which they escaped medical authority and the rules of appropriate use. To benefit from the civilizing effects of colonial medicine, colonized patients were seen as requiring preparation and education in the rules of hygiene, to ultimately obtain the status of "biomedical citizens."[51] At least until the 1910s, medicines were seen a threat: they might deviate attention and resources from hygiene and preventive public health and, furthermore, reinforce the "bad influence" of Vietnamese medicine, in which drug therapy played a central role. Particularly ineffective or toxic medicines, of course, were even more directly *counter-civilizing* and threatening to the image of European superiority and the legitimacy of colonial domination.

Some medical practitioners saw the problem of drug toxicity as further modulated by the specificity of what they called the *"constitution indochinoise"* ("Indochinese constitution") – that is, the distinctive predispositions, strengths, and vulnerabilities of local bodies. For example, in 1912, Dr. Legendre reported that he reduced "normal" doses of 606 in the treatment of relapsing fever because the average body weight of his subjects, soldiers of the Native Guard, was about a third less than the average

---

[48] "Rapport sanitaire annuel de la province de Vinh Yen, 1913," ANOM, RST NF 4014.
[49] "Rapport sanitaire annuel de la province de Bac Giang, 1913," ANOM, RST NF 4014.
[50] "Rapport sanitaire annuel de la province de Ninh Binh, 1914," ANOM, RST NF 4015.
[51] Warwick Anderson, *Colonial Pathologies. American Tropical Medicine, Race, and Hygiene in the Philippines* (Durham and London: Duke University Press, 2006), 9.

adult French male.[52] Other doctors pointed out the specific local forms taken by some diseases. Dr. Riou, director of the dermatology-venereology unit of the Protectorate's Hospital in Hanoi, stated in 1936 that "exotic syphilis" in Vietnam was similar to European manifestations of the disease several centuries earlier.[53] In 1942, Dr. Montel explained such differences to be the result of lack of effective treatment, poor hygiene, comorbidity (poverty and poor nutrition, hypotension, malaria, and intercurrent infections), as well as the effects of hot weather on the skin.[54] Combining biological, social, environmental, as well as historical and cultural considerations, these references to distinctive Indochinese biologies underpinned calls for the adaptation of therapeutic regimens. They formed a variant of more widespread and persistent doubts about the relatively recent idea of specific and universal drug effects, as we saw in Chapter 1. In the majority of cases, Vietnamese patients were seen as more sensitive to biomedical drugs, and thus requiring lower doses. Occasionally, however, they were observed to be surprisingly resistant and tolerant to medicines, for example, to emetine and the sulfa drug Dagénan, compared with Europeans.[55]

2.4   The Civilizing Potential of Arsenical Drugs

The first signs of change in the colonial discourse on medicines came after World War I. While many medical officers continued to see drug therapy as superfluous to the colonial health project, the first trials of arsenobenzols (in Europe and, shortly afterwards, in Vietnam) kindled enthusiasm among some AMI doctors. Yet doubts soon arose as to whether these costly and potentially toxic drugs were appropriate for a system short on both money and doctors. Despite demonstrations of their powerful effects on prevalent infectious diseases, these drugs failed to significantly change the role of medicines in colonial public health care. They were distributed with parsimony and provoked renewed calls for caution in using medicines as tools of medicalization. Surprisingly, the potential of

---

[52] Dr. Legendre, "Traitement de la fièvre récurrente par l'arsénobenzol: essais sur sujets militaires indigènes," BSPE 5 (1912): 339–42.
[53] "Rapport du Dr Riou, médecin chargé du service de dermato-vénérologie de l'hôpital du Protectorat au sujet de la syphilis tertiaire, héréditaire et latente," ANOM, RST NF 3686.
[54] Dr. M.L.R. Montel, "La syphilis dite exotique chez les Annamites de Cochinchine," BSPE 35 (1942): 132–50.
[55] J. Grenierboley and Nguyễn Hữu Phiếm, "Au sujet de l'utilisation des sulfamidés dans la blennorragie masculine et féminine," Revue médicale française d'Extrême-Orient (RMFEO) 17 (1939): 603–14; Drs. M. Alain and Ch. Ragiot, "De la diminution des effets toxiques de l'émétine par l'emploi de la vitamine B1 (essais effectués au cours du traitement de l'amibiase)," BSPE 32 (1939): 300–3.

medicines as civilizing forces instead emerged in trials of leprosy therapy. While these provided equivocal evidence of efficacy, they allowed for the cultivation of the figure of the "good (colonial) experimental subject," a template for that of the "good (colonial) consumer" of medicines. The cases of both arsenical drugs and leprosy treatments illustrate how therapeutic hopes were generated by the uses of medicines, but only under conditions of strict medical supervision, that might mitigate some of the earlier therapeutic skepticism.

Arsenical compounds stimulated the first real debates about drug efficacy in the colonial medical press. The earliest reports of trials with Atoxyl for malarial and relapsing fever in Indochina were published in 1908, at the same time as the drug's efficacy, and low toxicity, were being shown in the treatment of a range of infectious diseases, including sleeping sickness, in African colonies.[56] By 1911, experiments of Compound 606 (Salvarsan) had begun in Vietnam, only two years after the first clinical trials in Europe. A first test was conducted at Hanoi's Hôpital indigène on ninety-seven syphilis patients and twenty-nine who suffered from other conditions, under the supervision of the auxiliary doctor Nguyễn Xuân Mai.[57] Nguyễn Xuân Mai reported one case of death and another of toxic effects, but concluded that these risks were not serious enough to justify the "rejection" of a medicine that gave "such marvelous results." Soon afterward, a second trial in the same hospital led to similar conclusions. Its supervisors, however, insisted on administering lower doses to limit side effects, noting that 606 alone could not cure syphilis and thus needed to be complemented with mercury therapy.[58] They were not the only doctors to express ambivalence about arsenical drugs. Many warned of toxic risks and reported side effects that were sometimes lethal.[59] Still, these drugs' spectacular effects on deadly epidemics and highly prevalent endemic diseases impressed doctors in Indochina.

[56] Dr. Joseph Vassal, "L'Atoxyl dans le traitement de la fièvre paludéenne," BSPE 1 (1908): 539–44; Gaide, "Rapport sur les épidémies." On the history of Atoxyl, see Steven Riethmiller, "Ehrlich, Bertheim and Atoxyl: The Origins of Modern Chemotherapy," *Bulletin of the History of Chemistry* 23 (1999): 28. On the sleeping sickness trials, see Eckart, "The Colony as Laboratory."

[57] Nguyễn Xuân Mai, "Note sur l'emploi du dioxydiamidoarsénobenzol à l'hôpital indigène du protectorat," BSMI 3, 1 (1912): 35–36.

[58] Drs. Roux and Tardieu, "Ulcérations balaniques syphilitiques avec phagédénisme et onyxis du gros orteil gauche rebelles au traitement mercuriel et guéris par le 606," BSMI 3, 1 (1912): 37–39.

[59] See, for instance, in the BSMI: Dr. Le Dantec, "Traitement de la filariose par les injections intraveineuses d'arsénobenzol," 3, 5 (1912): 295–98; H. Dupuy, "Accidents mortels consécutifs à une deuxième injection de 606," 3, 8 (1912): 514–17; Drs. Ferris and Le Dentu, "Neuro-récidives et neurotropisme," 3, 8 (1912): 542–47.

Syphilis, ranked as the second highest cause of morbidity in Indochina, was the first and main target of arsenical drugs. Epidemics of relapsing fever in Tonkin in the early 1910s were also occasions for trials, which, it was reported, gave remarkable results in terms of mortality rates and recovery times.[60] Arsenical drugs were also experimented with in the treatment of a range of other diseases, including dengue fever, amoebic dysentery, malaria, yaws, and even mumps, chickenpox, and phagedenic ulcer.[61]

In 1913, Dr. Clarac, the inspector general of health services, reported to his colleagues at the third meeting of the Far Eastern Association for Tropical Medicine (FEATM) in Saigon that the use of arsenical compounds for the treatment of syphilis was largely responsible for a drop of ten thousand days of hospitalization between 1911 and 1912.[62] Clarac's statement suggests that, fewer than two years after the first trials of 606, the drug was being used more widely than just in Hanoi's biggest hospital. The drug was soon blamed for serious adverse effects, including nerve damage.[63] By then, however, Compound 914, which was deemed to be less toxic, was already in use in several facilities. The number of scientific articles on arsenical drugs in Indochina dwindled over the next few years, indicating, perhaps, that their use had become routine. Routine use, however, is not to be confused with "common" use, as health reports indicated. The nomenclature of usual medicines for AMI facilities in 1915 set a very low limit on the quantity of arsenical compounds. Nonetheless, by the 1930s, a significant quantity of 914 was listed in the inventories of Central Supply Pharmacies, alongside other arsenical drugs. These included newer pentavalent compounds, considered less toxic than the older trivalent arsenicals, such as Treparsol (Lecoq et Ferrand), Arsaminol (Clin, Comar et Cie), and Rhône-Poulenc's Stovarsol and Acétylarsan.

By the 1930s, there were enough arsenical drugs in the public health care system (and outside it, as we will see in Chapters 5, 6, and 8) for concerns to be raised anew about their toxicity and misuse, provoking a new wave of articles in the local medical press. In 1931, Dr. Nguyễn Văn

---

[60] Legendre, "Traitement de la fièvre récurrente"; Dr. Joseph Vassal, "Troisième congrès biennal de médecine tropicale. Compte-rendu," AHMC 17 (1914): 741–42; ANOM, RST NF 4018; Dr. Pierre Mouzels, "La fièvre récurrente au Tonkin," AHMC 16 (1913): 279.

[61] The phagedenic ulcer or tropical ulcer was a common chronic condition in Indochina. It generally presents as a deep wound in the lower limbs caused by the introduction of bacteria.

[62] Cited by Vassal, "Troisième congrès biennal," 731–32.

[63] Drs. Roux and Tardieu, "Neurotropisme et Salvarsan," BSMI 3, 1 (1912): 346–50; Dupuy, "Accidents mortels"; Ferris and Le Dentu, "Neuro-récidives."

Tùng wrote that the inadequate consumption of arsenical drugs, particularly in too-low doses, could lead to nervous complications associated with advanced stages of syphilis.[64] The same year, a spirited, even turbulent, debate flared up among the members of the French Société de pathologie exotique (Society of Tropical Medicine) in Paris on this potential connection between the use of arsenical drugs and cases of neuro-syphilis. In response to this debate, some colonial doctors reaffirmed their skeptical stance toward therapeutics, raising doubts about the use of synthetic drugs "as medical propaganda," and emphasizing instead the primacy of preventive health action in colonial contexts.[65] By this time, arsenical drugs provoked criticism internationally, particularly with respect to their presumed "abusive use" in the colonies. In Vietnam, the issue of iatrogenic complications evoked frequent and firm reminders of the need for strict medical supervision, and thus of the impossibility of distributing arsenical drugs widely, beyond doctor-staffed facilities. By the 1940s, arsenobenzols were definitively abandoned in both Paris and Hanoi due to their toxicity.[66]

The high cost of arsenical drugs, relative to the amounts in colonial "materials" budgets, also raised doubts about their potential for revolutionizing the Vietnamese therapeutic landscape. Doctors in Indochina had experimented with, and praised the effects of, arsenicals in treating prevalent endemic diseases such as syphilis or amoebic dysentery – a condition that, unlike bacillary dysentery, can lead to serious complications and may have been the most frequent cause of hospitalization in Cochinchina in the 1920s. Yet they continued to seek and use cheaper medication. Although colonial doctors declared, in the 1920s, Stovarsol and Treparsol to be safer and more effective than emetine hydrochloride in the treatment of dysentery, they warned that these drugs were too expensive and difficult to use routinely in the AMI system.[67] While, by the late 1930s, some arsenical compounds specifically indicated for the treatment of dysentery were stocked by the Central Supply Pharmacies, these were likely reserved for the larger hospitals.[68] Most small rural facilities continued to use only emetine hydrochloride, despite the high number of side effects recorded.[69]

[64] Nguyễn Văn Tùng, "Note sur la syphilis nerveuse en Cochinchine à propos d'un nouveau cas de tabès," BSMI 9, 2 (1931): 125–29.

[65] Dr. Thiroux, "Le rôle des médecins coloniaux," Hygiène sociale 61 (1931): 1072–73.

[66] "Cession de médicaments pour Dalat, juin 1943," RST NF 6441.

[67] E. Marchoux, "Action du Stovarsol sur le parasitisme intestinal," Paris médical, November 22, 1924, reprinted in Annales de médecine et de pharmacie coloniales (AMPC) 22 (1924): 430–31; Dr. Lecomte, "L'Assistance médicale en Cochinchine pendant l'année 1924," AMPC 26 (1926): 137.

[68] ANOM, Gougal SE 2920.

[69] ANOM, RST NF 3710 and Gougal SE 3142.

In 1923, the inspector general of health services, Gaide, recommended, by circular letter, the routine use of bismuth subsalicylate therapy for the treatment of syphilis, following the method developed by an AMI doctor named Lenoir. This substance, experimented on thousands of patients, was easy to produce and particularly cheap.[70] At 1 cent per injection, it cost on average 10 cents for a full therapeutic course, while a single injection of 606 was reported to cost 1.50 piasters. Outside large urban hospitals, arsenical drugs seem to have been distributed widely only during epidemic outbreaks, as emergency and experimental solutions. This was the case of relapsing fever epidemics in the early 1910s. Even for this disease, however, emetine hydrochloride remained a popular treatment.

There is also evidence of hierarchies in the allocation of public medicines within the AMI. On the eve of World War I, Governor General Albert Sarraut recommended that arsenical drugs, given their high price, be reserved for "exceptional cases."[71] Arsenical drugs, and several other expensive medical specialties, were, at least initially, limited to a small circle of elite patients – Viêt and white urban wealthy minorities who were able to pay for them. In 1914, for example, the head doctor of Ninh Binh Province stated that "common" patients were treated for syphilis with bi-iodide of mercury, while private patients, those who were not classified as needy, received arsenobenzol injections.[72] Conditions were also discriminated as worthy or not of the best available treatment. For example, arsenical compounds were hardly ever used to treat phagedenic ulcer. Not only was this affliction considered to be nonfatal; it was also seen as too widespread, especially among the poor, workers, and prisoners – who were often accused of inflicting it upon themselves to avoid work duties. Despite proof of the efficacy of arsenical drugs, the recommended treatment remained either tartar emetic, which was cheap and easy to handle although potentially toxic, or Pommade Ballot, an affordable bismuth-based ointment invented by a colonial pharmacist.[73]

---

[70] Several scientific publications suggest this directive was followed, despite adverse effects: P. Guillaume and La Cam Tuyen, "Contribution au traitement du pian par le salicylate de bismuth," BSMI 4, 9 (1926): 449–58; Dr. Decay, "Le salicylate de bismuth dans le traitement de la syphilis," AMPC 34 (1936): 74–85.

[71] "Hôpitaux. Réglementation des cessions de médicaments et objets de pansements par les formations sanitaires. Nomenclature des médicaments et objets de pansement, 1915," ANOM, Gougal 16368.

[72] ANOM, RST NF 4003. Yet some doctors attempted to persuade health authorities that even expensive drugs, if they were truly effective, were worth investment since they would ultimately reduce health care costs, for example by reducing hospitalization time (Mouzels, "La fièvre récurrente," 282).

[73] Dr. Ricou, "Traitement des ulcères phagédéniques et autres plaies infectées par la Poudre et la Pommade Ballot," BSMI 9, 10 (1931): 803–7.

The use of Pommade Ballot and of a similarly-named powder as affordable alternatives points to the role played by colonial pharmacists in producing what we might call "AMI specialties." These products were easier to use, and especially cheaper, than imported drugs, and could therefore be widely used in the public system (see Chapter 4). A few colonial doctors also invented medicines: Collyre Vert du Dr. Motais, a zinc and copper sulphate-based eye lotion to treat conjunctivitis and trachoma, was named after an ophthalmologist posted in Cochinchina in the 1920s. Another eye remedy, Collyre Jaune selon la Formule du Dr. Casaux, was named after another ophthalmologist who worked in Tonkin. Pandermyl, a cream "to heal wounds and relieve skin discomfort" was credited to a colonial doctor called Honnorat. Along with colonial pharmacists' work on the development of medicines from local plants and Vietnamese recipes (for example, chaulmoogra oils for treating leprosy, as will be seen in the next section), this local development of specialties shows how health care professionals, often at their own initiative, sought to expand the range of available therapeutic options through innovation. As mentioned previously, this pursuit of innovation sought to palliate gaps in the public system. However, some of the resulting products, notably Collyre Jaune, also became very popular in the private market (see Chapter 6).

2.5   Experimentation and the "Good Patient"

The use of arsenical drugs was never significantly scaled up in Indochina. There is little specific information about the rationing of public arsenical supplies, other than hints that some patients and conditions were more "worthy" of their use than others. Yet these clearly remained *elite drugs*, largely confined to wealthy, urban, or experimental populations or to emergency (and experimental) uses during deadly epidemics. They were acknowledged to be highly effective, yet they were not invested in, financially or ideologically, as tools capable of transforming Vietnamese bodies and habits. By contrast, trials of leprosy therapies, even before the introduction of the first truly effective curative drugs (sulfone-based antibiotics such as Dapsone) in the 1940s, forged a tentative association between medicines and civilization. Among the earliest therapeutic trials on leprosy were conducted by Dr. Montel, who, before World War I, experimented with subcutaneous injections of an iodoform-based antiseptic oil and noted objective improvements in the skin condition of three subjects.[74] From the 1920s, experimentation intensified as a result of

---

[74] M. L. R. Montel, "Notes de thérapeutique sur la lèpre," BSPE 4 (1911): 48–56.

renewed scientific interest in the pharmacological and therapeutic activity of chaulmoogra oils. Despite their equivocal results, these experiments index the changing, if still very ambiguous, role of medicines in the French Empire during the interwar period.

Long used in South and East Asia as a remedy for skin disorders, chaulmoogra oils were "rediscovered" by European doctors around 1850, becoming the main ingredient of Bayer's Antileprol, which was launched in 1908.[75] In Vietnam, trials involved thousands of individuals who, by law since 1912, were confined to leprosaria and agricultural colonies.[76] Efforts to reduce the side effects of the oil – which included nausea, fever, and intense pain – stimulated pharmacological research and clinical experimentation. Ethyl esters of the fatty acids of the oil were developed to allow for intramuscular injections. Attempts were made to produce this injectable form in Ernest Fourneau's lab at the Institut Pasteur in Paris, as well as in Indochina, including with a chaulmoogric species native to Cambodia called krabao.[77] A pill form was then developed from the sodium salts of fatty acids, which, from 1929, were prepared by the Institut Pasteur of Saigon. These pills were initially experimented, with the permission of the governor of Cochinchina, on volunteer patients. Trials were then extended to several leprosaria in Vietnam and at the Institut Pasteur's specialized weekly outpatient consultation.[78]

Leprosy patients were also, at the same time, subjected to a range of experimental medicines, from older preparations such as emetics and Lugol's iodine, an antiseptic solution of iodine and potassium iodine, to synthetic drugs such as arsenical compounds (Neosalvarsan and Eparséno). During a time of broader interest in the bactericidal action of dyes, methylene blue was also tried.[79] Only the latter seemed to have any measurable effect. Several publications in 1935 and 1936 were hopeful, despite a lack of knowledge about the dye's mechanism of action, but

[75] John Parascandola, "Chaulmoogra Oil and the Treatment of Leprosy," *Pharmacy in History* 45, 2 (2003): 47–57.

[76] Laurence Monnais, "Leprosy and Lepers in Vietnam: Could Confinement be 'Humanized'?," in *Public Health in Asia and the Pacific. Historical and Comparative Perspectives*, ed. Milton Lewis and Kerrie McPherson (London and New York: Routledge, 2008), 122.

[77] L. Alexis and B. Menaut, "Recherches sur le traitement de la lèpre par le krabao," AMPC 23 (1925): 201–26.

[78] Drs. Souchard and Ramijean, "Contribution à l'étude du traitement de la lèpre par les savons de krabao," *Archives des Instituts Pasteur d'Indochine* (AIPI) 18 (1933): 187–266.

[79] M. L. R. Montel, "Traitement de la lèpre par le bleu de méthylène en injections intraveineuses," in FEATM, *Transactions of the 9th Congress of the Far Eastern Association for Tropical Medicine Held in Nankin, China* (Nankin: National Health Administration, 1935), 753–75.

most insisted that good results could only be obtained by combining it with chaulmoogra oils. None of the trials concluded to any clear curative action on leprosy. At best, chaulmoogra oils might slow or stop the progression of the disease, perhaps even obtain *blanchiment*, a state of noncontagiousness that, in the case of leprosy, manifested as the disappearance of skin lesions. Still, the proliferation of trials, in which so much energy was apparently invested, is in itself suggestive of an emerging stance of therapeutic hope. This optimism was stimulated by the drug industry, but also by research conducted by several colonial chemist-pharmacists. It was eloquently expressed in a 1921 report on the Union's leprosaria:

The leprosarium must not be [. . .] merely a nursing home but [rather] a true place of treatment. According to studies conducted in various countries, it seems that iodide ester acids of chaulmoogra oil [. . .] have given very encouraging results in the treatment of leprosy [. . .] If it were to be proven that we have here a truly effective means of treatment, the leper might become an ordinary patient, one we might treat during periods of contagiousness and return to his family and work as soon as he ceases to be a threat. The possibility of improvement and even of cure would bring him towards our health facilities of his own will, instead, the prospect of prolonged or indefinite confinement brings him to hide his condition.[80]

The report also suggests that this optimism depended in part on patients "of good will" – those who cooperated with experimental treatment that was sometimes long and painful, or who asked to be treated after witnessing therapeutic effects in fellow patients. By contrast, the report harshly condemns those who refused, abandoned, or even escaped treatment.[81] It is well known that colonies served as laboratories for experiments, including therapeutic trials, conducted far from metropolitan scrutiny. The tight links between the colonial administration, industry, and public hospitals described earlier surely facilitated the overseas trial of some new medicines. Yet it is also interesting to consider experiments as potential sites for the emergence of novel therapeutic experiences and representations. Experimental drugs were potentially dangerous, but their first clinical uses could also create positive experiences of access, effect, and learning for experimental subjects. Indeed, colonial authorities pointed out that experiments, as potential sites for "witnessing efficacy," might give medicines civilizing effects. In March of 1924, the Minister of Colonies Albert Sarraut addressed the heads of each colony in a circular:

---

[80] "Essai d'un médicament sino-annamite pour la lèpre," ANOM, Gougal 65331.
[81] ANOM, RST NF 3683.

The experiments that have been undertaken in most of our colonies following the instructions contained in the circulars of 30 September 1921 and 10 January 1923 to evaluate the efficacy of new leprosy medications have resulted in some very interesting observations [. . .] [I] call your attention especially to the need to pursue these studies and research, methodically and with perseverance [. . .] Our dominant strategy of leprosy prevention must be treatment itself. There is no more powerful prophylactic weapon, none which can so directly strike the mind of the natives, than a truly active therapy.[82]

This is perhaps the first articulation of an explicit, official association between medicines, medicalization, and civilization, suggesting that the prospect of a drug treatment might lead to earlier intervention and, eventually, to reduced transmission, and even eradication, of a disease. By 1931, the president of the Société de pathologie exotique, the Pastorian Marcel Léger, could state that medicines had become an "excellent tool of medical propaganda in all colonial environments."[83]

There were, however, two implicit provisos: that these be the "right" kind of medicines (French drugs), and be consumed by the "right" kind of person. A segment of the Vietnamese press had made a similar distinction between categories of medicine as suited for proper medicalization in its promotion of Westernization as the path toward Vietnam's future. With the blunt title of "The Crisis of Medicines," an article published in the Saigon newspaper *La tribune indigène* in March 1918 declared that it was time for medicines to become an AMI priority, and demanded that this prioritization be reflected in budgets, particularly in hospital budgets. The shortage of French medicines in Vietnam was presented as a profoundly political problem, which "would surely cause grave prejudice to the Assistance [. . .] The consequence will be that foreign products [. . .] take advantage of this unique opportunity to invade the market of the colony and supplant [French products] in the minds of the masses. It is obvious that all these foreign products do not have the same therapeutic value as French medicines."[84]

The distinction between good and bad consumers of care also arose in a broader sense in the 1920s, and was further clarified in the 1930s. Medical professionals and authorities sorted the Vietnamese population on the basis of how well they accepted AMI medicines, and especially how closely they complied with biomedical therapeutic rules. A good consumer did not expect quick therapeutic solutions at the last minute; he or

---

[82] "Circulaire du Ministre des colonies au sujet de la prophylaxie et du traitement de la lèpre (24 mars 1924)," AMPC 22 (1924): 125–33.
[83] Marcel Léger, "Les dangers de l'abus des arsénobenzènes dans les colonies françaises," BSPE, 24 (1931): 266.
[84] N. H. Y., "La crise des médicaments," *La tribune indigène*, no. 60, March 28, 1918.

she did not resort to traditional remedies or self-medicate. Instead, one should consult willingly and at the right time, surrender to medical authority without question, and faithfully follow prescribed therapeutic regimens. Medical supervision and adherence were particularly crucial for the proper use of potentially toxic drugs.[85] Thus, despite chaulmoogra's lack of therapeutic efficacy, it was seen as a controllable medicine that was administered to controllable patients, and thus one suited to the goals of colonial medicalization.

The official, public role played by medicines in medicalizing projects in Vietnam, at a time of rapid and profound change in biomedical therapies, is difficult to pin down precisely. What is clear, however, is that this role was limited. There seems to have been no colonial consensus on the potential of medicines as vehicles of modernization, or even as tools for improving population health. In addition to the therapeutic skepticism prevalent among the French medical profession, the conditions of Vietnam's medicalization and the objectives of its colonization acted in concert to prevent any clearly articulated ideological, and much less practical, project of colonial pharmaceuticalization. This is certainly true at the level of discourse, in which medicines were represented as a last recourse, a default option, marginal despite the confirmed limits of preventive measures and the glaring need for essential care. It is also evident in meager and uneven budgetary allocations for medicines. By the late 1930s, medicines continued to be objects of both hope and fear; they were praised and vilified, as well as often accused of being ill-suited to local conditions of health care – that is, to the financial and structural realities of the public system, local pathological environment, and indigenous bodies. To these limiting factors we might add the presumption of a "cultural" tendency among the colonized to be "bad" patients, and therefore likely to jeopardize their own therapeutic outcomes. Thus medicines could only, in the end, tarnish the reputation and good intentions of the colonizers. There were, perhaps, some exceptions: when medicines were suited for mass distribution with little infrastructure and medical supervision and thereby had the capacity for large-scale prevention of morbidity and mortality, or might compensate for the lack of health care in rural areas. These *idealized* medicines, and the realities of their distribution, are the topic of Chapter 3.

---

[85] Edouard Sambuc and Hà Văn Sua, "Note sur les accidents dus aux injections de composés arsenicaux dans le traitement de la syphilis en Cochinchine," BSMI 4, 8 (1926): 409–12; Drs. Guérin, Borel, and Advier, "Stovarsol et paludisme," BSPE 20 (1937): 331–32; Nguyễn Văn Tùng, "Note sur la syphilis"; Alain and Ragiot, "De la diminution des effets toxiques."

3 The Mirage of Mass Distribution: State Quinine and Essential Medicines

While many medicines and issues related to their accessibility were met with prevailing indifference in colonial budgets and medical discourses, there were some exceptions to this trend. Some medicines do seem to have been invested in as tools that, if made sufficiently widely available, could have an impact on disease control and on the reach of colonial health care. This was the case for two initiatives that promised to "democratize," or at least to broaden and ruralize access to modern medicines in Vietnam: the creation of the State Quinine Service in 1909 and the authorization of *dépôts de médicaments* (medicines outlets) in 1920, whose function was to stock and distribute *médicaments essentiels* (essential medicines) in areas devoid of pharmacies and public health care facilities. Yet these efforts focused on limited categories of medicines – in the first case, on a prophylactic drug slated for mass distribution, and, in the second case, on basic, cheap, nontoxic medicines that excluded many of the most effective drugs available. They also failed to fulfill their stated objective: the expansive and equitable provision of (some) free or affordable medicines across the territories of the Union. This chapter describes the ideals and failures of these projects for QE and essential medicines, identifying the specific problems they encountered, as well as more generalized constraints on access to public medicines in and beyond the colonial or public health care infrastructure. This reveals many gaps between the discourse of medicalization and its day-to-day practice, as well as the complex relationship between medical imagination and action.

3.1 A Malarial Landscape and the Imperative of (Preventive) Control

From their first incursions in the Indochinese peninsula, the French military saw malaria as an omnipresent threat to the strength of their troops. Military doctors' reports and memoirs of Cochinchina in the 1860s pointed out the relentless ravages caused by "malarial miasmas."[1] To novelist and journalist Jules Boissière, posted in Annam and Tonkin for military service in 1866, malaria was the personification of evil, afflicting European and indigenous populations indiscriminately. Only opium was known to bring ephemeral relief.[2] By 1892, a report on the health situation of Tonkin stated that malaria was responsible for a third of the overall mortality rate.[3] The magnitude of the malaria problem was soon confirmed. In 1904, Édouard Jeanselme declared, "malaria is [one of the main] factors impeding the development of the native element."[4]

During the decades of conquest, colonial interventions against malaria were sporadic and uncoordinated, mostly responding to impending outbreaks or epidemics. Quinine was distributed regularly only to the French community and to Vietnamese soldiers. Since the 1850s, quinine had been used as a specific treatment for fever and as a prophylactic for malaria, despite the lack of precise knowledge about the etiology of the disease.[5] The discovery, in 1880, of malaria's causative agent, the Plasmodium protozoa, in Constantine, Algeria, and then of its vector, the female anopheles mosquito, in 1897–98 on the basis of studies by the British tropicalists Ronald Ross and Patrick Manson, kindled greater optimism about quinine as a disease-control weapon.[6] While environmental sanitation remained a priority, quinine was now seen as a potential tool of mass prevention on the basis of its capacity to neutralize the human "virus reservoir."[7] Coinciding with the end of Indochina's pacification, this shift was perfectly timed for quinine to be included in colonial malaria control policies.

In Vietnam, some of the earliest uses of quinine as a collective prophylactic occurred in large-scale construction projects. Meanwhile, in France, experts debated the appropriateness of European, notably

---

[1] Monnais-Rousselot, *Médecine et colonisation*, 35–37.

[2] Jules Boissière, *Dans la forêt*, in *Un rêve d'Asie*, ed. Alain Quella-Villégier (Paris: Omnibus, 1995 [1896]), 12–13.

[3] Dr. de Fornel, "Etat sanitaire du Tonkin pendant l'année 1889," *Archives de médecine navale* (AMN) 57 (1892): 244–62.

[4] Dr. Édouard Jeanselme, "Les principaux facteurs de la morbidité et de la mortalité indochinoise" (paper presented at the Congrès colonial français, May 29–June 5, 1904).

[5] This calls into question Daniel Headrick's argument about quinine's crucial role in the conquest of Sub-Saharan Africa in the nineteenth century: Headrick, *Tools of Empire*, 12.

[6] Alphonse Laveran identified Plasmodium Falciparum (or Praecox), which causes a particularly malignant form of malaria, with high rates of complications and death. During the colonial period, three other protozoa causing more benign forms of malaria were identified: Plasmodium Vivax, Plasmodium Malariae, and Plasmodium Ovale. In Vietnam, the Falciparum and Vivax parasites are present.

[7] Although a protozoa is a parasite rather than a virus, this term was commonly used in colonial health reports to denote a population harboring a transmissible disease-causing agent.

Italian, malaria control models for the colonies.[8] In the first years of the twentieth century, investigations of public works sites such as the Nha Trang-Dalat road in Annam and the Yen Bay-Lao Kay railway in Tonkin revealed shocking levels of malaria morbidity among workers.[9] Their conclusions recommended systematic and monitored distributions of quinine, complemented by measures such as: removal of vegetation around camps, limitation of working hours, adequate food rations, water purification, and repatriation of workers presenting anemia. Uncertainty about the effective dosage of quinine, and difficulty mastering seasonal variations in disease prevalence, limited the impact of these measures. The first collective uses of quinine among soldiers encountered similar problems, yet they obtained better results. M. L. R. Montel reported that the daily administration of quinine-fortified wine to a contingent of forty soldiers in Ha Tien Province (Cochinchina), where he was head doctor, brought the number of sick days down from fifty-nine to fourteen per month.[10] In Tonkin, military posts were supplied with malaria tablets from 1908 onward. By 1914, a TC doctor reported a 20 percent drop in malaria morbidity in Tonkin's European soldiers, and a "nearly identical" reduction among its Vietnamese soldiers.[11]

Alongside these interventions on targeted groups, there were attempts to broaden the distribution of preventive quinine in the general population prior to the formal establishment of QE. In a few highly malarial provinces in Tonkin, including Ha Dong, Hai Duong, and Thai Binh, *dépôts de quinine* (quinine outlets) were created to sell the substance at low cost.[12] The success of these initiatives, along with the recent establishment of the AMI, persuaded Tonkin's superior resident that the time was right to begin organizing quinine distribution on a larger scale.[13] In 1909, a Union-wide government service to manage quinine provision was

---

[8] Alexandre Kermorgant and Alphonse Laveran, "Sur les mesures à prendre pour développer dans les colonies françaises l'usage préventif de la quinine contre le paludisme," BSPE 2 (1909): 225–34.

[9] Joseph Vassal, "Géographie médicale de Nha Trang," AHMC, 9 (1906): 481–511; Noël Bernard, "Rapport médical sur l'application du programme d'organisation ouvrière aux chantiers de la ligne de Yen Bay à Lao Kay, Tonkin, 1er octobre 1904–1er octobre 1905," AHMC 10 (1907): 432.

[10] M. L. R. Montel, "Un essai de quinine préventive à Hatien (Cochinchine)," BSPE 3 (1910): 626–28.

[11] Dr. Boyé, "Relations entre la consommation de quinine et la fréquence de la fièvre bilieuse hémoglobinurique au Tonkin," AHMC 17 (1914): 71.

[12] "Gouvernement général de l'Indochine, Direction générale de la santé, Fonction des services de la direction générale de la santé pendant l'année 1907, Hanoi 1er août 1908," ANOM, Gougal 65324.

[13] "Vulgarisation de la quinine, 1908" and "Rapport à M. le Gouverneur général au sujet de l'institution d'un service de quinine d'état," ANOM, Fonds des Amiraux (hereafter Amiraux), Box 189, Folder 2787.

created by a governor general's decree. The QE service was defined as an "enterprise of social prophylaxis"; its mandate was to coordinate, rationalize, and oversee the drug's supply and distribution. Distribution would take place through a network of central and subsidiary outlets, to be managed by intermediaries accredited by the administration and monitored by each Local Directorate of Health. The core objectives of the service were to centralize control over the quality and sales price of QE, which would be set annually, and to facilitate wide and easy access to the drug. Conditions of purchase and use should, it was stated, remain flexible, to avoid all "unnecessary formalities and undue distance." State quinine was to be distributed in zones identified as malarial and used only for malaria prophylaxis, except in cases of major epidemics – only then could it be provided for curative purposes. It was to be free of charge for indigents in these malarial zones. The dispensation of QE was, however, explicitly restricted to the "medicinal dose," defined as the dose to be taken over a period of twenty-four to forty-eight hours.

The parameters set out by this initial decree continued to define the system throughout its existence. The modifications made were minor, despite recurring issues ranging from the difficulty of determining high-priority zones to the challenge of controlling drug quality. The QE system was structured by the cartography of malarial contamination. Its purpose was to prioritize populations most at risk. Vietnam had long been seen as made up of high- and low-risk zones for malaria. From at least the late 1880s, the high river valleys and the Dong Trieu mountain range in Tonkin were considered to be hyperendemic foci. In the North, only the provinces of the Red River Delta were thought to be free of contamination. The incidence of infection in the Annamite Range was estimated to range from 80 to 100 percent. In Cochinchina, the most heavily affected provinces were those of forested areas along the eastern and western borders. In 1907, Paul-Louis Simond, a doctor, medical geographer, Pastorian, and future inspector general of health services, wrote of Indochina as being "divided into two regions of which one is slightly, the other highly, malarial." The first was made up of low-lying and densely populated areas in river and coastal valleys and deltas. The second included all forested areas and uncultivated mountainous zones.[14] There were many further attempts to refine this epidemiological picture. Yet not only is malaria a remarkably complex disease; its distribution in Vietnam was also modulated, inadvertently, by population mobility and economic development. As early as 1904, Dr. Jeanselme remarked that malaria was depopulating "formerly prosperous"

[14] Cited in Monnais-Rousselot, *Médecine et colonisation*, 53.

provinces. In 1930–31, an investigation by the Institut Pasteur of Saigon confirmed that all of Annam's provinces were now contaminated: unevenly, to be sure, but with epidemic outbreaks even in the coastal areas.[15] In comparing Simond's 1907 geography of malaria with another dating from 1937, Annick Guénel found differences that, she argues, cannot be accounted for solely by the use of more sensitive indicators, such as the splenic index used to create the later map. She concludes that this major public health problem was also a dynamic one, representing a significant challenge for health authorities.[16]

A 1912 decree introduced a first classification system for determining which provinces of Tonkin should be prioritized by the QE service. Category A provinces, classified as "highly malarial," were to receive the most abundant and regular, year-round supplies of quinine. The category initially included Son la, Lai Chau, Ha Giang, Hoa Binh, and Tuyen Quang. "Moderately malarial" provinces were listed as Category B: in 1912, they were Lao Kay, Yen Bay, Thai Nguyen, Quang Yen, and Bac Kan. Such categorizations, for Tonkin as well as for other territories, were revised many times. In general, the malarial map was expanded to cover additional provinces. Most often, this reclassification resulted from the efforts of head doctors, who gathered up local epidemiological data and requested a reevaluation of the malarial status of the province they were responsible for. Yet the procedure for such requests was unnecessarily complex, requiring several levels of rubber-stamping prior to submission for final approval. The lack of sensitive tools for measuring malaria prevalence – splenic index examinations were quite easy to conduct but less reliable than indices based on the more costly and tricky detection of parasites in blood by microscopic examination – as well as its complex and moving epidemiology also constrained efforts to accurately map malaria risk. In addition, as several doctors recognized, there were variations in risks of infection even within provinces, which this system was not designed to take into account. Some provinces categorized as high risk contained malaria-free zones and vice versa. These discrepancies between an official cartography of malarial provinces and the realities of disease ecology made the criteria for preferential access to quinine inequitable from the outset.

---

[15] "Rapport au Grand conseil des intérêts économiques et financiers de l'Indochine sur le fonctionnement des services sanitaires et médicaux de l'Indochine, juin 1930 à juin 1931," ANOM, Gougal 47474.

[16] Annick Guénel, "Malaria, Colonial Economics, and Migrations in Vietnam" (paper presented at the Fourth Conference of the European Association of Southeast Asian Studies, Paris, France, September 1–4, 2004). The splenic index is compiled from palpations examinations to detect enlarged spleens, an indicator of malaria infection.

3.2   Distributing QE: From Constraints on Supply to Lazy Distributors

Factors other than classification as a low-prevalence province impeded the reliability, quality, and regularity of the QE supply. As for other public medicines, there were direct and indirect import circuits, as described in Chapter 2. In 1912, when the QE system was set up in Annam, the importation of quinine was managed by a private retail pharmacy on the basis of an agreement with the Local Directorate of Health, which thereby obtained a rate of 192 francs for a thousand tubes of quinine tablets –this was considered to be a very good price. Similarly, in Tonkin, the Hanoi-based pharmacist Édouard Brousmiche imported the drug for AMI authorities in two forms: preconditioned (as tablets) and in bulk (as powder). Over the 1920s and 1930s, an increasingly large share of public quinine stocks was imported in bulk, directly from France.

In their effort to rationalize drug imports, the new Central Supply Pharmacies provided the equipment, personnel, and know-how, such as adding talcum powder to quinine salts, needed to press tablets and package these in tubes of ten.[17] Direct imports and local conditioning capacity provided greater control over the quality, distribution, and price of QE.[18] Still, international production and trade networks for the drug imposed constraints on supply. The Dutch East Indies' monopoly over cinchona, which caused occasional spikes in world prices, hampered the French colonial administration's attempts to reduce quinine's cost. There were, from the 1880s, numerous yet unsuccessful attempts to acclimatize cinchona in Indochina in the hope of bypassing the monopoly of the Amsterdam-based Kina Bureau.

The availability of funds to purchase QE also was very uneven. The 1909 decree placed the financial burden of QE on local budgets. This meant that each province, according to its malarial status, was responsible for allocating a lump sum of its annual budget to the purchase of quinine. In principle, most of this money would be recovered through the sale of QE to those who were not entitled to free quinine. In a few provinces, this system seems to have worked. In Nghe An (Annam), for example, which was served by 20 outlets, the amount allocated to QE jumped from 150 piasters in 1911 (enough for about 1,500 tubes of quinine) to 1,000 the following year. Other provinces struggled to sell the drug in 1912:

---

[17] "Organisation du service de la quinine d'état dans les provinces du Tonkin, 1908–1912," VNA, centre no. 1, Fonds de la Direction locale de la santé (hereafter DLS) 581.

[18] One advantage of this method was to avoid the risk of acquiring an older stock of tablets that might have lost some of their bioactivity over time: Drs. Guillon and Keruzore, "Quelques précisions sur la quinine et ses sels et leur emploi en thérapeutique coloniale," AMPC 24 (1926): 516.

a meagre 1,000 tubes of QE were supplied to Phan Rang's 10 outlets, not one of which, according to the province's head doctor, had managed to sell out its stock. Of the 100,000 tubes sold across the entire protectorate over an 8-month period, 66,000 were purchased in the province of Binh Dinh.[19]

The supply problems that arose with World War I delayed any plan to improve this system: in 1917, only 294 kg of quinine were distributed in Indochina (in comparison with 1,638 in 1921 and more than 3,000 in 1930).[20] In his 1917 health report for Tay Ninh Province, Cochinchina, Dr. Havet was particularly bitter about the disproportion between paltry quantities of quinine (which had just fallen from 7 to 2 kg per year) and a large at-risk population (80,000, all exposed to malaria). He concluded: "One cannot [. . .] compare the means to the ends without being struck by the quasi futility of this enterprise."[21] Because of the war, the QE service simply did not exist before the 1920s in some areas, such as the provinces of Ninh Binh, Vinh Yen, Kien An, and Phuc Yen in Tonkin. On the scale of Vietnam, the size and distribution of the outlet network remained, throughout the 1920s and 1930s, inadequate in relation to the cartography of malaria infection. Furthermore, existing outlets were not always, as Havet pointed out, adequately supplied (sufficiently, and in a timely manner) with quinine by the central depots.[22] This is hardly surprising, given the burdensome procedures for renewing stocks: First, outlet managers were required to transmit to local authorities both a notice that their stocks were sold out and the money collected from quinine sales. Notices then had to make their way up the hierarchy before a new order could be submitted, but only if there was a sufficient sum allocated to QE in the local budget. It is easy to see how this system might create bottlenecks and delays.

Complaints were frequent. For example, in August of 1912, the head doctor of Lai Chau, a Category A province, repeatedly enquired about a quinine order submitted the previous April. He had received only a third of the order (2.5 out of 7.5 kg), and had to borrow another 500 gr from his

---

[19] Dr. Allain, "Paludisme et quinine d'état en Annam pendant l'année 1912: rapports des provinces collationnés," BSPE 6 (1913): 730–44. A significant portion of this QE (46,290 tubes) was sold in the district of Phu My, where an epidemic of malaria had broken out at the time: Dr. A. Bordes, "Les premières recherches sur le paludisme en Indochine," AIPI 12 (1930): 11–12.

[20] Dr. Audibert, "Les maladies endémo-épidémiques observés en Indochine pendant l'année 1921," AMPC 21 (1923): 64; ANOM, Gougal 47474.

[21] Dr. Havet, "Rapport médical concernant la province de Tay Ninh," Bulletin de la Société des études indochinoises (1916–17): 190–91.

[22] In the 1920s, Central Supply Pharmacies served as central outlets, while provincial capital hospitals, under the control of the head doctor or AMI, often served as intermediary outlets.

colleague in Lao Kay before the order was finally completed in late August.[23] When the Customs Agency was put in charge of QE supply in 1922 – an odd decision, which will be further explored later – the system became even more burdensome and arbitrary. AMI doctors openly criticized this transfer of responsibility. Putting orders through the administrative hierarchy, which now involved several ministries, required an extra dose of patience and tenacity. The system clearly ran counter to the principle of flexibility announced by the 1909 decree. Supply was further threatened by the hazards of transportation, especially for getting quinine to remote areas and/or during the rainy summer months, when malaria transmission rates were generally high.[24] In the late 1930s, many provincial health officers still reported failures in the provision of QE to local outlets.

Concerns about the quality and bioactivity of QE also arose. In the 1920s, a few doctors expressed doubts about the distribution of quinine in tablet form, pointing to several studies demonstrating that it was more effective when consumed as dissolved powder. Tropical humidity further affected the solubility of tablets.[25] Quinine sulfate, the cheapest salt, which was widely used at the time, was accused of being less effective and more toxic than the hydrochloride salt. The use of sulfate by the QE service was blamed for cases of severe hemoglobinuric fever (a complication of malaria infection, also known as blackwater fever) and for the failure of malaria control in some regions.[26] Sulfate was only gradually replaced by the hydrochloride salt, which was more soluble, less irritating to the stomach, richer in quinine, and made it easier to prevent toxic side effects. The former was formally banned in the French colonies in 1926. It took more than fifteen years from the creation of the QE service to standardize quinine in content and form, and to thus tighten control over its safety and efficacy. Yet complaints persisted about the quality (and solubility) of tablets in some outlets, suggesting that counterfeit and falsified products also circulated within the system. Such products indicate a popular demand, at least a perceived one, for the drug, yet they

---

[23] VNA, centre no. 1, DLS 581.

[24] "Rapports mensuels et statistiques de l'Assistance médicale de Langson, 1920," VNA, centre no. 1, DLS 379.

[25] M. Blanchard, "Les insuccès de la quinine préventive dus à l'insolubilité des comprimés," BSPE, 15 (1922): 293–95. On the other hand, reports from the mid-1910s contained requests for QE in tablet forms due to the inconvenience and poor quality of liquid and powder forms: Havet, "Rapport médical," 190–91.

[26] Boyé, "Relations"; L. Normet, "Le traitement du paludisme," AMPC, 19 (1921): 202–7; J. Legendre, "A propos de l'efficacité de la quinine préventive," BSPE 18 (1925): 272. Hemoglobinuric fever has since been linked to the inadequate or irregular use of preventive quinine or other antimalarial drug treatment.

could also, if less effective, damage people's trust in QE and confer a lower degree of protection from malaria (see Chapters 5 and 6). Indeed, there are reports of individuals giving up on QE to seek more reliable drugs in private pharmacies.[27]

The outlet system prioritized accessibility, at least in theory, by widening the distribution of QE beyond the network of private pharmacies and health care facilities. From the outset, however, the system was beset by problems, among which was the question of how to identify and recruit outlet managers. The 1909 decree was vague on this issue. In 1910, the governor of Cochinchina proposed that private pharmacists be authorized to dispense QE, allowing them a 5 percent profit margin. AMI authorities then turned their attention to outlet managers, emphasizing these should be competent, honest, diligent, and have the "natives' best interests" at heart. Yet the selection process could be haphazard and indiscriminate. An early plan was to entrust the responsibility of distributing QE mainly to colonial agents such as employees of the postal or customs services and members of the Native Guard. Those authorized as distributors of other state-controlled products such as opium and alcohol were also considered to be reliable candidates. Colonial agents were seen as particularly easy to control and to impose additional tasks upon. Some officials claimed that village-level colonial agents were ideal "ambassadors" of QE because of their proximity to the population, with many working in their village of origin.[28]

With the exception of Native Guard soldiers (who, in the end, had little involvement in QE distribution), all of these categories of agents were, from 1921, under the supervision of the Customs Agency. The agency took over responsibility for the monitoring, resupply, and distribution of stocks, and for the application of set sales prices. However, doubts were soon raised about its capacity to broaden access to the drug, pointing to a drop in the volume of QE distribution following the transfer of responsibility that was blamed in large part on popular mistrust of designated outlet managers.[29] Criticism of QE distributors was also expressed in provincial health reports. Customs agents were accused of being overly rigid, or lazy, and of failing to disseminate information and quinine beyond a restricted circle. Distributors of state-controlled alcohol and opium were said to charge too much for QE, and to refuse coupons for free QE presented by those entitled free health care (which they were under obligation to accept, and then put in a claim for reimbursement

[27] Guillon and Keruzore, "Quelques précisions," 530–31.
[28] Following this logic, local schoolteachers, Vietnamese mandarins, and communal chiefs were sometimes also enlisted to distribute QE.
[29] Audibert, "Les maladies endémo-épidémiques."

from the provincial treasury). Such negligent, greedy, and illegal attitudes, said the head doctor of Binh Dinh, were to blame for the fact
that fourteen of its seventeen outlets had not dispensed a single tube of
quinine over a three-year period.[30]

If distributors did not seem eager to boost the distribution of QE, their
enthusiasm may also have been dampened by the conditions imposed on
them by supply procedures. Although they were granted a 10 percent
profit on quinine sales as an incentive, distributors were sometimes
required by the local administration to pay up front for the renewal of
their drug stock. They rarely, as some distributors stated openly, had
sufficient cash funds to cover even a small supply.[31]

3.3   Quinine Consumption at Any Cost?

While AMI monthly reports contain some statistics on the volumes of QE
sold and provided free of charge, these are not reliable or comprehensive
enough to precisely map out distribution.[32] Furthermore, data on circulation can obviously only be taken as a proxy for the amount of quinine
actually consumed. These figures do, however, suggest significant fluc-
tuations in consumption between provinces as well as over time, with
a substantial but unsurprising dip in 1914–18. A few data sets compiled
from different sources from the 1930s also give a clearer picture of disparities and trends during this period.

From January to June of 1939, the recorded amount of QE distributed
in Tonkin was 69 kg. Of these, nearly 25 kg were sold by customs agents
and nearly 18 kg by other agents. Only 27 kg, less than 40 percent, were
distributed free of charge. In 1930, 80 percent of all QE was provided for
free in Indochina; this proportion was as high as 95 percent in
Cochinchina and as low as 35 percent in Annam.[33] There were also

---

[30] "Rapport annuel sur le fonctionnement de l'Assistance médicale dans la province de Binh
Dinh, 1921," VNA, centre no. 1, IGHSP 34. The 1926 health report for the village of
Song Cau (Phuc Yen) states that some outlets, many of which were managed by persons
of Chinese origin, sold Chinese antimalarial drugs instead of QE (VNA, centre no. 1,
IGHSP 36).

[31] A decree of January 1922 stated that distributors were to be advanced, free of charge, an
initial stock of quinine for which they were accountable. It does not specify how, and by
whom, subsequent stocks would be paid for. Nor can we be sure this measure was
consistently applied.

[32] Research in the archives of the Customs Agency has not located any further statistical
information about QE. Even if complete data series on QE consumption were available,
the work required to link consumption patterns to distribution networks and epidemiological information would be daunting.

[33] Annam was clearly disadvantaged compared with the other territories. In the late 1910s,
only 14 percent of its volume of QE was distributed free of charge, and only in three of its
twelve provinces (ANOM, Gougal 65327, 65328, 65329, and 65330).

wide disparities between provinces. For example, 87 percent of QE was provided for free in Lang Son during the first semester of 1939, while every gram of QE dispensed in Phu Ly was charged for. These interprovincial differences obviously resulted in varying levels of financial accessibility. This likely means that overall consumption rates were also very uneven. For example, according to reports for 1939, 15.6 kg of quinine were consumed in Lao Kay versus 0 kg in Quang Yen, even though both provinces were classified as "moderately malarial." Furthermore, over a six-month period in 1939, some Category A provinces consumed negligible quantities of QE: 1,795 gr in Hoa Binh and only 87 gr in Son La! In such provinces, there was clearly a huge gap between the risk of malaria infection (and perhaps the demand for protection) and the consumption of QE. Yet it is difficult to pinpoint the specific and direct cause(s) of these discrepancies. Was it the result of problems in supply to outlets or in distribution to consumers? Or were clients unable or unwilling to obtain QE due to problems of access, lack of information, or popular mistrust?

As we have seen, very poor individuals residing in provinces classified as malarial qualified for free quinine. Some groups judged to be at high risk also received quinine free of cost, mainly laborers in large-scale public works.[34] All others were required to pay. The sales price of QE was first set at the central level of the Union, in Hanoi, and then adjusted by the representative of the governor general for each territory. Thus prices not only changed over time, but also varied from one colony or protectorate to another. In 1912, the governor general's price was of 0.10 piasters for a tube of ten tablets, each containing a dose of 0.25 gr of quinine. Between 1922 and 1930, the price of a tube remained stable at 0.18 piasters in Cochinchina. Over the same period, in Tonkin, it rose from 0.08 (dropping from 0.10 in 1921) to 0.15 piasters, ending up at the same price as in Annam. These prices, especially in Tonkin, seem relatively low, if somewhat erratic. Yet the quantity of quinine required to comply with the recommended preventive regimen remained unaffordable for a large majority of the population up to the end of the QE service.

The recommended dosage, frequency, and duration of treatment were also readjusted over time, according to official epidemiological parameters for each region.[35] When the QE service was launched, the daily

[34] According to several texts of law, it seems that large private employers had to pay for preventive quinine for their workers, but the QE service could sell them the drug at a preferential rate, while the colonial administration had the right to control the application of prophylactic measures. The impact of this policy was mixed. Records of worksite inspections from the 1930s reveal that quinine prevention was often inadequately applied or not at all.
[35] ANOM, Amiraux, Box 189, Folder 2787.

dose recommended for malaria prevention was the equivalent of two tablets for adults (0.50 to 0.60 gr) and one for children. In Haut-Tonkin (Upper Tonkin), a region of mountains, forests, and low population density, individuals were advised to take this dose for ten days during the first month of their annual treatment, and eight days during the second and third months. Treatment was to be resumed the following year. In the Red River Delta, however, the advice was to take a double dose (four tablets) every second day of the first month, every eighth day of the second and every day of the third. By the 1930s, some malariologists argued that, in high-risk regions, adults should take one gram of quinine (four tablets) every day for at least a month.[36] To follow these instructions, an individual would need to purchase five tubes per year (during the period of treatment) in 1909 and twelve tubes per year in 1930. If a tube cost on average 0.15 piasters, then a month of intensive prophylactic treatment in 1930 would add up to 1.80 piasters per person. For a whole family, the cost could easily reach 10 piasters. This was a significant sum, particularly in rural areas where such amounts were rarely available in cash.[37]

Health officers denounced the high cost of QE on a regular basis. Even high-placed colonial officials complained of high sales prices and overly complicated regulations for QE. In 1924, local director of health in Cochinchina Dr. Lecomte stated that the state service only worked thanks to the "personal initiatives" of administrators and doctors who "dared to modify [its] rules of operation." He pointed to the exemplary case of the province of Baria, where village-level communal budgets subsidized QE to cut its sales price by half.[38] Conversely, around the same time, the entomologist and Pastorian Joseph-Emile Borel and the AMI doctor Pierre Dorolle both observed, in Chau Doc (Cochinchina) and in Ha Giang (Tonkin), respectively, that the unaffordability of QE restricted its impact on the human reservoir for the malaria parasite.[39] Another indicator of financial obstacles to consumption was the reported inability of outlets to sell off their stocks. The outlet in Lang Son, a province classified as moderately malarial, managed to sell only 170 gr of its rather substantial stock of 5.2 kg in 1921, a problem that persisted for at least five

[36] Émile Farinaud, C. Toumanoff, and Hoàng Thuy Ba, "Le paludisme à Tuyen Quang. Enquête malariologique," BSMI 10, 1 (1932): 66–128.

[37] At this time, the average annual tax burden for a peasant family of five was evaluated to fall between 25 and 30 piasters. This represented between 15 and 30 percent of the household income (Brocheux and Hémery, Indochine, 96–97, 257–60).

[38] Lecomte, "L'Assistance médicale," 137.

[39] M. Borel, "Anophèles et paludisme dans la région de Chaudoc (Cochinchine). Résultats d'une enquête faite du 16 au 21 janvier 1926," BSPE 19 (1926): 806; Dr. Pierre Dorolle, "Le paludisme à Ha Giang (Tonkin)," BSPE 20 (1927): 921.

years.[40] In 1926, Song Cau's head doctor reported that a rise in the price of QE – for reasons he does not specify – made it unaffordable even for those who had previously purchased it regularly.[41]

The lack of clear information about QE, which was often confusing and/or poorly disseminated, was another obstacle to widespread and effective prophylactic consumption. AMI authorities insisted from the outset that persuasion, rather than compulsion, be used.[42] Informing the population about the virtues of prophylactic quinine was thus essential to the success of the service. Furthermore, because most QE was distributed by nonprofessionals, it was mainly used without direct medical supervision. In the service's early years, tubes of QE were distributed with an instructional leaflet, written in both quốc ngữ and Chinese characters.[43] In parallel, advertising was used to relay messages about the benefits of quinine, as well as information about where to obtain it and how to use it properly. Posters and placards were displayed near sites of sale; pamphlets were distributed in busy public places. The following is an example of a publicity text from 1912:

Message to quinine buyers. Quinine is the best medicine we have for fever. The government provides this medicine to the population at the lowest possible price. It will be sold in tubes of 10 tablets; each tube will cost 10 cents.

Those who want to cure a fever must take the medicine in the following way:
For 4 days, 2 tablets each day; for 3 days, no quinine.
For 4 days, 2 tablets each day; for 3 days, no quinine.
For 4 days, 1 tablet each day.
For children, give only one tablet per day.

The medicine will work better if, to swallow it, it is crushed and dissolved in one cai-chen of tea. The fever will not go away in a single day; one must take the quinine for a long time[44]

What is striking about this text, besides its didactic tone, is that its instructions are for treating fever rather than for preventing malaria. This was likely an attempt to make quinine more attractive. Commenting on the text, Dr. Hermant recommended that the population be gradually persuaded to accept quinine prophylaxis, a goal that justified lowering

[40] VNA, centre no. 1, DLS 380.
[41] "Rapports mensuels et statistiques de l'Assistance médicale de Langson, 1926," VNA, centre no. 1, DLS 385.
[42] Most instances of compulsory prophylaxy I found were in worker communities or during epidemic outbreaks. Private company doctors usually ensured that workers took the drug, some going as far as to analyze workers' urine to ensure the presence of quinine: "Les coolies et leur médecine," *La tribune indochinoise*, no. 176, October 14, 1927.
[43] VNA, centre no. 1, DLS 581.
[44] Dr. Hermant, "A propos d'une note récente sur la quinine d'état," BSMI 3, 6 (1912): 344.

doses, at least temporarily, below those official prescribed.[45] There were other attempts to market QE. For example, in 1931, at the request of the Instituts Pasteur d'Indochine, "a color poster, a product of the talent of Mr. Pia, professor of drawing at the Lycée of Saigon, was printed and widely disseminated. It shows a coolie who, having failed to take quinine, is obviously ill and cannot [bring himself to] touch the food that is being eaten, visibly with the greatest pleasure, by his companions who, the legend in quốc ngữ tells us, have taken their preventive quinine" (Figure 3.1).[46]

Outlet managers, however, were frequently criticized for the lack of effort they put into promoting QE. Evoking the inadequacy, and some-times the absence, of their efforts, some of Cochinchina's elected colonial counselors[47] signed an open letter in the newspaper *L'Écho annamite* (hereafter *L'Écho*) in September 1927, in which they demanded "that the sale [. . .] of QE tablets [. . .] be entrusted to teachers or retail merchants [. . .]; that the dissemination of advice on antimalarial prophy-laxis be intensified by conferences given by auxiliary doctors, by messages in quốc ngữ posted in schools, in public buildings and in markets."[48] The governor released a statement in which he promised to make improve-ments, but there is no record of the implementation of concrete measures.[49]

3.4   The Limits of Mass Quininization as Malaria Control

As knowledge of the etiology and epidemiology of malaria grew, doubts arose as to whether mass drug prophylaxis alone, or even with supportive measures, could have a significant impact on disease prevalence. By 1936, twenty-seven years after the State Quinine Service was created, malaria remained the most frequently reported cause of consultation in the AMI, accounting for 15 percent of all hospital admissions (52,196 cases) in Indochina. Many more were probably admitted for other reasons, but were also infected with malaria, while others did not come to hospital at all. It accounted for a stable proportion, 10 to 13 percent, of the total mortality rate.[50] A few surveys of malaria-carrying mosquitoes and of splenic

---

[45] Hermant, "A propos d'une note récente," 345.
[46] H. G. S. Morin and L. Bordes, "Développement de la lutte anti-malarienne en Indochine," AIPI 12 (1931): 81.
[47] The Conseil colonial (Colonial Council) in Cochinchina was an elected assembly of French representatives who participated in the management of the colony from 1880.
[48] "Contre le paludisme," *L'Écho*, no. 983, September 23, 1927.
[49] "Pour la santé publique en Cochinchine. Distribution de la quinine d'état," *L'Écho*, no. 1360, January 3, 1929.
[50] Monnais-Rousselot, *Médecine et colonisation*, 389.

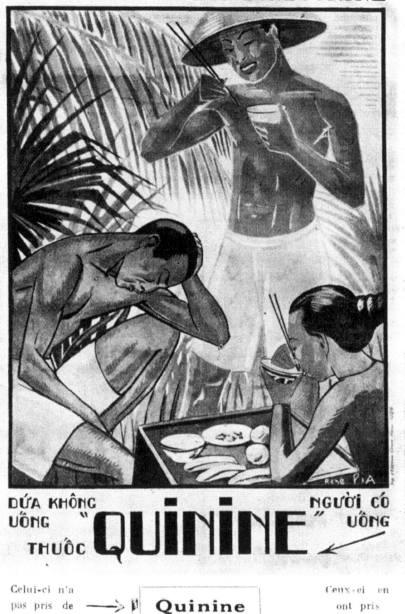

Figure 3.1 Poster Promoting Quinine Consumption, 1931 (reproduced in Henri G. S. Morin, *Entretiens sur le paludisme et sa prévention en Indochine* [Hanoi: Imprimerie d'Extrême-Orient [IDEO], 1935])

indices conducted in the 1920s and 1930s suggested that malaria prevalence was, at least in some areas, much higher than health care facilities' data suggest. Blood tests conducted in South Annam and Cochinchina under Dr. Borel's supervision in 1926 showed that 50 to 70 percent of some populations carried the parasite, while in the fertile Terres Rouges (Red Lands) region, where intensive land-clearing and agricultural colonization campaigns were carried out in the 1930s, malaria was reported to be the top cause of infant mortality and was even accused of lowering birth rates.[51] Only a handful of provinces reported reductions in malaria prevalence, such as Can Tho, Bac Lieu (Cochinchina), and Nghe An (Annam). These were exceptions.[52]

Several experts, especially Pastorians, warned that it would be impossible to bring prevalence rates down without a significant investment in vector control measures. Such warnings were voiced especially when malaria posed a threat to a region's economic development, or when intensified economic activity caused ecological disruption resulting in the proliferation of mosquitoes. Increased mobility, particularly the migration of workers (moving, with no immunity, from low to high risk areas or in the other direction, carrying the parasite back home) modulated the cartography of malaria endemicity. The colonial administration lacked the means to gain control over what the Pastorian Léon Bordes called, in 1931, "a generalized experience of transmission."[53] This implied not only that mapping the distribution of the parasite requires massive screening of spleens and blood samples, but also that any form of effective action would necessitate the wide implementation of a multipronged strategy across the entire Union.

Yet measures such as larval control by drying or filling bodies of water or the generalization of screened or glass windows to protect against mosquito bites were seen as expensive and unfeasible. Such broad-based strategies were only implemented in delimited places and populations where there was much to be gained, such as large rubber plantations.[54] On the basis of a formal agreement made in 1923 between the governor general and the Instituts Pasteur d'Indochine, malaria research was entrusted to a team of Pastorians. At the plantation of Suzannah An Loc (Cochinchina), for example, they tested a multipronged attack on malaria that included biological and chemical

[51] M. Borel, "Résultats d'une enquête épidémiologique à Yaback (Annam)," BSPE 19 (1926): 845–52.
[52] Guénel, "Malaria, Colonial Economics."
[53] Exposition coloniale internationale, Paris, Louis A. Bordes, Le paludisme en Indochine (Hanoi: IDEO, 1931), 14.
[54] ANOM, Fonds de la Commission Guernut (hereafter CG), Box 22, Folder Bb.

larval control as well as comprehensive drug treatment and prevention. This resulted in a 50 percent drop in parasite prevalence in children.[55] In 1938, Pierre Hermant, the inspector general of health services who had earlier overseen mass quinine prevention in Annam, called this strategy a "solution for the wealthy."

French colonial authorities' emphasis on quinine prophylaxis, despite its problems, may have inhibited efforts to develop alternative control measures, and thereby contributed to a neglect of socioeconomic factors in malaria epidemiology. Historian Randall Packard explains this neglect, which was common in many tropical countries, as a product of the predominance, until the 1950s, of a biomedical approach to the disease that focused on the parasite or the vector.[56] Yet Indochina did lag behind some of its neighbors, such as British Malaya and the Dutch East Indies, with respect to the development of broader-based strategies of malaria control.[57] And, as we have seen, the Indochinese administration failed even to generalize access to quinine prophylaxis. According to an investigation mandated by the League of Nations in 1932, Indochina's estimated prevalence rate would have required the consumption of at least thirty tons of quinine per year – ten times the amount it reportedly consumed at the time.[58] The introduction of synthetic antimalarial drugs in the 1930s kindled hope for more effective and accessible drug-based prophylaxis. Yet if the new drugs opened the possibility of alternative supply circuits, they were, at first, no cheaper than quinine, nor was their therapeutic action any more specific or more versatile.

Some synthetic drugs, like quinine, acted only on the schizont phase of the parasite's life cycle, as was the case of quinacrine (mepacrine), commercialized as Atabrine (IG Farben). Others, such as praequine (branded Plasmochine by Bayer) and Rhodoquine Rhône-Poulenc, destroyed the Plasmodium only in its gamete phase, and thus had only a curative effect. Because of this, these drugs were often combined with quinine; in addition, they required a lengthy therapeutic regimen that was potentially

[55] M. Borel, "Paludisme en Cochinchine. Résultats de mesures prophylactiques à la plantation de Suzannah (11 au 13 août 1926)," BSPE 19 (1926): 811–15.

[56] Randall Packard, *The Making of a Tropical Disease: A Short History of Malaria* (Baltimore: Johns Hopkins University, 2007), 7–8, 102, 113.

[57] Annick Guénel, "Malaria Control, Land Occupation, and Scientific Developments in Vietnam in the twentieth Century" (paper presented at the Fifty-First Annual Meeting of the Association for Asian Studies, Boston, March 11–14, 1999); Pierre Hermant, "La lutte contre le paludisme dans les États malais fédérés," *La Presse médicale*, no. 84, October 18, 1930.

[58] Société des nations (SDN), *Enquête sur les besoins en quinine des pays impaludés et sur l'extension du paludisme dans le monde* (Genève: SDN, 1932).

toxic.[59] In Vietnam, trials were conducted in circumscribed populations that could be monitored closely – for example, in work and military camps or in agricultural and penal colonies. Some obtained spectacular results. For example, the distribution of quinacrine over a six-month period to the prisoner population of Poulo Condore in 1937 was reported to have reduced cases of malarial fever twenty-five-fold to thirtyfold relative to the previous year, thus preventing the loss of 7,231 work days. While the Institut Pasteur's Malaria Control Service in Saigon obtained excellent results from the systematic treatment of mountain-dwelling communities in late 1935, it concluded that synthetic drugs were no better than quinine for preventive treatment.[60]

Drug combinations were tried out with the aim of improving efficacy and safety. Rhône-Poulenc's combination drug Prémaline (Plasmochine, quinacrine, and Rhodoquine), introduced to the French market in 1934 and to Vietnam three years later, was the first to really compete with quinine. Although it was only distributed to targeted populations and sold at a high price to private companies by the administration,[61] there were hopes that its use would be broadened to a large scale. In late 1938, the local director of health for Tonkin, Dr. de Raymond, initiated an experimental protocol in a group of 2,500 soldiers of the Native Guard and 3,000 civilians, including civil servants, prisoners, colonists, and students. A significant advantage of the recommended treatment was that it cost 15 percent less than quinine. Its therapeutic results, however, were inconclusive.[62]

Further research was stalled by the outbreak of World War II, and postponed the possibility of adopting synthetic antimalarial drugs for use in systems of mass distribution, even though their production was stepped up in response to the Japanese takeover of cinchona plantations in the Dutch East Indies. For AMI authorities, synthetic antimalarial drugs were still to be seen as experimental drugs. This was corroborated by

[59] "Plasmochine et 'composés' dans le traitement de la malaria par M. Freiman," *Journal of Tropical Medicine and Hygiene* (June 1929), cited in AMPC 27 (1929): 477–78.
[60] Drs. Émile Farinaud and P. Moreau, "La prophylaxie du paludisme par médicaments synthétiques en Indochine. Expériences en zone hyperendémique," BSPE 39 (1937): 2908–15.
[61] "Assistance médicale. Divers" and "Lettre du Directeur local de la santé aux médecins de l'AMI, Hanoi, 22 novembre 1937," ANOM, RST NF 3710; "Cession de Prémaline aux émigrants de Nam Dinh venant s'installer à Yenbay, 1938," and "Cession de Prémaline aux exploitations agricoles, 1938," ANOM, RST NF 3783.
[62] "Lettre du Directeur local de la santé du Tonkin concernant un essai de prophylaxie par la Prémaline, 1938, 16 novembre 1938," ANOM, RST NF 3829; J. Genevray, C. Toumanoff, and Hoàng Tich Tri, "Essai de prophylaxie du paludisme par la Prémaline dans une localité du Tonkin et son effet sur le degré d'infection naturelle du vecteur majeur," RMFEO 17 (1939): 397.

the Malaria Commission of the League of Nations, which continued to assert that "quinine remain[ed] the first choice [of treatment], given its clinical efficacy and lack of toxicity, but also widespread knowledge of its use and posology."[63] By 1941, there were severe constraints on the supply of QE, and by 1942, synthetic antimalarial drugs were no longer available in the region.[64] Ultimately, the QE system probably had a negligible impact on malaria prevalence in Vietnam. The failure of this pseudo-public system also suggests that controlling malaria in the general population, beyond the communities directly involved in colonial military or economic enterprises, was never a real priority for the French colonial state.

3.5   The Prehistory of Essential Medicines

Reorientations in the AMI system in the early 1920s brought greater, if belated, attention to medicines as potentially valuable weapons on the frontlines of colonial medicalization. A sharpened focus on urban-rural disparities led to efforts to increase the accessibility of health care via the distribution of medicines. However, only a limited number of innocuous drugs were targeted by these measures. These viewed as stopgaps – that is, as a form of minimal care that might be extended toward people and places not yet reached by the health care system.

According to the regulations of the AMI and, more generally, on medical prescriptions, AMI facilities not staffed by a doctor were held to a distinct drug nomenclature that excluded any medicine containing substances defined as toxic by law. Thus the majority of small rural health posts and infirmaries, most of which were headed by a nurse or midwife, could not dispense the new, highly active synthetic antimicrobials. Given these legal restrictions and, above all, the AMI's resource limitations, one solution that was attempted was to make a substantial investment in health care professionals' mobility. Medical mobility was key from as early as the 1870s, when the first smallpox vaccination campaigns were organized. Yet, as we saw in Chapter 2, many doctors protested the official 1907 proposal for medical tours meant to ensure a minimal medical presence at the village level. The principle of the tour system was to "put the AMI within the reach of all natives" by dedicating a time and space in each village for a doctor to hold consultations, "open to all, with

---

[63] E. Sergent, G. Balfour, O. Pittaluga, and J. Sinto, "Étude de la thérapeutique et de la prophylaxie du paludisme par les médicaments synthétiques comparés à la quinine. Rapport général de la commission du paludisme de la SDN," BSMI 14, 4 (1938): 458.

[64] "Lettre du Directeur local de la santé au Résident supérieur du Tonkin, Hanoi, 19 janvier 1943," ANOM, RST NF 3783.

no administrative formalities," every thirty to forty days. This directive gave local authorities much latitude in organizing the service, while its implementation depended on individual doctors – that is, on the time and means at their disposal,[65] but also on their motivation and vision of what counted as "good medicalization."

While this system was therefore implemented unevenly, it foreshadowed another initiative for a *medicine of proximity*. During the course of medical tours, some doctors began placing stocks of medicines in villages they visited regularly to avoid the burden of transporting them. By 1914, Dr. Constant Mathis, head doctor of Cao Bang, had placed nine fixed crates of medicines around the province. They contained remedies for common symptoms, infections, and fevers: quinine sulfate, sodium sulfate, bismuth subnitrate, iodine tincture, santonin, ipeca pills, as well as some eye drops and morphine solution. Mathis inspected them, he reported, at six-month intervals, obtaining new supplies from the Local Directorate of Health or, in urgent cases, from the closest public facility or pharmacy.[66] During his absence, the AMI doctor put local notables in charge of dispensing emergency medicines. Elsewhere, similar stocks were supervised by militiamen or forestry agents.[67] In 1915, the head doctor of Binh Dinh praised such "emergency stocks" for allowing him, "while chatting about hygiene advice, to extract a tooth [. . .], to rid others of the parasites that torment them, [. . .] to [inject] morphine to someone who suffers from atrocious pains, in sum to show them how we take pains to provide care in order to attract their attention."[68] These localized initiatives aroused the interest of health authorities. An early plan was to dispatch "mobile health teams" to diagnose and prevent diseases, particularly conditions defined as social such as trachoma. They would also distribute medicines. While in Tonkin a team was created for each province, Annam and Cochinchina each obtained only three teams. Furthermore, these operated erratically. By the late 1930s, they seem to have disappeared entirely.[69]

Another strategy was to spread stocks of essential medicines across the countryside.[70] The 1919 decree on pharmacy and toxic substances

---

[65] Vinh Yen's provincial medical officer, for example, had access to a motorized vehicle beginning in 1913 (ANOM, RST NF 4014).

[66] Constant Mathis, "L'helminthiase, le goitre, la lèpre dans la Haute région du Tonkin (Langson-Caobang)," AHMC 17 (1914): 204.

[67] ANOM, Gougal 65324.

[68] ANOM, RST NF 4003.

[69] "Rapport au Grand conseil des intérêts économiques et financiers de l'Indochine sur le fonctionnement des services de l'hygiène et de la santé publique de l'Indochine, de juin 1937 à juin 1938," ANOM, nouveau fonds Indochine (hereafter NF Indo), Box 410, Folder 3569.

[70] It is interesting to note that the term "essential medicine" was in use in the 1920s. While its definition differed from the one given by the WHO in 1977 ("of utmost importance,

introduced the term *dépôts de remèdes officinaux* (officinal remedy outlets). These were peripheral stores authorized to sell, but not to prepare or package, "officinal remedies and simple, nontoxic drugs" in localities situated at least ten kilometers from the nearest pharmacy. This outlet system was formalized in April 1920 by decree of the governor general. The decree reiterated the conditions stated in 1919: minimal distance, no pharmaceutical manipulations, and no sale of toxic substances. It specified that outlets could not be located within a shop that also sold "any medicine from the traditional Sino-Annamese pharmacopoeia, any food, any beverage." It also described those who might be authorized to create and manage these outlets as "diploma-holding indigenous doctors and pharmacists [. . .] not employed by the administration," or individuals, French, Vietnamese, or other, having "successfully passed a probationary examination" and obtained "a certificate of aptitude to manage a pharmacy depot." Every new outlet and outlet manager had to be authorized by the local administration with the approval of the Directeur local de la santé. These outlets were also subject to the same inspection rules imposed on pharmacies since 1908.[71]

The original 1920 list of essential medicines tells us that about forty-five substances and preparations were authorized for sale in these dépôts (Table 3.1). For the most part, these were medicines indicated for symptomatic relief (pain, coughing, fever, diarrhea, and constipation), the treatment of common infections (notably of the skin and eyes), and the disinfection of minor wounds. The large majority were not considered to be specific curative drugs. Rather, they were intended for use as symptomatic treatment, or as adjuvant therapies for diseases such as malaria, dysentery, syphilis, gonorrhea, and even tuberculosis. Many, such as Antipyrin, quinine, or potassium iodide, had multiple indications, qualifying, if not quite as panaceas, as highly versatile remedies. Although this list was revised on several occasions, the changes made were minor.[72]

By 1934, thirty-nine of these essential medicines outlets existed in Tonkin; a year later there were forty-four. They were unevenly spread across its territory: five in some provinces (Phu Tho, Ninh Binh, and Thai Binh) to one in others (Ninh Giang, Phu Ly, Hon Gay, Sept Pagodes,

basic, indispensable, and necessary for the healthcare needs of the population": http://apps.who.int/iris/bitstream/handle/10665/153132/WHA32_10_eng.pdf;jsessionid=F0C288ECE791E6357DB4A797941AFC31?sequence=1), initiatives aiming to expand access to basic drugs in the interwar period are indicative of the new roles and meanings given to medicines in the improvement of human health.

[71] "Au sujet de la constitution à Diên Bien Phu d'un dépôt de médicaments les plus usuels, 1920," VNA, centre no. 1, RST 20744.

[72] For example, santonin would replace semen-contra powder, a substitution enabled by its shift from schedule A to schedule C drugs in April 1921.

Table 3.1 *Medicines Authorized for Distribution in Officinal Remedy Outlets, 1920*

Properties	Product	Main Therapeutic Indications
Antiseptic/ Antibacterial/ disinfectant	Boric acid	Ear, nose, and throat infections
	Bismuth nitrate	Dressing of wounds
	Potassium chloride	Various indications
	Copper sulfate	Inflammations of the mouth and gums Various dermatological conditions
	Zinc sulfate (eye drops)	Eye conditions (conjunctivitis)
	Cresyl	Disinfection of buildings
	Dermatol	Dressing of wounds and burns
	Iodoform	Dressing of wounds, venereal diseases
	Potassium iodide	Syphilis, asthma (and leprosy)
	Potassium permanganate	Gonorrhea, disinfection of hands and water
	Quinine (salts)	Malaria
	Sulfur	Disinfection
Parasiticide	Crysophanol	Skin conditions (eczema, psoriasis, herpes)
	Helmerich's ointment	Scabies
Anthelmintic	Semen contra powder	Ascaris lumbricoides (giant roundworm), Enterobius vermicularis (pinworm)
Sedative	Camphor spirit	Neuralgia, bruises, rheumatic pain
Analgesic	Antipyrin	Various painful symptoms
	Chloroform water	Stomach pains
	Pyramidon	Nevralgia (facial nerve pain), migraine, tabetic ocular crises, neuritis
	Quinine (various salts)	Pneumonia, flu, whooping cough
Cholagogue	Sodium bicarbonate	Digestive problems
Astringent	Zinc sulfate (eye drops)	Conjunctivitis
	Copper sulfate (eye drops)	Trachoma
Revulsive	Mustard seed powder	Painful symptoms (nevralgia), states of inflammation (pulmonary congestion, acute bronchitis)
Resolutive	Iodotannic liquor	Engorgement, chronic inflammation of bones, joints or skin, bronchitis (brushed on skin)
Stimulant	Camphorated oil	Antispasmodic, pneumonia, acute lung edema, cardiovascular collapse, asthenia
	Cod liver oil	Appetite stimulant
Tonic	Powder/tincture/wine of cinchona	Infectious fevers, wasting afflictions (tuberculosis, diabetes), recovery from serious and infectious diseases; cases of anemia, paleness, and weakness; adjuvant to quinine for the treatment of febrile convulsions
	Rhubarb	Lack of appetite, gastrointestinal atonia

Table 3.1 *(cont.)*

Properties	Product	Main Therapeutic Indications
Substances altering bronchial secretions	Expectorant syrups	Coughing
	Syrup of tolu	Chronic bronchitis
Purgative/ laxative/ diuretic	Castor oil	Constipation, diarrhea, gastric discomfort
	Linseed meal	Various
	Lactose	Various
	Rhubarb	Various
	Magnesium sulfate	Gastric discomfort, febrile conditions, dysentery
	Sodium sulfate	Idem
Siccative (moisture absorbents)	Zinc oxide (ointment)	Skin conditions (impetigo, eczema, pruritis), chapped and scratched skin
	Talcum powder	Perspiration and weeping skin
Softener	Regular/borated vaseline	Sunburns, burns, wounds
Multiple uses	Alun crystals	Sore throat (pharyngitis or amygdalate), to stop minor hemorrhaging (nose bleed), dysentery, gonorrhea
	Officinal ether (diethyl ether)	Analgesic (topical), local and general anesthetic, antispasmodic, sedative
	Ipeca powder	Emetic, tonic (digestive), dysentery
	Tincture of iodine	Antiseptic (various uses), engorgement, inflammation

Tuyen Quang, and Vinh Yen). In between, some provinces had three (Cao Bang, Ha Dong, Lao Kay, and Mon Cay) or two (Bac Giang, Hung Yen, and Thai Nguyen) outlets.[73] One can guess, if not say for sure, that provinces with more outlets were seen as offering a better market for medicines because they were more densely populated and/or because they lacked professional retail pharmacies and AMI facilities. Provinces that bordered China, or had a strong military presence, also had more outlets. Outlet networks in other territories cannot be mapped out due to lack of data. The persistence of propharmacy, which remained legal in Vietnam until the end of colonial rule, is a sign that this network was not extensive enough to provide universal access to basic medicines even by 1940.[74]

[73] "Direction locale de la santé, rapport sanitaire annuel, 1934," ANOM, RST NF 3684.
[74] One archival file (ANOM, Fonds des affaires politiques [hereafter Aff Po] 3242) reveals that the list of these outlets was among the documents that vanished from the IGHSP archives during World War II. One can suggest, though, that some of these outlets were

It seems to have been difficult to attract health care professionals to the task of managing these outlets. I found a single mention of a Vietnamese auxiliary pharmacist, by the name of Trần Văn Bình, taking up the role of manager, in Tonkin in 1935.[75] Most were managed by laypersons who were required to submit a certificate of good conduct and a criminal record check to qualify for eligibility; they then had to pass an aptitude test and complete a training course in which they were taught to dispense "emergency medicines."[76] Not all distributors went through all of these steps, however, which may indicate a scarcity of candidates. Some were approved on the basis of their status, as local dignitaries, for example, and underwent only minimal training at the nearest provincial hospital. Others were already authorized as distributors of QE.[77] Of the thirty-nine persons listed in 1934 as managers in Tonkin, thirty-seven had names of Vietnamese or Chinese origin (the remaining two names were French sounding, but may have been Franco-Vietnamese métis).[78]

Although it was prohibited to hold dual posts as outlet manager and civil servant, distributors could, and many probably did, engage in other professional activities, especially commerce. For example, Mr. Beauvoir explained in his request for an aptitude test in 1924 that he ran a small shop in Nam Dinh City and wanted to sell medicines alongside other common consumer goods in order to please his customers, who, he specified, were both European and Asian.[79] Outlets that were not integrated into existing shops were placed in public buildings, usually in the đình, the village communal house, which had both religious and secular functions. A decade later, two Vietnamese men of Chinese origin, Alim and Macca, who were already authorized to sell state opium and Sino-Vietnamese remedies, obtained a license to sell

displaced from the late 1920s by private pharmacies managed by Vietnamese pharmacists (as discussed further in Chapter 4).
[75] ANOM, RST NF 3685.
[76] "Examen pour la tenue des dépôts de remèdes officinaux et drogues simples, 1929," VNA, centre no. 1, Fonds de la mairie de Hanoi, 7831. In 1944, the examination included a written test, including French spelling and an arithmetic problem; an oral test on toxic doses and the use of medicines authorized for sale by the outlets; and a practical test on the identification of some of these medicines ("Avis d'examen," L'Écho, no. 15, June 8, 1944).
[77] "Lettre du lieutenant-colonel commandant du 2ᵉ territoire militaire (Lu Py) au médecin-capitaine chargé des service extérieurs à Cao Bang, Cao Bang, 11 octobre 1938," ANOM, RST NF 3719.
[78] ANOM, RST NF 3684.
[79] "Demande formulée par Beauvoir en vue d'être autorisé à vendre des médicaments à Nam Dinh, 1924," VNA, centre no. 1, RST 48323.

colonial medicines in the frontier town and military garrison of Sapa (or Chapa, Lao Kay) – the initial law forbidding this combination had been altered in 1927.[80]

By the late 1930s, several vaguely defined categories of outlets coexisted: *dépôts de médicaments non-toxiques* (outlets of nontoxic medicines), *dépôts ruraux de médicaments* (rural medicines outlets), *dépôts de pharmacie ruraux réduits* (reduced rural pharmacy outlets), and *dépôts de spécialités* (specialty outlets). The list of drugs authorized for sale in these outlets seems to have varied according to their distance from the nearest pharmacy; however, there is a lack of clear information about this. Analgesics, digestive aids, tonics (such as iron-based preparations and cinchona wines), and purgatives (such as magnesium sulfate) were nevertheless listed among the "most common" products in "facilities without doctors" in 1940.[81] But unlike public pharmacies and, to some extent, QE outlets, these outlets did not dispense free medicines, and thus did not comply with AMI regulations on access to free care. They did, however, sell their products very cheaply, usually by the unit or the dose. A tablet of Antipyrin cost, on average, from 0.10 to 0.20 piasters; it was a few cents more for copper sulfate eye drops. One might wonder how they were able to maintain such low prices, regardless of whether they were supplied by public hospitals or private pharmacies (both were probably common), and whether they made any profit. One possibility is that very low prices were displayed to attract customers, but higher prices were often charged. Another is that, in the case of "mixed" businesses, profit was made on other products. A third is that these nominally public drug outlets were appropriated by urban private pharmacies to create publicity and liquidate stocks (see Chapter 4).

What is clearest and most important here is that these dépôts operated on the margins of the public health care system and, as with QE, largely beyond medical supervision – which is, in a way, indirectly illustrated by the lack of official sources on how they were run. There is also evidence that, from 1921, most essential medicines distributors had to obtain their own drug supplies and increasingly did so through private retail pharmacies. This abandonment of outlets by the AMI can be taken as an additional sign of the low priority of both medicines and rural health in the colonial medicalization project.

[80] ANOM, RST NF 3684.
[81] Dr. Henry Angier, *Guide médical. Formulaire pratique de thérapeutique et de pharmacie à l'usage des postes dépourvus de médecin*, 6th ed. (Saigon: Portail, 1940).

3.6   When There Is No Doctor (or Pharmacist)

It should be clear by now that contrasting regimes of pharmaceuticals and public health care were created in colonial Vietnam: an urban and a rural one. The cases of QE and essential medicines highlight the failure of specific initiatives to democratize access to medicines. The vast majority of the Vietnamese population still could not obtain, at least not close by or for free, drugs that were, in the interwar period, identified as the only truly effective disease therapies. To end this chapter, I take a step back to examine the broader underlying synergy of human, material, and legal constraints on the availability of public medicines, and to describe their combined impact for potential consumers. The infrastructural gaps as well as the recurring staff and material shortages faced by the AMI form the first axis of a systemic set of constraints on drug accessibility. These interacted with a second axis: a legal framework for the circulation and distribution of medicines that, paradoxically, became increasingly strict just as new plans emerged to expand access to primary health care. As objects of historical inquiry, colonial medicines illuminate these disparities with particular clarity, opening an analysis of the realities and consequences of inequalities in public as well as biomedical care.

The most obvious gap in the provision of AMI care was at the level of its clinical infrastructure. By the turn of the 1920s, Vietnam's public health care facilities were undeniably clustered around cities and in densely populated provinces. Most of Tonkin's hospitals were in and around Hanoi, with about fifty facilities (general and maternity hospitals, and infirmaries) located within its perimeter. The majority of Annam's facilities were small health posts and dispensaries, and were either lined up along the coast or served provincial capitals; there was little penetration of the hinterland. In Cochinchina, the axis formed by road and river routes connecting Saigon–Ben Tre–My Tho–Sa Dec–Long Xuyen–Chau Doc was particularly well-served by about sixty facilities. Further from the Mekong, toward the Cambodian border, the network became sparse.[82] There were disparities both between and within provinces.

In the conclusion of an investigation conducted in Ha Dong in 1926, Henri Marcel, the Vietnamese (or perhaps métis?) head doctor of the province, strongly criticized the growing gap in services between the capital and other areas. Although it was one of the most densely populated provinces in Vietnam, there were only three maternity hospitals and a handful of medicines outlets.[83] In the late 1920s, Dr. Lavau pointed out

[82] Monnais-Rousselot, *Médecine et colonisation*, 116–21, 207–21.
[83] Henri Marcel, "L'hygiène publique dans une province du Tonkin (Ha Dong)," BSMI 4, 2 (1926): 40–57.

that the average AMI facility served a restricted perimeter. Using outpatient consultation figures from Sa Dec (Cochinchina) covering a one-month period, he calculated that 1,109 of 1,442 patients (nearly 77 percent) resided within a five-kilometer radius: this was what he called the facility's "zone of influence." Lavau thus calculated that only 3.6 percent of the population within this perimeter (a total of 30,650) was receiving care.[84] In 1932, Dr. Chesneau made a similar estimate for Thanh Hoa (Annam), and concluded that rural infirmaries had an "attraction perimeter" of no more than ten kilometers.

All three of these doctors emphasized the need for mobile health teams and for distribution of medicines in rural areas, in addition to efforts to create more facilities. Despite a clear increase in the number of infirmaries and rural consultation services in the 1930s, these remained strikingly unevenly distributed and resourced.[85] In 1936, Tonkin, with nearly 300 facilities, of which 250 were dispensaries and small consultation centers, was the best-equipped territory of the Union. Cochinchina had almost 200 facilities, of which 110 were dispensaries, 20 were rural infirmaries, and 35 were stand-alone maternity hospitals. Annam, however, relied on only 160 facilities; 110 of these were small infirmaries, and very few were maternity hospitals and dispensaries. To palliate Annam's infrastructural gaps, the program of Assistance rurale was launched in 1937 under the direction of the colonial doctors Terrisse and Chesneau. Seen as highly innovative, this program divided the territory into twenty-two decentralized sectors of rural health care. By late 1938, however, only three such sectors were functional.[86] Many Vietnamese, in Annam as well as in Tonkin, thus fell into the vast gaps of this infrastructural network; they were visited only erratically, if at all, by mobile medical personnel. The closest medicines outlet could very well be several kilometers away, and the pharmacy even further. In 1933, for example, the residents of La Xa (Hai Duong) petitioned the superior resident of Tonkin to maintain their village outlet, even though a new pharmacy had opened seven kilometers away, in the provincial capital.[87]

Health care facilities were, on the whole, inadequately maintained and supplied with equipment, medicines, and staff. Small rural facilities were especially thinly stretched. Year after year, head doctors of provinces

---

[84] Dr. Lavau, "La zone d'action d'un hôpital d'Assistance," BSMI, 5 (1928): 235–58.

[85] "Assistance médicale en Annam. Autorisation d'exercer la médecine libre, d'ouvertures de maternités, de vente de produits pharmaceutiques non toxiques, etc., 1936," VNA, centre no. 2, RSA 3704.

[86] "Organisation et fonctionnement médecine rurale en Annam 1938," VNA, centre no. 2, RSA 37911.

[87] "Lettre du Ly truong de La Xa (Hai Duong) au Résident supérieur du Tonkin, 6 janvier 1933," VNA, centre no. 1, RST 47835.

complained that their buildings were dilapidated, and that they disposed of too few nurses to send them on tour or even to maintain daily consultation services. Drs. Terrisse and Chesneau's 1938 report also complained of a generalized shortage of medicines and especially of insufficient staff ("ninety-two nurses for [. . .] ninety-seven infirmaries").[88] Rural consultation rooms were often described as small and bare, contrasting with spacious and well-equipped urban facilities. Their value was mainly based on their strategic locations near public spaces or in transport hubs.[89] Many opened no more than two to three hours a day if a nurse was stationed there, or, if the nurse was responsible for several facilities, only one or two days a week. Some health posts offered consultation services intermittently over the year, such as the service in Tam Dao (Vinh Yen), which was open only from June until October.[90] The patients who did make it to a working consultation service might not, however, obtain medicines for free; they might be given only a shortened course of treatment or no medicines at all. There is evidence that the conditions of access to free consultations and medicines were not always respected. Some head doctors of provinces were accused of "mistreat[ing]" their patients during free consultations in order to "sell" them services.[91] In 1937, the residents of Rach Gia Province complained to the governor of Cochinchina that their head doctor, Dr. Nguyễn Kien Ba, and one of his deputies, Doan Van Khiem, had, for several years, been making patients pay for interventions and medicines.[92]

Doctors also worried about the cost and unavailability of medicines. While some complained that drugs ate up health care and hospital budgets, thus suggesting that resources would be better allocated elsewhere, others were concerned about the effects of cost and availability on patient treatment. Some even improvised to mitigate the lack of means. In a few cases, they simply used their own money to buy specialties from the nearest pharmacy, or borrowed medicines from colleagues. Indeed, this is what Dr. Henriette Bùi Quang Chiêu, the first female Vietnamese doctor, who worked at Cholon's maternity hospital in the late 1930s, did. Told by the hospital pharmacist that her requests were "excessive," she most often gave up and borrowed medicines from the neighboring Hôpital indigène.[93]

[88] VNA, centre no. 2, RSA 37911.
[89] Mathis, "L'helminthiase"; La tribune indigène, no. 113, October 22, 1918.
[90] ANOM, RST NF 4021.
[91] Du'o'ng Văn Lợi, "La vénalité des médecins français de l'Assistance. Les certificats médicaux," La tribune indochinoise, no. 30, October 15, 1926; "Le mercantilisme médical," La tribune indochinoise, no. 242, March 30, 1928.
[92] "Plainte contre M. Nguyen Kien Ba, médecin-chef de l'Assistance médicale de Rach Gia, 1937," VNA, centre no. 2, Goucoch 3086.
[93] Interview with Dr. Henriette Bùi Quang Chiêu, Paris (France), January 16, 1997.

Others, however, reduced the duration or dosage of therapies, or they diluted medicines, sometimes to the extent of dropping below "minimal active levels." Sometimes they could not even offer a dose of Aspirin or emetine.[94] Shortages might thus jeopardize therapeutic efficacy, both materially and symbolically, affecting the population's interpretation of colonial health care and biomedical drugs. AMI staff constantly warned the authorities that they were forced to practice "a cut-rate [brand of] medicine [. . .] which would eventually [make them] lose what they had gained, driving away dissatisfied patients [. . .]," but to no avail.[95]

Staff shortages, specifically the lack of staff qualified to prepare or to prescribe drugs, formed another significant barrier to broadening the accessibility of medicines. Brick-and-mortar facilities could perhaps be dispensed with, but qualified professionals could not. The law defined medical doctors and pharmacists as gatekeepers to the majority of effective drugs, notably the growing number of medicines defined as toxic or to be administered by injection. Only a small minority of the AMI's staff, however, held full rights to prescribe and dispense medicines for most of the colonial period. Pharmaceutical legislation had its reasons: to protect French colonial professional and commercial interests, and to protect the Vietnamese population from the risks of badly handled and dangerous drugs. Yet it was totally incongruous with the realities of public health care in Vietnam, impeding its reach and probably its success, whether measured as positive perception or as material effects on health.

According to the *Annuaire statistique de l'Indochine*, 114 European doctors and 220 Vietnamese doctors worked for the AMI in 1931.[96] There was, on average, 1 doctor per 100,000 Tonkinese, and this was one of the highest ratios in the Union. In 1937, the ratio had grown to 1 per 40,000, including private practitioners.[97] Around the same time, there were nearly 3,000 indigenous nurses and about 1,000 midwives.[98] For a population estimated at around 23 million inhabitants, staff numbers were decidedly inadequate. The AMI failed even to reach the ratio of nurses (1 per 3,000 inhabitants) estimated as minimal by the colonial health administration.[99] Furthermore, nurses and midwives were not

[94] "Rapport sanitaire annuel de la province de Hung Yen, 1913, " ANOM, RST NF 4014.
[95] "Rapport sanitaire annuel de la province de Bac Giang, 1915, " ANOM, RST NF 4003.
[96] Gouvernement général de l'Indochine française, *Annuaire statistique*, 100.
[97] In France, the ratio was of 1 doctor per 2,000 and in British Malaya 1 per 22,000. By contrast, the Dutch East Indies had only 1 doctor per 110,000 people: Annick Guénel, "The Conference on Rural Hygiene in Bandung, 1937: Towards an New Vision of Health Care?," in Laurence Monnais and Harold J. Cook, ed., *Global Movements, Local Concerns. Medicine and Health in Southeast Asia* (Singapore: NUS Press, 2012), 70.
[98] Monnais-Rousselot, *Médecine et colonisation*, 242, 300.
[99] ANOM, RSA S1.

authorized to prescribe,[100] while Vietnamese doctors' prescriptions rights were highly restricted until the 1930s. According to the French law of 1892, which was quickly applied in Indochina, the authority to prescribe was reserved to fully qualified doctors holding a *doctorat d'état* (state doctorate). This authority was thus de facto long withheld from the vast majority of Vietnamese doctors – that is, the auxiliary doctors who graduated from the Hanoi Medical School, which, until 1935, did not grant its own doctorates in medicine. When the AMI was created in 1905, the first cohort of auxiliaries had just graduated from the three-year program in Hanoi. These auxiliaries were placed under the authority of French doctors of medicine, and were only authorized, under well-defined conditions, like the officiers de santé of the metropole prior to 1892, to dispense "some medicines," mainly products that were prepackaged and nontoxic, which they were allowed to stock "in their place of residence."[101]

The status of auxiliary doctors did improve, but slowly. For a long time, they were forbidden from private practice, while restrictions on their right to prescribe were only very gradually lifted. During World War I, Vietnamese doctors compensated for the absence of mobilized French doctors, pushing the colonial administration to loosen these restrictions.[102] The governor general examined the issue of prescribing rights when the 1916 metropolitan law on toxic substances was being transferred to Indochina. In 1920, he authorized auxiliary doctors to "prescribe medicines containing toxic substances included in the regulatory nomenclature intended for AMI facilities staffed by a doctor." Yet they were allowed to prescribe any schedule A or B substance only in "doses [no] higher than the maximal doses set by the pharmacopeia for twenty-four hours." Even when, in 1922, the category of médecin auxiliaire was renamed *médecin indochinois* (Indochinese doctor) in recognition of the high quality of the local training program, limitations on the right to prescribe were maintained.

These restrictions were criticized in an open letter to the governor general, dated March 1924 and signed by Henri Marcel, then president

---

[100] Midwives were authorized to dispense only corrosive sublimate (mercury bichloride), an antiseptic used in obstetrics, and a solution of silver nitrate to prevent neonatal eye infections.

[101] "Rapport sanitaire annuel de l'Indochine, 1906," ANOM, Gougal 6742.

[102] It seems that they also bent the rules with their supervisors' approval. Paul-Louis Simond remarked in his personal notes that in October 1915, an auxiliary doctor in Binh Dinh had prescribed strychnine ampoules, having first asked the AMI pharmacist to prepare these for him and ensured that he would not be reprimanded ("Carnets, 1913–1917," Archives scientifiques de l'Institut Pasteur de Paris, Fonds Simond SIM.2).

of the Association des médecins auxiliaires d'Indochine (Association of auxiliary doctors of Indochina), created in 1918. The letter not only claimed equal competence to prescribe with French doctors; it also argued that restrictions jeopardized the success of French medicalization by penalizing (potential) patients:

Mr. Governor General,
    [. . .] At the medical school, students must learn how to utilize all medicines that are routinely used in hospitals. At the end of the fourth year of study, they must pass a test in materia medica before a jury made up of professors of pharmacy and of therapeutics. Granted the title of auxiliary doctors [. . .] these students holding diplomas that recognize their competence to practice medicine are restricted in this practice by some current laws [. . .] By limiting the range of medicines and the dose of toxic substances, the administration is taking a cautious approach, aimed at protecting patients from the risk of accidental poisoning. I can only commend this [intention]. However, I take the liberty to very respectfully draw your benevolent attention to the fact that this limitation, wise as it is, entails impediments to the penetration of French medicine in native environments [. . .] When the latter must make daily trips to the pharmacist to have their potion renewed, they find eventually that all this travel is really exasperating and expensive. As for unwell people from remote provinces lacking a European pharmacy! [. . .] They will certainly prefer to go to empirics. This puts both French therapeutic methods and the interests of auxiliary doctors at a disadvantage [. . .] Yet, if the same medicine prescribed by a European doctor to the same patient does not cause toxic effects, we cannot understand why these would result if the medicine was prescribed according to the rules, by the auxiliary doctor.[103]

Marcel's demand was for auxiliary doctors to be allowed to prescribe *any* medicine in the French pharmacopeia, without distinction, and at doses adjusted to the patient's state and distance of residence rather than at the medicinal dose. This was granted a few weeks later, in April 1924, by decree.[104] By then, the system had nevertheless, for many years, been denied a substantial number of "prescribing arms." And still, by 1930, there were fewer than four hundred doctors with full prescription rights serving more than five hundred public health care facilities. Authorities were not oblivious to the consequences of these severe and chronic health staff shortages on access to medicines, as evidenced by the creation and extension of the network of essential medicines outlets. Yet beyond their practical failures, these solutions could only ever be partial since they could not provide access to the pharmaceutical specialties that had been

---

[103] Henri Marcel, "Projet de lettre au sujet de la prescription des médicaments par les médecins auxiliaires," *Bulletin de l'Amicale des médecins auxiliaires de l'Indochine* 3 (1924): 34–35.
[104] Not until 1936 did a decree of the minister of colonies modify the 1892 metropolitan law in order to give French subjects full rights to practice medicine.

proven to be effective against the region's most prevalent and deadly infectious diseases.

The shortage of pharmacists in the AMI system is even more striking and puzzling. Unlike doctors who worked for the Assistance, pharmacists never joined an official civilian medical corps. The category "AMI pharmacist" simply did not exist. Of the few who worked in the public system, nearly all were military pharmacists who had been lent to the AMI by the TC.[105] Civilian pharmacists were rarely employed, and only on a limited contract basis. There were Vietnamese auxiliary pharmacists. Yet in addition to restrictions on their field and rights of practice, they joined AMI's staff belatedly and in small numbers. Opened in 1914, the pharmacy section of Hanoi's medical school produced its first four graduates in 1917, and only three to five graduates per year up to the end of the 1920s (during the same period, eleven to twenty-five doctors graduated each year). In 1922, no more than thirty pharmacists were listed on the AMI staff for all of Indochina; twenty-two of these were auxiliary.[106] By 1931, official figures had grown, respectively, to forty and thirty-four. Yet not all pharmacists on the books were in active service: in Annam, in 1931, only three of eleven were on the ground; the others were on leave or about to resign. Moreover, they were concentrated in urban areas, where they worked for the larger hospitals, government laboratories, Central Supply Pharmacies, or the Pharmacy Inspection Service.

The conspicuous lack of pharmacists in the AMI, as well as of information in the colonial archives on their roles and activities, is difficult to explain. This may be indicative of the very minor part these actors were expected to play in colonial public health. Given that, by law, pharmacists were indispensable preparators and distributors of medicines, their small numbers in the AMI can be taken as yet another sign of the marginal role of medicines in colonial medicalization. Whereas the distribution of small volumes of public medicines came up against the human and infrastructural limits of the AMI, a restrictive legal framework further impeded efforts to broaden access to effective drugs. Revolutionary medicines largely remained elite medicines, since large urban hospitals not only had bigger pharmaceutical budgets; they were also better equipped to manipulate these medicines as well as to oversee trials and supervise treatment.

---

[105] For a general overview of colonial (military) pharmacists, see Pierre Pluchon, *Histoire des médecins et des pharmaciens de Marine et des Colonies* (Toulouse: Privat, 1985), 281–300.

[106] "Rapport sur le fonctionnement de l'Assistance médicale au Tonkin, 1922," VNA, centre no. 1, RST 32026; ANOM, Gougal 47474.

The two initiatives described in this chapter promised to broaden the distribution of medicines beyond the confines of a public health care system in which (limited) resources were concentrated around the places (and people) considered to be important to the colonial economy. These initiatives might have given medicines a key role, a symbolic and practical value, in colonial medicalization. The principles underlying the QE service put mass drug therapy at the heart of a major public health goal: the collective prevention of one of Vietnam's main causes of sickness and death. Alongside vaccines, quinine was the first medicine in which the Indochinese government made a significant investment, orchestrating its distribution and consumption on a large scale. The authorization and expansion of an outlet network made essential medicines a potential vehicle for the provision of basic universal care beyond the limits of the AMI's material and human presence. Instead, both distribution networks reveal ambivalence toward medicines and their accessibility. Authorities made little effort to resolve the many practical problems that arose in the supply and provision of QE; they largely abandoned the persons they put in charge of basic drugs distribution, giving them very little material support and supervision. In many places, the provision of free medicines was an empty promise. QE and essential medicines were not, in the end, public medicines; instead they were marginalized drugs. Is it surprising, then, that many Vietnamese did not, as AMI doctors often lamented, rush to be treated in colonial health care facilities? Is it not plausible that recourse to Vietnamese medicine was often maintained out of lack of alternatives rather than by conviction? We will return to these two fundamental questions, about the possible relationship between problems of accessibility to medicines in the colonial health care system and this observed reluctance to seek public biomedical treatment paired with persisting recourse to Vietnamese remedies. For we must first examine the very different set of dynamics that governed drug distribution in the colony *beyond* the AMI, by looking at private distributors and distribution channels of colonial medicines.

4 The Many Lives of Medicines in the Private Market

Despite the limits of the public system, it seems to have stimulated, according to some reports, a growing and indeed avid demand for pharmaceuticals. AMI distributions of medicines occasionally turned into riots. There are also reports of regular drug thefts from the stocks carried by nurses traveling to remote villages.[1] In some regions, QE was sold so quickly it was hard to maintain stocks, and some distributors sought to stimulate sales by selling it by the tablet instead of the tube.[2] An even more striking sign of the popularity of pharmaceuticals is the significant number of drugs that appear to have circulated in Vietnam *only* outside the AMI. Of the 1,121 medicines in my database, more than half were never mentioned in AMI reports or in the medical press, nor were they listed in the pharmaceutical nomenclature for public medical facilities. The majority of these were commercial specialties that could be sold OTC but only by qualified pharmacists. The high number of these hints at the significance of private channels of drug distribution in shaping pharmaceutical circulation and consumption in Vietnam. They raise a new set of questions about what counted as a colonial medicine, and about who could produce, distribute, and gain access to this category of drugs. In fact, as they moved through vibrant private, sometimes illicit, networks of pharmaceutical production and distribution in Vietnam – the focus of this chapter and Chapter 5 – colonial medicines became increasingly difficult to circumscribe as objects of competing, but also intersecting, commercial, as well as consumer logics and actors. Although colonial law sought to distinguish between "European-style" pharmacies, which

---

[1] "Organisation de l'Assistance rurale en Annam, 1935–1937," VNA, centre no. 2, RSA 3362.

[2] "Rapport sanitaire annuel de la province de Bac Kan, 1915," ANOM, RST NF 3829; "Commande annuelle de médicaments pour le Tonkin, 1938"; "Lettre de l'Inspecteur général de l'hygiène et de la santé publique Hermant au Gouverneur général de l'Indochine, Hanoi, 28 octobre 1937," ANOM, Gougal SE 2931; VNA, centre no. 1, IGHSP 4. Allain, "Paludisme et quinine," 643; Audibert, "Les maladies endémo-épidémiques," 64. The practice of selling QE by the tablet was prohibited since it could increase the risk of treatment interruptions and thus of jeopardizing its efficacy.

were owned and managed by pharmacists, and "Asian" sites and actors, these commercial and therapeutic worlds often collided on the ground. Intense competition existed between traders in medicines, but there were also surprising connections cutting across networks, making it difficult, and unproductive, to fully untangle them. I thus approach the private medicines market as a whole, crossing over legal demarcations, to describe its many lives and layers, and attending to the points of contact that mutually shaped diverse production and marketing strategies. This resulted in innovative pharmaceutical representations and practices, giving colonial medicines multiple and hybrid identities that blurred the lines between qualities and identities: foreign and local, Western and Asian, traditional and modern, as well as licit and illicit.

4.1   The Field and Business of Private "Western" Pharmacies

Two hundred and eighty: this is the number of qualified pharmacists (whether holders of a state diploma from a French university or a diploma delivered by the Hanoi Pharmacy School), both military and civil, who I identified as having worked in colonial Vietnam before 1940. One hundred and ninety of these, or nearly 70 percent, were in private practice. These numbers are probably underestimated, given that pharmacists and private health care professionals are not mentioned very often in colonial sources. While many opened, bought, or joined private pharmacies as soon as they arrived in Vietnam or graduated in Hanoi, some did so only after they resigned from military/public service. These figures are surprisingly high, especially relative to those for AMI personnel (provided in Chapter 3). What does this discrepancy mean?

In the early decades of French administration in Indochina, French pharmacists' clientele was largely restricted to colonial society. This was the case for the two pharmacists who set up in Hanoi at the end of the nineteenth century, as it was for the city's one plumber, two booksellers and shoemakers, three tailors, four bakers and barbers, five butchers, and fourteen baristas. As more French colonists and civil servants arrived with their families, the number of pharmacies gradually increased. By 1910, there were fourteen "European pharmacies" across the Union: six in Tonkin (three in Hanoi, two in Haiphong, and one in Nam Dinh), five in Cochinchina (all in the Saigon area), and three in Annam (in Hué, Tourane, and Vinh).[3] Because initially they did not count Vietnamese

---

[3] "Pharmacie. Exercice de pharmacie, M. Raymond, arrêté du 4 octobre 1910," ANOM, Gougal 17171; "Demande de renseignements sur l'installation d'une pharmacie en Indochine formulée par M. Matet, 1911–1912," ANOM, Gougal 17168.

population as a potential client pool, colonial authorities considered the market for medicines to be saturated. Even the prospect of operating a pharmacy in a provincial capital was excluded at the time. Competition was already fierce, and some pharmacies, facing bankruptcy, had closed their businesses.[4] By 1918, however, Hanoi and Saigon, whose European population was still no more than a few thousand, accommodated from about fifteen to twenty "Western pharmacies."[5] It seems clear that these urban pharmacies had begun attracting an indigenous clientele.

Three other factors catalyzed the growth of private pharmacy during the war. Two are related to the development of AMI: the opening of the pharmacy section at the Hanoi School of Medicine and health authorities' reluctant reliance on private pharmacists to help supply the public system in the face of high drug costs and obstacles to importation (see Chapter 2). The third factor is connected to the growth of a local Vietnamese economy, and an increase in the number of Vietnamese businesspeople and professionals. Between 1900 and 1912, the number of small French firms registered in Indochina jumped from twenty-three to seventy-eight, while small businesses grew from three hundred in the late 1880s to one thousand in 1910. From 1915, however, this number began to drop due to local competition, particularly from Asian businesses – Chinese, Viêt, and Indian.[6] During the same period, a growing number of biomedically trained pharmacists competed for customers. The Vietnamization of the pharmacy profession, like the medical one, accelerated in the 1920s, and even more so in the 1930s. Of the 280 pharmacists in my repertory, about half were of Vietnamese origin (including a dozen women), and 65 percent of these were in private practice. By 1944, seventeen (or 71 percent) of twenty-four pharmacists with state diplomas practicing in Saigon-

---

[4] "Pharmacie. Demande de renseignements sur les conditions d'installation d'une officine de pharmacie formulée par MM. Rouzet et Moggi, 1907," ANOM, Gougal 1716; "Pharmacie. Demandes formulés par MM. Quihou et Sylvestre, pharmaciens, en vue d'être mis en relation avec ceux de la colonie, 1910," ANOM, Gougal 17169 and 17168.
[5] In the early 1920s, there are about 25,000 French people living in Vietnam; the population of Saigon was estimated to be between 200,000 and 400,000 inhabitants, of which only 4,000 were European. The colonial capital was smaller but its European population was similar in size.
[6] Vorapheth, *Commerce et colonisation,* 56, 59, 70. The Indian migrant community in Indochina (of several thousands) was a thriving community. The vast majority, of Tamil origin, were French citizens who migrated from the French Establishments in India and settled in Cochinchina. Many worked for the colonial administration while others were active in economic activities, especially trade, including the drug trade: Natasha Pairaudeau, *Mobile Citizens: French Indians in Indochina 1858–1954* (Copenhagen: NIAS Press, 2016).

Cholon were Vietnamese.[7] In 1942, so were seventy-one, or nearly 90 percent, of the eighty members of the Association professionnelle des pharmaciens d'Indochine (APPIC; Professional Pharmacists' Association of Indochina).[8]

While there are major differences between the histories of Vietnamese pharmacists and of doctors, both are marked by a similarly slow accession to parity with French graduates. A few Vietnamese trained in France in the 1910s, and were thus able to obtain the status of first-class pharmacist. The first to do so was André Lê Văn Minh, son of an important landowner from the South, which allowed him to be naturalized as French, and thus to study in France and obtain a state diploma. He graduated from the Faculty of Pharmacy of Paris in 1918.[9] Pharmacy graduates of Hanoi were, like auxiliary doctors, initially confined to civil service, but they were authorized sooner, by a 1925 governor general's decree, to enter private practice. At first, restrictions applied: they could open businesses only outside a fifteen-kilometer radius from a practicing French pharmacist and could not sell narcotics (and had to comply with general regulations on the sale of other toxic substances). But while Vietnamese doctors "owed" a number of years of practice to the state upon graduation, this condition was never applied to Vietnamese pharmacists. A governor general's decree dated August 1933 expanded the dispensing rights of "Indochinese pharmacists," and in 1935 the Hanoi School of Pharmacy, like the medical school, obtained the authority to grant its own doctorates of pharmacy.[10]

The number of private pharmacies in Indochina, under both French and Vietnamese ownership, rose from fourteen in 1910 to eighty-four in 1942 – a 600 percent increase. For the period from 1880 to the 1930s,

[7] "Liste nominative des pharmaciens diplômés d'état exerçant leur profession à titre privé sur le territoire de Saigon-Cholon en 1944," VNA, centre no. 2, S09-6, Tòa đại biểu chính phủ Nam Việt, Bang kê nhung y si baò chê su và nha si dông duong tôt nghiêp tu 20 dên 50 tuôi không phap tich, cu ngu tai dô thành Saigon-Cholon. Note that the proportion of Vietnamese who owned pharmacies was higher outside of Cochinchina, where colonial commerce and professional presence were better established.

[8] "Groupements professionnels. Association professionnelle des pharmaciens de l'Indochine, 1942," ANOM, Gougal SE 158. While we lack detailed data on this topic, it seems that pharmacists in Indochina began organizing to defend their professional rights in the 1930s. The APPIC was the form taken by this first syndicate under the Vichy regime.

[9] *La tribune indigène,* no. 159, April 10, 1919.

[10] From that year, pharmacists who graduated earlier could obtain a certificate proving their aptitude to exercise pharmacy in order to establish businesses wherever they liked; several would grab this opportunity: "Liste des pharmaciens indochinois, nr 19/4, DB du 21 juin 1945 (Saigon) à Monsieur le Gouverneur général, Hanoi," VNA, centre no. 2, S09-7, Bảng kê các bào chê su dông dương tôt nghiệp thuốc hà nội cu, 1945.

I identified a total of about 170 different businesses.[11] Unsurprisingly, the majority continued to be concentrated around big cities, particularly the twin cities of Saigon and Cholon, which, by the interwar period, already had twice as many pharmacies as Hanoi. Within these urban areas, they were clustered around the busiest roads. Three of Hanoi's biggest pharmacies (Blanc, Montès, and Chassagne) had addresses on Paul Bert Street (numbers 31, 54, and 59), at the heart of the colonial administrative district. In the 1930s, seven Vietnamese-owned pharmacies were established in the city's older commercial district, alongside colonial trading companies, on streets such as Chanvre (Hemp), Soie (Silk), Chapeaux (Hats), and Changeurs (Moneychangers). In Saigon, four of the oldest and best-known French pharmacies were located on the vibrant Catinat street, Vietnam's own Champs Elysées: the Pharmacie Principale Solirène, established in 1856 on the Place du Théâtre across from the Hôtel Continental; the Pharmacie de France, with the address 109-12; the Pharmacie Normale, at 119-23; and the Pharmacie Centrale, on 195-201. Seven pharmacies, five of which were Vietnamese-owned, were established on Spain Street and four were on Bonnard Boulevard (Figure 4.1).

About a quarter of the colony's pharmacies were established outside these two agglomerations, but either in economically important cities (nine in Haiphong, five in Hué, four each in Vinh and Tourane, three in Dalat) or in the most densely populated and vibrant provincial capitals, such as Vinh Long and My Tho (three each), Soc Trang, Quang Yen, Can Tho, and Bac Ninh (two each). By the 1930s, an additional twenty-one provinces had at least one Western pharmacy.

How similar were pharmacy businesses in Vietnam and in France? Did pharmacists in Vietnam face the same issues, and engage in the same strategies, as pharmacists in the metropole? Information on pharmacists' activities is available mainly for a handful of individuals, mostly French (Table 4.1). Some left traces because they were public figures. We know, for example, that Victor Holbé and Louis Sarreau were members of the Colonial Council. Pharmacists also served as mayors of Saigon (Lourdeaux in 1872–74 and J. Guérin in 1884), while Gabriel Renoux was deputy mayor for several years. Others held high positions in local chambers of commerce. We can also find information on pharmacists who owned some of the larger, longer-lasting businesses. These were well

---

[11] The higher number of pharmacists surveyed is explained by the presence of a number of military and AMI-employed pharmacists who never owned a private pharmacy but also, to a lesser extent, by succession at the head of the largest pharmacies and their employment of salaried pharmacists.

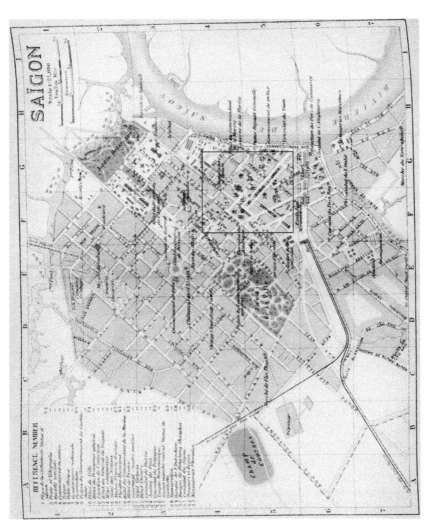

Figure 4.1 Saigon Therapeutic Landscape in the Interwar Period (adapted from a map of Saigon printed in Tetsudosho, *An Official Guide to Eastern Asia*, vol. 5 [Tokyo: Department of Railways, 1920], 222)

Table 4.1 *Principal Pharmacies of Vietnam, 1900–45*

	Name of Business	Name of Owner
Hanoi	Pharmacie française et étrangère de l'Indochine (or Pharmacie Blanc)	Noël Reynaud
		Julien Blanc
		Louis Blanc
		Louis Guillou
	Pharmacie Maire then Montès	Adrien Maire
		? Montès
		Pierre Domart
	Pharmacie Chassagne	Edmond Chassagne
		E. Lafon and E. Lacaze
		E. Lafon
Saigon	Pharmacie Principale	Victor Holbé (and Gabriel Renoux)
		Gabriel Renoux
		Louis Solirène
		Maurice Heumann
	Pharmacie Normale	F. Berenguier, Molinier and de Mari
		? Dourdou
		Louis Sarreau
		Jean Roux
		Paule Guignet
	Pharmacie Centrale	André Lê Văn Minh
		J. Mus
		R. Bonniot
		Henri-Francis Gamby
	Pharmacie de France	Marcel Collet
		Marcel Mercier
Haiphong	Pharmacie Brousmiche then Grande pharmacie centrale Brousmiche	Édouard Brousmiche
		? Bourguignon
		René Lagauzère
Hué	Pharmacie centrale de l'Indochine	François Imbert

known; they had visible, spacious buildings, a large, competent, and welcoming staff, and were also heavily advertised.

For these flagship pharmacies, it is possible to get a glimpse of their owners' activities, the marketing tools they used, their relations with the administration, and the issues they faced. Most striking is how diverse their activities were. In addition to the retail sale of medicines, cosmetics, toiletries, and disinfectants, many also sold chemicals (for artwork, industry, and especially agriculture) and household products; provided industrial and medical analysis and sterilization services; and sold medical, surgical, and dental supplies and accessories. Some even sold medicinal plants, perfumes, and stationery; ran labs to test new medicines; and offered optometry and photography services.

The publicity for some of these pharmacies emphasized the broad range of products and services they offered, not all of which pertained to health. A few pharmacists also imported chemical and pharmaceutical products in bulk for resale to smaller pharmacies. One early such initiative was the Droguerie commerciale de l'Union, founded by André Lê Van Minh in 1919. Although it was short-lived, it is still notable for its Vietnamese management, including several Vietnamese businesspeople on its board of directors.[12] François Imbert, who took over the Pharmacie centrale de l'Indochine of Hué in 1929, soon became one of Indochina's main exporters of papain.[13] Import-export, however, required substantial capital and networks, and most pharmacies preferred to use the services of well-established commercial firms such as Bourgouin-Meiffre, Descours & Cabaud, and Denis Frères. An Office des spécialités pharmaceutiques (Office of pharmaceutical specialties) was established in Saigon in 1933. It took care of "all operations of representation, commission, brokerage of pharmaceutical specialties and products, chemical and household products, pharmacy accessories, etc."[14] In the 1930s, while still relying on various suppliers and intermediaries in Europe and sometimes also in North America, pharmacies in Vietnam could also call on the branches of some metropolitan firms, such as Rhône-Poulenc and its subsidiaries from 1936, or on the representatives they sent.[15] In 1939, the pharmacist Lucien Gamby established a Comptoir pharmaceutique d'Extrême-Orient (Far-Eastern Pharmaceutical Trading) in central Saigon, from which he traveled across Southeast Asia, including Thailand (Siam), the Philippines, and Malaysia, as a "general agent of pharmaceutical firms."[16]

After a visit to Indochina to assess its pharmacy sector in the late 1940s, Professor Charles Bedel was pleasantly surprised to find busy and well-established businesses that had "quite the same appearance as our top pharmacies in France." He also noted that the owners appeared to be less

[12] *La tribune indigène*, no. 225, November 13, 1919.
[13] "Documents sur les exportateurs de papaïne en Indochine, 1935," ANOM, AFOM, Box 240, Folder 313. Papain (an enzyme present in the papaya trees) was then used for various industrial purposes as well as therapeutically for its digestive, anti-inflammatory, and antiseptic properties.
[14] Gouvernement général de l'Indochine, Direction des services économiques, *Répertoire des sociétés anonymes indochinoises* (Hanoi. IDEO, 1944), 177–78.
[15] "Indochine, Plantes médicinales. La noix vomique, 1919–1936," ANOM, AFOM, Box 240, Folder 311, "Plantes médicinales en Indochine, plantes à chaulmoogra, du XVIe au 30 novembre 1937," ANOM, AFOM, Box 240, Folder 308.
[16] "Produits toxiques. Autorisation personnelle et permanente d'importer en Indochine des substances toxiques du tableau B, 1937–1940," ANOM, Gougal SE 217.

commercially oriented than their French counterparts and more invested in "the scientific side of their profession."[17] Publicity for pharmacies placed in the local press often emphasized the quality of prescription-filling services, as well as the availability of the latest pharmaceuticals. There seems, however, to have been much variation in the range and type of products sold by each pharmacy. At the turn of the 1930s, for example, 60 percent of the Pharmacie Chassagne's stock was made up of commercial specialties, against 35 percent at the Pharmacie Blanc.[18] Pharmacie Chassagne sourced its commercial and medical specialties from at least thirty-five firms; most were French, an origin that was presented in its publicity as an implicit guarantee of quality, including Laboratoires Robin, Produits Scientia, Clin, Comar et Cie, and Hoffman, Laroche et Cie. The Pharmacie Montès, however, mainly distributed Rhône-Poulenc products (including several synthetic antimalarial drugs) and Roussel products (of which the sulfonamide Rubiazol from the late 1930s). Whereas a few pharmacies obtained exclusive rights to distribute a specific product or brand in Indochina,[19] some highly popular products (at least they were popular in the "West"), such as Ricqlès Peppermint Cure, Pilules du Dr. Dehaut, Dr. William's Pink Pills for Pale People, and Foster's Mecca Ointment, were advertised as being available "in all good pharmacies."[20]

This wide range of products and services suggests a willingness to please (and to attract) a heterogeneous and demanding clientele. Not all pharmacies were equally successful. And, even into the 1940s, there were still few pharmacies per capita relative to European countries, for example. Still, their growing presence in urban areas, as well as their efforts to expand their clientele, are indicators of their important role in the history of colonial medicines in Vietnam, especially in the 1920s and 1930s. Publicity for both French and Vietnamese-owned pharmacies also underlined the competence and availability of staff and the continuity and convenience of the service they offered. Some pharmacies opened seven days a week and even "during nap time and night-time." The Pharmacie Principale offered a rapid mail delivery service

---

[17] Charles Bedel, "La pharmacie en Indochine. Impressions de mission," *La libre pharmacie*, 43 (1949): 3–6.

[18] This assessment is based on the identification, with no claim to statistical representativity, of about eighty products known to be sold by each of these pharmacies.

[19] Such as the Jemalt-brand cod liver oil and Jamet-brand baby cereals for the Pharmacie Centrale in the 1920s advertised in *L'Écho*. Rudy products (ten commercial specialties that included various tonics and a cough syrup) were sold solely by the Pharmacie Normale under the Sarreau's ownership according to ads in several newspapers.

[20] There is also evidence of commercial agreements between pharmacies to maximize the distribution of some products and share the dividends.

and the Pharmacie Chassagne had a correspondence service from 1926, and a car delivery service from 1930, to serve clients on the outskirts of the city.[21] From 1940, a night and holiday duty system was even organized by the APPIC to provide year-round, twenty-four-hour access to a designated pharmacy in Saigon.[22] The pharmacy market was a space of fierce competition and of intense energy and will to innovate. Indeed, the pressures of competition stimulated strategies to expand and take over clienteles, but also to reduce the number and power of competitors.

4.2 Competition and Its Consequences: The Politics of Denunciation and Advertising Strategies

Pharmacies varied widely in size and profitability. Among the most prominent was the Pharmacie Blanc in Hanoi, which, from the 1900s, had a fifteen-meter-wide façade on Paul Bert Street and Rivière Boulevard, and a staff of about twenty, mostly Vietnamese, employees.[23] Under Louis Solirène, in the late 1930s, the Pharmacie Principale in Saigon was said to directly employ three hundred individuals, and contracted another hundred as salespeople, representatives, clerks, manual laborers, assistants, as well as several salaried pharmacists, and even an optician.[24] Solirène had additional staff members who managed his warehouse and his pharmaceutical research and drug production laboratory. Qualified pharmacists' annual trading license dues (*patente*), which were set in proportion to the trade volume of each business, show that some pharmacies were highly lucrative and that others struggled. For example, the owner of the Pharmacie Montès paid 1,000 piasters in 1939, while in the provincial capital of Soc Trang, Lê Quan Trọng paid 192 piasters. The dues owed by most other pharmacists in Hanoi varied from 400 to 700 piasters.[25] By comparison, the annual trading licenses of private doctors during this period cost between 50 and 400 piasters; the French commercial company Descours & Cabaud paid 3,000 piasters, while traders of Chinese or Vietnamese medicines were charged from 50 to 100 piasters.[26]

[21] Advertisements, *La tribune indigène*, no. 1, August 20, 1917; *L'Écho*, no. 944, August 6, 1927; VSB, no. 56, September 15, 1930 and no. 57, October 15, 1930.
[22] "Pharmacie de nuit," *L'Écho*, no. 265, January 8–9, 1941.
[23] Villemagne-Renard, "Les commerçants."
[24] Vorapheth, *Commerce et colonisation*, 183, 205.
[25] VNA, centre no. 2, S09-7, Tòa đại biểu chính phủ Nam Việt.
[26] "Ville de Hanoi. Service des contributions directes. État nominatif des Européens patentés en 1939 pour servir à l'établissement de la liste des électeurs consulaires de 1940," ANOM, RST NF 2836.

In comparison with other dimensions of the pharmacy business, the colonial archives are quite informative on problems of, and responses to, intra-professional competition. In the early years of colonial rule, even the handful of pharmacists must have competed for the very small market of mainly European consumers in Vietnam. This might explain why they were so keen to bid for public service contracts and to create other types of connection with the AMI. As the offer (and the demand, as we will see) for medicines grew, competition persisted. But its nature changed. Pharmacy owners regularly complained to colonial authorities about losing business to other pharmacies, as well as to other types of French or Asian business.[27] From the early years of the AMI and the creation of the Pharmacy Inspection Service in 1908, pharmacists occasionally denounced each other or Asian traders for the illegal practice of pharmacy. In this, they sought legal intervention that would eliminate, or at least tarnish the reputation of, an overly "greedy" competitor. Pharmacists also fought against the loss of market shares to traders who did business in non-prescription pharmaceutical products, called *parapharmacie* in France. They accused department stores of illegally selling antiseptics, bandages, and toiletries such as toothpaste and soap, and then turned on smaller grocery stores and shops specializing in household supplies. They claimed that some of these goods were within the purview of their expertise and, therefore, their monopoly.[28] Most accusations involved the sale of foreign specialties prohibited from importation or toxic products sold without prescription.

In the summer of 1908, the denunciation of two French pharmacists, Louis Blanc and a Mr. Serra, led to the closure, by decree of the municipality of Hanoi, of their colleague Adrien Maire's *comptoir de spécialités japonaises* (Japanese specialty counter).[29] Unsuccessful in his appeal, Maire then informed on Édouard Brousmiche for owning three pharmacies in Haiphong, Tourane, and Hanoi, a practice forbidden by law in both France and Vietnam. As this affair shows, pharmacists were willing

---

[27] "Dépôts de pharmacie, 1933," VNA, centre no. 1, RST 47835; "Au sujet des réclamations de Che Quang Thuong, pharmacien à Sontay sur sa situation difficile par la concurrence des marchands de drogues sino-annamites, 1933," VNA, centre no. 1, RST 47935.

[28] Pharmacists were calling for a strict application of the decree of July 1919. The Pharmacy Inspection Service seems to have been particularly intransigent with regards to the sale of sterile bandages and other hygiene products by non-pharmacists. Pharmacists were nevertheless forced to share the market for many products that fell in the fuzzy space between food and drug (for example, Nestle's milks, which were also distributed directly by the Swiss company which had several branches in Indochina from the 1920s), aperitif wines, and digestive drinks, as well as cosmetics and optometry.

[29] "Lettre de M. Maire au Gouverneur général de l'Indochine, Hanoi, 15 juillet 1908," ANOM, Gougal 17166.

to denounce each other. In parallel, they promoted their businesses aggressively and sometimes quite creatively. The pervasive presence of publicity for pharmacies, at least for the pharmacies listed in Table 4.1, and for their products in the local popular press (both in French- and Vietnamese-language newspapers) is in itself an indication of intense competition in the market for medicines. One of the most active advertisers was the Pharmacie Principale, under Solirène and then Heumann. Its publicity appeared in most issues of *La dépêche d'Indochine*, whose readership was mainly French, but also in *L'Écho*, *La tribune indochinoise*, *La tribune indigène*, *Công luận báo*, *L'Opinion*, and *Le progrès annamite*, as well as more specialized newspapers written in quốc ngữ, such as the women's magazine *Phụ nữ tân van. La nouvelle revue de la femme* (PNTV). Other active advertisers were the Pharmacie Normale, under Dourdou then Sarreau, and the Pharmacie Centrale under Mus and Lê Văn Minh.

Over time, pharmacists refined their marketing strategies. For example, they offered discounts on selected products, free shipping, and gifts to new or loyal clients, announcing these perks in the press. Readers of *La tribune indigène* learned in 1922 that any client making a purchase at the Pharmacie Normale during the Christmas holiday period would receive a liter of tonic wine, while, in *L'Écho*, the owner of the Grande Pharmacie de France announced in 1925 that, for its opening, he offered free samples of "the famous vin tonique Quina Laroche [a tonic wine]" to its first clients.[30] Louis Solirène (Pharmacie Principale) as well as E. Lafon and E. Lacaze (Pharmacie Chassagne) also publicized their donations, in drugs and tonic wines, in support of charitable and fundraising activities, such as a raffle for the construction of a memorial in Saigon in 1920, or a trachoma outpatient consultation service championed by the governor general's wife in 1935.[31] Maire, it was revealed in the aftermath of the 1908 scandal, had used a wide variety of strategies to promote his Japanese products, including posters, prospectuses, announcers, and commercial representatives who crisscrossed the area around Hanoi.[32] From the 1920s, some pharmacists also produced almanacs and catalogues containing, alongside health advice, publicity for the

---

[30] *La tribune indigène*, no. 522, December 22, 1921; *L'Écho*, no. 175, January 3, 1925, and no. 176, January 4, 1925.

[31] *La tribune indigène*, no. 283, April 15, 1920; BAYB, no. 10, April 1935.

[32] There was also a seizure from someone named Nguyễn Văn Hoàn of 406 boxes and 92 sachets of medicines, as well as advertising material that included a pack of posters ("Vente de médicaments japonais par des Japonais non munis de diplômes français, 1908," and "Procès-verbal de la saisie chez Nguyen-Hai-Hoan dont l'inventaire est déjà rapporté ci-haut," ANOM, RST NF 894).

products they sold. A few also invested in the health magazines that will be described in greater detail in Chapter 6.[33]

Seeking footholds outside the main urban centers, some pharmacists quickly took advantage of the opportunity offered by the authorization, by a decree of January 1910, of outlets for the private sale of European pharmaceutical products and QE.[34] In the following years, Brousmiche opened several of these in Tonkin as well as in Vinh.[35] In 1930, the pharmacist Imbert advertised outlets in Quang Tri and Tam Ky (Annam), and in 1932, the pharmacy of Khương Bình Tịnh (Can Tho) published an advertisement for its outlets in Long Xuyen and Sa Dec.[36] The line between these small legal outlets and illegal ownership of multiple pharmacies is hard to draw, and was probably easy to cross. Some pharmacists did operate several businesses, often under the discrete management of other pharmacists who had no ownership. Dourdou and Solirène, for example, were both officially owners of pharmacies in Saigon but also operated branches in Cholon from the late 1910s.[37] Others appear to have also maneuvered to use the AMI essential medicines outlet network to liquidate stocks and advertise their pharmacies, as suggested in Chapter 3.

As early as 1924, the inspector of pharmacies for Tonkin remarked on the sale of specialties in outlets across Vietnam that had been provided by city pharmacists, who had failed to take adequate precautions (many medicines lacked labels or posology information) for the protection of consumers.[38] On the eve of the Japanese occupation of 1940, it was discovered that some of these outlets were so well stocked that even the directors of the AMI's best hospitals would have been envious.[39] Recall that outlet managers, receiving little support from the

---

[33] *La tribune indigène*, no. 688, February 21, 1923; VSB, no. 47, December 15, 1929; VSB, no. 57, October 1930. It was unfortunately not possible to locate these publications.

[34] Like the essential medicines outlets that would be created in 1920, these outlets could not sell toxic products.

[35] ANOM, RST NF 3684.

[36] Advertisements, *Trung Kỳ vệ sinh chỉ nam. Moniteur d'hygiène de l'Annam* (TKVSCN), no. 5, May 1930; PNTV, no. 151, June 24, 1932.

[37] Solirène's branch was called the Pharmacie franco-asiatique du marché, while Dourdou's was the former Pharmacie Laurens whose eponymous owner died in 1915 and had not been replaced ("Rapport de la commission d'inspection des pharmacies à Saigon, année 1915," ANOM, Gougal 17174). Both were located on Sailors' Street, Cholon's busiest commercial street.

[38] "Lettre de M. Bloch, inspecteur des pharmacies du Tonkin et de l'Annam au médecin-inspecteur général des services sanitaires et médicaux de l'Indochine, Hanoi, 31 mars 1924," ANOM, RSA S1.

[39] And thus the stocks were promptly requisitioned: "Tournées d'inspection de M. le Directeur local de la santé et de l'Inspecteur général de l'hygiène et de la santé publique, 1943," ANOM, RST NF 6432.

AMI, were forced to rely on private pharmacies for their supply. It was probably easy for pharmacists to make use of these connections to expand their business and attract a clientele outside the crowded market of urban enclaves.

4.3 The Production of Local and Hybrid Specialties

A few pharmacists also began producing their own pharmaceuticals – "house" drugs. This was probably, in part, a marketing strategy; indeed, these products were generally heavily advertised. Yet we should also consider how these initiatives might have reflected the emergence – as well as the changing nature – of a local demand for modern medicines. Notably, among these *local specialties* were a number of what historian Sherman Cochran, for early twentieth century China, calls "new medicines," and which I call *hybrid specialties*. I use this term to emphasize the incorporation, in the content and representation of these medicines, of elements associated with more than one therapeutic tradition that were identified with both "tradition" and "modernity." Thus, the specific interactions that took place within the Vietnamese therapeutic market under colonial rule gave rise to a new type of medicine – one that can also be defined as a type of colonial medicine.

Among the earliest initiatives to produce local specialties among both European and Western-trained pharmacists were anti-opium preparations, which, as their name suggests, were meant to cure opium addiction. The first of these was Holbé's anti-opium solution, invented by the French military pharmacist Victor Holbé in the late 1880s. Sold in the form of a liqueur or drops, it contained morphine and cocaine hydrochloride (combined with cherry laurel water and rum).[40] It was apparently an instant success. Taken up by Holbé's successors, including Renoux, the specialty was sold under different names (Solution R., Solution Renoux, SR no. 1 Holbé) during the entire colonial period. The pharmacist Trombetta had his own formula for anti-opium pills, as did Dourdou with his Solution Anti-opium. By the early twentieth century, there was a clear demand for such aids from the urban elite, particularly the southern Chinese elite, despite international movements to control and criminalize drug use, as well as professional framings of drug

---

[40] Laurent Gaide, "Le visage inconnu de l'opium," *Bulletin des amis du vieux Hué*, 2–3 (1938): 198. Thomas-Victor Holbé arrived in Cochinchina in 1881 as a pharmacist of the Marine Corps. After a short stint at the hospital of Phnom Penh, he returned to France in 1886. In 1888, he resigned from the Marine Corps to practice privately in Saigon, where he took over Lourdeau's pharmacy.

addiction as both a disease and a social ill.[41] Thus, they attracted the attention of pharmacy inspectors, particularly after the promulgation of the 1916 French law on toxic substances, as we will see in Chapter 5. Similar preparations were popular in China at the time, and were sold in Indochina by both Chinese and Vietnamese druggists. Among the products advertised in several newspapers were Alcool Qui Chánh Thánh Dược Tửu, Bà Ngọc Dương's Con O, and Hồng Lạc Dường; this last product was said to cure addiction in only twenty-four hours!

Besides these highly visible and contested products, I was able to identify seventy to ninety local specialties, some of which were widely advertised.[42] These do not form a homogeneous or stable category. While some of these products were akin to the artisanal secret remedies of the nineteenth century, they were joined, from the time of World War I, by commercial specialties that were distinguished by the use of innovative ingredients (including synthetic substances) and modern forms of conditioning and packaging. For example, Renoux inherited from Holbé an anti-cholera elixir, a mint extract, and various expectorant syrups and pills. In the 1910s, he, and later Solirène, also developed, owned, and advertised Acryptol, a medicine for asthma; Nucléophytase, for digestion; two tonics (Trikinal and Vin 33.500); and a Dépuratif Asiatique, "unparalleled in cases of scrofula and chronic, tenacious eczema." Montès produced antiseptic tablets (Cachets Montès), a restorative (Hémoglobine Montès), a urinary tract antiseptic and gonorrhea remedy (Ablennol), as well as a peptone with iron, a "triple" digestive elixir, and a tonic wine called Vin Tonique Tonkinois. Louis Blanc advertised his own cod liver emulsion, a tonic wine, a depurative, and a remedy "for anemia and malaria" (Mixture J. B. S. L. F.).[43] Imbert owned at least three products, including Junase "for the relief of painful menstruation." As for the Pharmacie Chassagne, it produced and marketed a house phosphated iodo-tannin syrup, a cod liver oil, a tonic wine, a peptone elixir, and the Collyre Jaune selon la formule du Dr. Casaux.[44] There is

---

[41] On opiomania in Vietnam, see Philippe Le Failler, "Le coût social de l'opium au Vietnam. La problématique des drogues dans le philtre de l'histoire," *Journal asiatique* 283, 1 (1995): 239–64.

[42] This figure must, of course, be treated with caution, since I was not able to identify the producer in all cases of specialties surveyed. While some pharmacists openly advertised specialties as their own (or made this ownership evident in their names), others did not, which creates uncertainty about their origins.

[43] The initials J.B. probably stood for Julien Blanc, owner of the Pharmacie française et étrangère de l'Indochine in the 1890s to 1910s.

[44] In the 1920s, the Pharmacie Chassagne also probably produced Tricarbine (for gastric problems), Poudre Saint André (for upset tummies), Laxosodyl (a laxative), Sirop Khol (a syrup aiming at fighting tuberculosis), Sirop Nofal, and Cachets Nofal (a syrup and tablets to cure the flu and common colds).

evidence that the commercial rights for Pandermyl were obtained by the Pharmacie Solirène from the inventor (Dr. Honnorat) himself in the late 1910s. However, there is no information as to how the Collyre Jaune's formula was passed on from its inventor, an AMI ophthalmologist, to Edmond Chassagne.[45] In the 1930s, the pharmacy also advertised its own pills for anemia and fatigue (Pilules Robur) and two products to treat gonorrhea, the Pilules Bleues Antiblennorragiques and La Rose du Dr. Aboud.

Chassagne is probably the most striking case of pharmacists' growing involvement in local pharmaceutical production. Yet the initiative taken by some Vietnamese pharmacists is also worth mentioning. André Lê Văn Minh, an astute businessman, began advertising a house line of specialties as soon as he opened the Pharmacie Centrale. I was able to identify at least five products under his label, including Quinium (a fever-reducing tonic), Gaduol (cod liver oil extract capsules), Purgose (a "synthetic purgative"), and the Tridigestif Lê Văn Minh (to aid digestion). Nguyễn Viet Canh, who graduated from Bordeaux and set up business in Vinh Long in the 1930s, advertised at least three house specialties: a tonic wine, a "baby" syrup, and a "baby" digestive wine. Phạm Đoàn Điểm was the owner of a "histogenic" elixir with iron, while Huynh Van Son (Saigon) lauded the merits of his Élixir Végétal as follows: "a pleasant hygienic infusion: tonic, stimulating, cordial and digestive [. . .] indispensable at home and away."[46]

Like commercial specialties produced elsewhere, the majority of these house specialties were indicated for a wide range of mostly benign ailments and common symptoms. Information about their ingredients is harder to find. Many were modeled on Western and especially French products, sometimes very similar to these in name and presentation, and raise the thorny question of counterfeiting and the limits of legality in the production of medicines in a colonized context. But a few were instead named to reflect their local provenance, or marketed using therapeutic references familiar to a local clientele. Some tonic wines and depurative medicines, for example, were said to restore equilibrium to an unbalanced organism, while Pulmocid (made by Barberousse's Grande Pharmacie de France) was described as allowing energy to circulate more freely.[47] Nguyễn Văn Tri, who owned a pharmacy in My Tho, "adapted" the specialties he marketed by giving them Vietnamese brand names: Rượu

---

[45] Nguyen Van Dinh, "Chronique médicale. Pommade Pandermyl," La tribune indigène, no. 210, October 7, 1919.
[46] Advertisement, L'Écho, no. 779, January 6, 1927.
[47] Advertisement, L'Écho, no. 1, March 15–16, 1939. The effects of this "energetic treatment" were represented by a highly schematic drawing of a radiating human body.

Bổ Lửa, a tonic wine for women's problems; Thuốc Suyễn, a potion for asthma; and Sirop Trị Ho Thật Hay, a pectoral syrup.[48] There are other intriguing examples of "localization": Khương Bình Tịnh, a Vietnamese pharmacist who owned a cholera elixir, also produced an anti-opium preparation that combined alcohol, opium, and Chinese plants.[49] This use of locally sourced ingredients was probably a convenient and money-saving strategy, but Khương Bình Tịnh openly advertised it, which suggests that he, and perhaps his customers, also saw it as a selling point.

The hybridity of some locally produced specialties was a product of various types of mixing. Some contained a combination of ingredients from European and Asian pharmacopeias; others were based on the application of modern production processes to "traditional" ingredients and recipes. They might also be manufactured and packaged using Western-style or modern material forms and aesthetics, or be described and promoted using scientific-sounding names and therapeutic indications, as well as innovative marketing methods. These *modes of hybridization* were not mutually exclusive, while forms of innovation also varied across time and place. This gave rise to a dizzying number of possible permutations, making it nearly impossible to define these medicines as a specific category, especially since non-pharmacists, including Chinese and Vietnamese manufacturers and druggists, also invented, produced, advertised, and sold medicines that can be described as hybrid. In 1921, a drugstore in Cholon, by the name of Pharmacie de Shanghai (though it was not, technically, a pharmacy), advertised several house specialties, including a tonic that was packaged in boxes of twenty tablets that were identical to contemporary French packaging.[50] Ông Tiên, Mr. Tiên, a druggist located on Spain Street in Saigon and the owner of several drugstores across Vietnam, even advertised a remedy for STIs in several newspapers in 1939 as having obtained a "French attestation" of efficacy. Regardless of the veracity of this statement, it is revealing as a marketing ploy.[51]

Remedies promoted as "traditional" were sometimes advertised in French, as was the case of the restorative Thuốc Mạnh Đại Quang, that

---

[48] It is also worth mentioning that French brand names were sometimes Vietnamized when they were advertised in the press, such as Santal Midy (San tan Mi Dy), Gastrol (Ga tò rôn), Morrhuol (Mo ru on), and Potion Maubar (Thuốc bổ Mô Ba).

[49] "Pharmacie: Importation frauduleuse. Demande autorisation de vendre pilules anti-opium. Demande d'autorisation pour ouvrir dépôts pharmaceutiques. Visite de dépôts. Mise en vente du produit chinois Élixir La Tuyên," VNA, centre no. 2, Goucoch, IA-8/237(4).

[50] Advertisement, *La tribune indigène*, no. 482, September 13, 1921.

[51] This "attestation" was in fact a letter from a satisfied client, who signed as Nourdine from Saigon, dated 1934 (*L'Écho*, no. 112, December 18–19, 1939).

Đại Quang, an impressive Asian drugstore established in Cholon in the 1920s and 1930s, marketed with the promise of "energy, vigour, health."[52] The text promoting Tay Dam Tiên Don Pills for constipation provides an example of the type of qualities that might be highlighted:

> If you do not pass stools at least once every day
> To remain in good health, it is essential to pass stools regularly, at
>   least once a day
> The irregularity of stools induces a great number of discomforts,
>   which result, if they are not treated, in real disease [. . .]
> Violent laxatives or brutal purgatives cannot bring about a durable
>   recovery, since constipation itself is almost always a consequence
>   of disorders of the LIVER, disorders that ordinary laxatives are
>   unable to correct.
> To eliminate disorders of the LIVER, nothing comes close to
> TAY-DAM TIÊN-DON Pills
> Made especially in this aim, with local pharmaceutical products,
>   TAY-DAM TIÊN-DON are always suited to the atmosphere of
>   the country. They are targeted to fight partial or chronic con-
>   stipation and to protect you even from many diseases of the
>   intestines and stomach[53]

Scientificity and modernity – whether of the manufacturing process, active ingredients, conditioning, or specific curative action – were the key features put forward in advertisements for hybrid specialties produced by pharmacists and local druggists alike. The Đầu Rồng Company repeatedly affirmed in the PNTV that its products were constantly being improved on the basis of up-to-date scientific research. From the early 1920s, many of these hybrid specialties were trademarked, taking advantage of the French law promulgated in Indochina in 1909. The term "trademark" was sometimes mentioned in publicity, even for products that in fact originated from old family compendia (*gia truyền*), but had been revamped by new packaging and serial production techniques. The 1940 prospectus for the antimalarial Phát Lành Hoàn, made by the Lôc Hà nhà thuốc, or Lôc Hà drugstore (*nhà thuốc* literally means "medicines house"), simultaneously emphasized its suitability to Vietnamese patients and its basis in the latest knowledge of etiology and transmission of the disease. The pamphlet, which addressed "workers," emphasized the "risks" of malaria and described the drugstore's

---

[52] Advertisement, *L'Écho*, no. 89, October 18–19, 1939. Several advertisements for this type of hybrid product mentioned that these were also consumed by French clients.
[53] Advertisement, *L'Écho*, no. 371, October 6–7, 1941.

"expertise" in preparing effective remedies for various intestinal parasites and puerperal fever.[54]

Local specialties were also often advertised as being well-suited to Vietnamese biologies and bodies, sometimes by explicitly listing the names or number of plants of the Vietnamese pharmacopeia as a guarantee of this compatibility. Lê Văn Minh emphasized the mildness of his Purgose and its particular suitability to the "Vietnamese constitution."[55] In numerous advertisements placed in *Báo đông pháp* (BDP) in the late 1920s, the Hanoi-based Tự Ngọc Liên drugstore advertised its range of products with the motto "Annamese remedies for the Annamese." The businessman Nguyễn Đức Nhuận, maker of Từ Bi Oil and owner of the PNTV, in which he frequently advertised his own products, even proposed a "third" therapeutic option for minor wounds and injuries. Issue after issue, readers of the women's magazine were invited to "Take neither traditional nor Western medicines: Take Từ Bi Oil."[56]

Even outside the drug business, combining references in product design and marketing seems to have been a strong selling point. Hybridization strategies were deployed to make and promote a wide range of consumer goods in interwar Vietnam, including clothes, foodstuffs, cosmetics, and toiletries, such as Đại Quang brand "antiseptic soaps."[57] By their very existence and the confusion they created, hybrid specialties flouted the dividing line between supposedly "Western" and "Sino-Vietnamese," and by extension between "traditional" and "modern" medicines – a line that colonial laws and regulation worked so hard to draw in order to maintain the purity and exclusivity of biomedicine. They also offer a glimpse into the complex networks and multiples actors of the drug business that did not fit colonial definitions of what a pharmacist, or a pharmaceutical, should be. The Vietnamese modern drug market (or perhaps, more accurately, markets) was a dynamic space that blurred boundaries between therapeutic systems and stretched beyond Indochina's borders.

4.4   Networks and Actors of Traditional Medicines

As Sherman Cochran has described so well, the commercialization of medicines in China was, from the nineteenth century, located at the heart

---

[54] "Demande de distribution de prospectus et de remèdes antipaludéens formulée par M. Ngô Lân, propriétaire du Loc Ha Duoc Phong, 1940" and "Lettre de Ngô Van Lân au Résident supérieur du Tonkin, Hanoi, 1er mars 1940," ANOM, RST NF 3829.
[55] Advertisement, *La tribune indigène*, no. 294, May 11, 1920.
[56] Advertisement, PNTV, no. 188, February 23, 1933.
[57] Advertisement, *L'Écho*, no. 104, November 27–28, 1939.

of an emerging, early, and distinctively Chinese consumer culture.[58] Commercial networks quickly reached beyond China's borders thanks to the long-standing presence of active Chinese communities across the Southeast Asian region – southern Chinese populations, the Hakka, are known to have settled in various parts of Southeast Asia, including Vietnam, as early as the seventeenth century, mainly as merchants.

Indeed, intense exchanges of ideas, knowledge, techniques, and consumer goods, including medical knowledge and therapies, had animated the region since the first wave of European expansion.[59] Vietnam, especially, was connected to China by deep-rooted networks of commercial and medical exchange. For more than one thousand years, when Vietnam was dominated by the Chinese imperial court, Vietnamese medicinal substances circulated northward, while prepared Chinese medicines made their way south.[60] Such exchanges are examined in Florence Yvon-Trân's study of artisanship and business in the Kinh Bac region of the Red River Delta. Strikingly, she reveals that one community, Ninh Giang, was engaged in the commercialization of local medicinal plants as well as the importation and resale of Chinese medicines to both consumers and therapists as early as the mid-seventeenth century. While Yvon-Trân was unable to determine how Chinese materials made their way south, she affirms that Ninh Giang's merchants did not need to travel to China.[61]

By the nineteenth century, according to early colonial accounts, significant quantities of medicinal commodities, including both raw substances and prepared medicines, entered Vietnam through well-established circuits. Likely from as early as the beginning of the eighteenth century onward, many were made into pill form, initially by using wax, partly in order to facilitate transportation. Itinerant merchants crossed from China into Vietnam near Lao Kay, by the Lô River (Rivière Claire), Mon Cay, or Ha Giang: "Caravans from Yunnan [. . .] once or twice a week [. . .] bring their merchandise by horseback [. . .]"

---

[58] Sherman Cochran, *Chinese Medicine Men. Consumer Culture in China and Southeast Asia* (Cambridge: Harvard University Press, 2006), 2–3.

[59] Anthony Reid, *Southeast Asia in the Age of Commerce, 1450–1680* (New Haven, CT: Yale University Press, vol. 2. Expansion and Crisis, 1993), and Harold J. Cook, *Matters of Exchange: Commerce, Medicine, and Science in the Dutch Golden Age* (New Haven, CT, and London: Yale University Press, 2007).

[60] On the historical influence of China over Vietnamese medicine, see C. Michele Thompson, *Vietnamese Traditional Medicine. A Social History* (Singapore: NUS Press, 2015).

[61] Florence Yvon-Trân, "Artisanat et commerce villageois dans le Viêt nam prémoderne, du XIe au XIXe siècle. Le cas de l'ancienne agglomération villageoise de Phu Ninh (région du Kinh Bac)," *Bulletin de l'École française d'Extrême-Orient* 88 (2001): 227–31, 240.

These Yunnanese exchange tea, opium, vegetables, chin-chai (Chinese medicines for rheumatism) for salt and cotton cloth."[62] These border areas, also used to traffic opium, weapons, and other illegal goods, were kept under close watch by colonial authorities from the 1860s.[63] Medicines containing plants harvested both locally and in China could also be purchased from Chinese residents established in the northern part of the country.[64] This busy trade in medicines provoked anxiety among colonial officials well before the 1908 Datura stramonium incident (see Chapter 1). Colonial correspondence from the late nineteenth century evokes Chinese, as well as Korean and Japanese, itinerant merchants who traveled with suitcases full of pills and tablets destined for shops and stalls across the territory.[65] With the development and equipment of the Red River Delta and the Mekong Delta with transport infrastructures, medicines and medicinal substances entered with increasing ease through the big ports, especially in Haiphong but also in Saigon.

In the first decades of the twentieth century, the border between China and Vietnam seems to have remained extremely porous. In addition, the Vietnamese increasingly participated in commercial exchanges with other Asian colonies: British Malaya, including the Strait Settlements of Singapore, Malacca, and Penang, as well as Hong Kong and British India, the Philippines, Korea, and the Dutch East Indies.[66] Products circulated through these networks because they were illegal (weapons, narcotics), because of high price differences between regions (rice, salt), but also because of the growing demand for new consumer goods, including alcohol, newspapers, cloth, and medicines.[67] Saigon and its twin city Cholon were key nodes in these increasingly diversified commercial networks. Northern locations in the Red River Delta and border provinces also continued to play an important role. As early as 1902, the unchecked circulation of medicines from Hong Kong in border areas prompted a request, by the Hanoi-based health committee of Tonkin, for an

---

[62] "Indochine. Les ressources du Haut-Tonkin," *La revue coloniale*, 10 (1895): 409.

[63] ANOM, RST NF 886, 4718, 4181, and 4182.

[64] Dr. Foiret, "Topographie médicale du poste de Haiphong," AMN (November 1878): 241–65.

[65] "Au sujet de la circulation au Tonkin de nombreux Chinois vendeurs de médicaments, septembre 1897," ANOM, Gougal 25900; "Surveillance des Chinois vendeurs de médicaments à Nam Dinh, 1909," VNA, centre no. 1, RST 8974; "Au sujet du passage de huit Chinois et d'un Coréen vendant des médicaments à Hoa Binh, 1924," ANOM, RST 48324.

[66] "Commerce. Les principaux produits d'échange de l'Indochine avec les autres pays d'Extrême-Orient (1er semestre 1903)," *La quinzaine coloniale*, April 10, 1904: 237–39.

[67] On these networks and traffics, see Eric Tagliacozzo, *Secret Trades, Porous Borders. Smuggling and States along a Southeast Asian Frontier, 1865–1915* (New Haven, CT: Yale University Press, 2005).

evaluation of the regulation of "Asian pharmacy."[68] The first pharmacy inspections in 1908 found that nearly all "Sino-Vietnamese pharmacies," particularly the "Chinese shops" of Cholon, sold products manufactured in China.[69] Inspectors described these products as highly diverse, with some being mass produced, and noted that some medicines traders had direct links with the emerging Hong Kong and Shanghai-based pharmaceutical industries.

By the late 1910s, according to diplomatic and consular documents, Asian non-Vietnamese firms that imported medicines, and in some cases manufactured them from imported raw products, were already well established in Cholon, Nam Dinh, and Haiphong.[70] Sam Nghiep Ltd., a drug company based in Korea, had a representative in Cochinchina by the name of Cao Ly Sam Tinh, as well as a distribution agency in Saigon beginning in the 1920s. Its medicines, including the Polar Star, were advertised in the popular press as "traditional" and sold by local druggists.[71] Some Asian companies even sought, rather naively, to have their products distributed by the colonial public health care system. In 1904, a Sumatra-based firm, Medicine Coy, sought permission to distribute its specialties via a Chinese merchant and the French consular services in the Dutch East Indies, in Batavia (Jakarta).[72] In 1919, a Chinese individual from Singapore by the name of Goh Lai Kang went as far as to ask the governor of Cochinchina to test his "infallible remedy" for cholera, named Queuesh, which, he claimed, was already authorized for sale in the British Straits Settlements.[73] Both requests were denied.

Products from the expanding Japanese pharmaceutical industry, some marketed as traditional medicines and others as innovative pharmaceuticals, appear to have been promoted in Vietnam with particular zeal from the 1900s. The investigation into the 1908 Maire affair revealed that a "Japanese medicines firm" had supplied not only Maire's Japanese clerk, Shigetaro Kuroshima, but also an impressive list of traders in Hanoi and other Tonkinese provinces.[74] In the 1930s, Nguyễn Pho, employed by the Hanoi-based An Hoa firm, acted as wholesaler for another Japanese company that dealt in traditional medicines, which he

[68] "Comité d'hygiène du Tonkin, 1902–1903," ANOM, Gougal 6707.
[69] ANOM, Gougal 17174.
[70] ANOM, RST NF 3684 and 4685.
[71] Advertisement, L'Écho, no. 779, January 6, 1927.
[72] "Consulat de France à Batavia. Offre de vente au gouvernement indochinois de médicaments faite par M. Fan, 1904," ANOM, Gougal 54243.
[73] Gougal SE 213 and 3160; "Pharmacie, importation frauduleuse, 1919," VNA, centre no. 2, IA8/237(4).
[74] ANOM, RST NF 894.

resold to several traders across the city.[75] By then, the Dainan Koosi firm had also established several branches across Indochina to distribute both Western and Asian, including "Sino-Japanese," specialties. Other commercial and shipping companies also invested in the importation of medicinal plants, such as Mitsui Bussan Kaisha Ltd.[76]

Medicines from Japan, however, had no legal status in Indochina, whether as modern drugs or as traditional medicines. Only medicines falling under the category of "Sino-Vietnamese remedies" could legally be imported from neighboring countries. China thus had an advantage over Japan in exporting its products to Vietnam until 1942, when a series of agreements with the Decoux' Vichy government legalized the presence of Japanese pharmaceutical firms.[77] Import circuits from Chinese, Japanese, and other Asian pharmaceutical industries in Indochina nevertheless brought, or attempted to bring, a wide variety of pharmaceutical specialties labeled as "traditional" to Vietnamese consumers. Some shops sold "exotic Anglo-Indian products" from Shanghai, which, according to *La tribune indigène*, were very popular in Saigon.[78] In 1934, the head inspector of pharmacies for Tonkin noted that a large number of traditional medicines were packaged to look like French specialties (one of the previously mentioned forms of hybrid specialty). He conceded that it would be extremely difficult to prevent this "progress."[79]

Archival information on druggists and sellers who were involved in these networks is profoundly marked by authorities' anxieties, but also by their ignorance. An apparent source of fear was the impressive quantity of such actors, in sharp contrast with the scarcity of biomedical health care professionals. In May of 1920, a bill was proposed with the rather naive objective of limiting the number of authorized "Sino-Vietnamese therapists" to 500 in Cochinchina (we will come back to this in Chapter 5). A recent nominative survey ordered by the governor general had estimated there were 1,660.[80] Seventy-five traders of Sino-Vietnamese medicines were spread out among 41 villages in the single province of My Tho; there were 152 in Ben Tre.[81] In 1931, an inspector of pharmacies

---

[75] "Demande d'importation et de vente de médicaments japonais formulée par M. Bui Duy Dan, Hanoi, 1939," ANOM, RST NF 3710.

[76] *L'Écho*, no. 152, April 1–2, 1940.

[77] Among these firms were Kichuchi Shikko and Dainan Koosi, which manufactured several sulfonamides at the time (ANOM, RST NF 3710; "Lettre confidentielle du délégué permanent du commerce colonial en Indochine au Directeur des services économiques, Saigon, 8 septembre 1942," ANOM, Gougal SE 213).

[78] Un médicastre, "Laboratoire d'analyse," *La tribune indigène*, no. 76, June 3, 1918.

[79] ANOM, RST NF 3684.

[80] ANOM, Aff. Po 3242.

[81] "Pharmacie. Pharmaciens chinois et indigènes. Etats nominatifs dans diverses provinces et ville de Saigon-Cholon, 1921," VNA, centre no. 2, IA-8/285(3).

estimated that 1,700 permanent shops (that is, excluding mobile stalls) sold medicines in Tonkin; 188 were in Thai Binh, 180 in Ha Dong and Hanoi, and 77 in Sontay, which explains why the only Western-trained pharmacist in Sontay City complained bitterly of their competition.[82]

Although I did not create a systematic repertory of these various traders, which would anyhow have been an impossible task (especially given that many traders escaped the trade license system, such as itinerant vendors, and that their practices and expertise were difficult for authorities to pin down using legal and biomedical criteria), I could easily identify thousands of names in my sources. These individuals were spread out widely across the territory – especially in comparison with AMI staff and private pharmacists – in both urban and rural areas. By the end of the 1930s (relatively reliable statistics are available for 1937), there was at least 1 traditional medicine shop for each 4,700 individuals in Ha Dong; 1 for 3,900 in Rach Gia; 1 for 3,800 in Son Tay; and 1 for 858 in Hanoi.[83] Recall that, in the same year, there was no more than 1 doctor for every 40,000 inhabitants in Tonkin.

Further information is provided in pharmacy inspection reports and applications for trading licenses – submitted in the wake of proposed laws to limit the number of authorized Sino-Vietnamese dealers in Cochinchina in 1920 and across the Union a year later. They reveal, notably, that a high proportion of these traders were of Chinese origin. Of the 21 "Asian pharmacies" inspected in Saigon in December 1915, 17 (about 85 percent) were Chinese-owned, another 3 were owned by Vietnamese individuals, and 1 was owned by a *minh hương*, a Sino-Vietnamese. By 1920, a list of 38 "Asian pharmacies" in Saigon, acknowledged in the source as a probable underestimation, attributes 34 to Chinese owners.[84] This predominance of Chinese-owned businesses was also observed in the provinces at the time, accounting for 60 out of 85 surveyed shops in My Tho (the rest were "Annamese," except one "European," named Tiêu Pham, possibly a naturalized métis), while Chinese applicants for trading licenses in 1920–21 account for 34 out of 38 businesses in Vinh Long, all of the 11 in Chau Doc, 90 out of 108 in Ben Tre, and 47 out of 60 in Rach Gia.[85] The situation was similar in

---

[82] VNA, centre no. 1, RST NF 3683 and RST 47835.

[83] VNA, centre no. 2, IA8/285(4).

[84] "Procès-verbal constatant la visite par la commission d'inspection des boutiques de droguistes, médecins et épiciers indigènes qui font le commerce des drogues et médicaments sino-annamites, Commissariat de police, Saigon, 2e arrondissement, 28 décembre 1915," ANOM, Gougal 17174; VNA, centre no. 2, IA-8/285(3).

[85] "Pharmacie – pharmacies chinoises et indigènes (dossiers individuels). Arrêtés autorisant ouverture dans diverses provinces, ville de Saigon (arrêté 23/5/21). Demande d'autorisations, 1921–1922," VNA, centre no. 2, Goucoch IA-8/ 285(4).

Tonkin, where not one of the twenty-three requests for legalization in Hanoi, Haiphong, and Nam Dinh made in 1921 was identified as having been submitted by an "Annamese."[86]

The connections available to the Chinese diaspora probably put Vietnamese traders at a disadvantage, and would explain the durability of Chinese dominance in the medicines business. The same documents, however, also reveal a marked Vietnamization of this trade beginning in the 1920s. This trend can be linked to the emergence of a Viêt middle class of small business-owners, as mentioned previously. An economic nationalist movement was also launched in Cochinchina in 1919, supporting the boycott of Chinese products and proposing viable alternatives to the importation of common consumer goods.[87] By the early 1920s, when the number of Vietnamese biomedically trained pharmacists and doctors was also growing, there were hundreds of Vietnamese-owned "traditional" medicines shops, thus signaling the start of a marked indigenization of the health sector as a whole.

A few of these Vietnamese drugstores quickly, in just a few years, acquired a reputation for the quality of their products, such as the Grande pharmacie sino-vietnamienne de Vinh, owned by Phó Đức Thành. Phó Đức Thành, author of an impressive number of drug catalogues and authoritative texts on Vietnamese therapeutics, regularly advertised his business in *Lực tỉnh tân văn. Gazette de Cochinchine* and *Đại Việt tạp chí. Revue indigène de l'Indochine. Organe de propagande de la pensée française.* Another drugstore owner, Đăng Thúc Liêng (Saigon) became, after writing a book that combined the genres of a scientific manual and a commercial almanac, the president of an influential group the Viêt nam y dược hội (Association of Sino-Vietnamese Doctors and Pharmacists; see Chapter 7).[88]

Also striking in the license applications of 1920–21 is that a considerable number of Chinese and Vietnamese traders reported that

[86] "Au sujet du commerce de médicaments de la pharmacopée indigène, 1921–1922," VNA, centre no. 1, RST 48311; "Demandes d'autorisation de faire le commerce de médicaments formulées par Lo Can Ky et Quan Ley Tching à Hanoi, 1921," VNA, centre no. 1, RST 48039; "Demande d'autorisation de faire le commerce de médicaments présentée par Lo Pock Tchi à Nam Dinh, 1921–1922," VNA, centre no. 1, RST 48319.

[87] Micheline Lessard, "Organisons-nous! Racial Antagonism and Vietnamese Economic Nationalism in the Early Twentieth Century," *French Colonial History* 8 (2007): 171–201.

[88] Đăng Thúc Liêng, *Tri y tiện dụng quyễn chi nhứt: biết đạo y cách dụng phuống tiện. Cuốn thú nhứt* (Sadec: Imprimerie Bao Tôn, 1931).On Đăng Thúc Liêng's professional and political activities, see Alexander Woodside, "The Development of Social Organizations in Vietnamese Cities in the Late Colonial Period," *Pacific Affairs* 41, 1 (1971): 43.

they had opened their businesses recently, after 1905, or even, in many cases, after the war. Of thirty-eight shops in Saigon, eighteen had opened between 1905 and 1918, and fourteen after 1919. More than half of the shops in Ben Tre had opened within the previous eight years: only two before 1905, seventy-two between 1905 and 1918 (of which forty-four opened during the war), and forty-three afterwards.[89] It is difficult to track this expansion in detail, but one thing is clear: the AMI did not reduce the presence of Chinese and Vietnamese drugs or druggists. Quite the opposite: wartime supply difficulties, shortages in both biomedical staff and medicines, and difficulties in accessing public and especially free treatment may have contributed to a densification of the offer for medicines labeled as "Sino-Vietnamese" or "traditional."

4.5   A Lucrative Trade: The Emergence of a "Small Pharma"

From the 1930s, overviews of the trade in Sino-Vietnamese medicines noted recent changes, both quantitative and qualitative. Writing in 1931, Dr. Albert Sallet, a keen observer of local medical and healing practices, observed an increase in the number of simple traders of medicines, although "pharmacy" and herbalism, in the markets and on the streets, also continued to thrive.[90] Among the hundreds of catalogues and almanacs produced by Vietnamese druggists and therapists at that time, many were used to promote a new, scientific traditional medicine.[91] In 1949, the pharmacist Bedel remarked on the popularity, in both city and countryside, of Sino-Vietnamese medicines, and described a lucrative trade of plants and simple remedies on the streets. He also noted that Vietnamese businesses were "catching up" with the "more advanced" Chinese pharmacies.[92]

Both Sallet and Bedel also pointed out the existence of enterprising new actors who lacked experience, and who were improperly trained and in some cases even unscrupulous and exploitative, and thus posed risks for the health of gullible clients. The AMI doctors Millous and Nguyễn Văn Hoành had already insisted in the BSMI in 1926 on the need to

[89] VNA, centre no. 1, IA-8/285(3); "Pharmacie – pharmacies chinoises et indigènes (dossiers individuels), Arrêtés autorisant l'ouverture dans différentes provinces, ville de Saigon (arrêté du 23 mai 1921). Demandes d'autorisation, 1921–1922," VNA, centre no. 1, IA-8/285(4).
[90] Albert Sallet, *L'officine sino-annamite. La médecine annamite et la préparation des remèdes* (Paris: Imprimerie nationale, 1931).
[91] Annick Guénel, "Nationalism and Vietnamese Medicine" (paper presented at the Eleventh International Conference on the History of Science in East Asia, Munich, Germany, August 13, 2005).
[92] Bedel, "La pharmacie en Indochine."

distinguish between an older, better-educated set of medicine traders who knew their "doctrine and materia medica and [sold] toxics with care," and a "new generation that is more ignorant and dangerous, causing a growing number of poisoning [incidents]."[93] Such comments and distinctions were echoed not only by pharmacy inspectors but also by associations of therapists who claimed to practice "true" Vietnamese medicine.[94]

Attacks on corrupt, greedy, and incompetent traders of Sino-Vietnamese medicines were not exclusively motivated by the protection of public health. Nor was this critique simply a product of colonial arrogance and ignorance. It also arose as part of some Vietnamese thera-pists' efforts to define and defend their profession against competition and a tainted reputation. Others criticized "bad" healers in the defense of nationalist pride or the goals of modernization, calling on the colonial administration to enforce the law more effectively and to improve access to biomedical care. In 1924, an auxiliary doctor, Lam Chan Manh, partly blamed the inaccessibility of Western medicines for the popularity, even in the countryside, of a growing range of aggressively advertised Chinese specialties "promising miracle upon miracle."[95] L'Écho, a tribune for progress and modernization, was particularly active in this crusade. In 1921, for example, the journalist Minh Nguyệt criticized Chinese mer-chants from Cholon for flooding the Vietnamese press with advertise-ments for Chinese drugs, intending only to "take advantage of the ignorance and misplaced trust of our compatriots."[96] In January 1923, an article described the death of the patient of a "pseudo" Sino-Vietnamese doctor caused by an excessive dose of purgatives combined with other plant-based remedies, which had been prescribed on the basis of an incorrect diagnosis – the "doctor" would be arrested and convicted of manslaughter.[97] A few years later, another victim, a "housewife in Binh Trao," was raped by a "Malaysian healer" who had promised to cure her, within three days, of "disappointments in love and hallucinations."[98]

[93] Pierre Millous and Nguyễn Văn Hoành, "Intoxication par usage prolongé d'une médication de droguiste sino-annamite contenant de la strychnine," BSMI 4, 1 (1926): 27–28.

[94] "Rapport sanitaire annuel du Tonkin, 1936," ANOM, RST NF 3686; T. L. "La querelle séculaire entre les anciens et les modernes. Les deux arts de guérir. Une science contre l'empirisme – il s'agit de leur donner des armes égales," L'Écho, no. 170, May 17–18, 1940.

[95] Lam Chanh Manh, "Médecine française et propagande," Bulletin de l'Amicale des médecins auxiliaires de l'Indochine 7 (1924): 149.

[96] Minh Nguyệt, "Médecine chinoise . . . et réclame," L'Écho, no. 201, June 16, 1921.

[97] L'Écho, no. 424, January 3, 1923.

[98] "Mytho. Charlatan et satyr," L'Écho, no. 1080, January 27, 1928.

Such reports of abuse were published up until the end of the colonial period.[99]

Regardless of its form, the trade in "old" and "new" Vietnamese medicines was clearly a lucrative and versatile one. The range of labels used to describe traders draws attention not only to their heterogeneity but also to their capacity for innovation. It also reveals the colonial government's struggle to impose a classification system on this complex therapeutic landscape. In addition to *pharmacien annamite* (Annamese pharmacist or Chinese pharmacist, native pharmacist, Sino-Annamese pharmacist), *droguiste* (druggist), and *herboriste* (herbalist), authorities used less specific terms such as *marchand de médicaments* (medicines trader) and *vendeur de pilules* (pill peddler). In the 1920s and 1930s, many businesses sold medicines alongside other products and services, announcing, for example, *imprimerie et pilules* (printing and pills), *pilules et pâtisserie* (pills and pastry shop), *nickelage et médicaments* (nickel-plating and medicines), *bijouterie et remèdes* (jewelry and remedies), or *horlogerie et épicerie* (clocks and groceries). Others, however, sold only a limited set of specific remedies, in particular to treat STIs.[100] In 1926, an inspector of pharmacies in Tonkin visited several *marchands de pilules contre la fièvre* (fever pill merchants). These were reported to mobilize clerks and produce attractive prospectuses, color catalogues, and eye-catching placards, reaching far into the countryside.[101] Thus both "Western-style" and "Sino-Vietnamese" drug distributors used the same type of publicity materials and strategies to attract clients, in particular by aggressively, and skillfully, promoting a few key products.[102] As new commodities, these neo-traditional, local, and hybrid specialties suggest that drug production processes had become increasingly industrialized, standardized, and serialized by the late 1930s.

[99] See also, in *L'Écho*: "Charlatan pincé," no. 298, June 5, 1925; "Serait-ce un phénomène de génération spontanée?," no. 1006, October 20, 1927; Nguyễn Phan Long, "Les docteurs d'Occident vont-ils relever le gant?," no. 1299, August 11, 1928.

[100] "Prophylaxie des maladies vénériennes, 1917–1940" and "Lettre de Terrisse, Directeur local de la santé à M. le Résident de France à Hadong, 19 mai 1937," ANOM, RST NF 3856.

[101] "Rapport de l'Inspecteur des pharmacies du Tonkin concernant l'inspection des pharmacies européennes, des boutiques de médicaments sino-annamites, photographes et tous magasins soumis au décret du 16 janvier 1919, 1927," VNA, centre no. 1, RST 32073.

[102] This marketing talent has been analyzed for other East and Southeast Asian countries: Cochran, *Chinese Medicine Men*; Sivaramakrishnan, *Old Potions*, 104–57; Wendy Suiyi Wong, "Establishing the Modern Advertising Languages. Patent Medicine Newspaper Advertisements in Hong Kong, 1945–69," *Journal of Design History* 13, 3 (2000): 213–26; Liew Kai Khiun, "Newspapers and the Communication of Medical Sciences in Colonial Malaya, 1840s–1941," *EASTS. East Asian Science, Technology and Society. An International Journal* 3, 2–3 (2009): 209–30.

The local proto-industry of hybrid specialties cannot be entirely separated from the emerging industrialization of the Western(ized) pharmaceutical sector. Several well-established and successful private "European pharmacies" had clearly, by 1940, been turned into sites of research, development, and production of prepared medicines that could no longer be called artisanal. While this embryonic industry remained fragile during a period of growing political and socioeconomic unrest, the outbreak of World War II appears to have accelerated its emergence. Major wartime shortages of both basic chemicals and pharmaceuticals created a pressing demand for local alternatives and innovation. From 1940, as colonial health authorities began to organize local pharmacological research, particularly into the composition of local cheap and/or available specialties and commonly used traditional remedies (see Chapters 5 and 8),[103] a few local chemical firms and pharmacies, which were equipped with research laboratories, launched private initiatives to produce medicines, including of synthetic drugs. Among these were French, Vietnamese, and a few mixed-ownership firms.

In the late 1920s, Chassagne's pharmacy housed, at its address, the Laboratoire du Collyre Jaune, a lab which produced the highly advertised eponymous eye drops. In 1936, an advertisement for La Rose du Dr. Aboud suggests that Chassagne's "Laboratoires R. E. L." had moved.[104] Was this a new name for the Laboratoire du Collyre Jaune, indicating an expansion in Pharmacie Chassagne's manufacturing activities? One cannot say. We do not know what became of the Laboratoires R. E. L. either, but in 1942, Jean Roux, owner of the Pharmacie Blanc in Hanoi, created one of the first real pharmaceutical laboratories in Vietnam in order to produce caffeine and several organotherapeutic specialties.[105] The Laboratoires Bonniot, of the name of the owner of the Pharmacie Mus in Saigon, which was directed by the pharmacists Henri-Francis Gamby and Nguyễn Văn Cao, also produced chemical products and specialties.[106] In 1943, René Clogne, of the Pharmacie Métropole in Saigon, founded the Usines Chimiques de la Pharmacie Métropole (Chemical Factory of the Pharmacie Métropole), which produced acetic acid, cresol, yellow mercuric oxide, as well as organotherapeutic products. Hồ Đắc Ân, a former AMI pharmacist

---

[103] Monnais and Tousignant, "The Values of Versatility."

[104] Advertisement, BAYB, no. 21, March 1936.

[105] This seems to have been one of the only French retail pharmacies that survived the war. Roux was apparently able to obtain supplies thanks to his privileged commercial links with Java in the Dutch East Indies.

[106] A. Bigot and Roger F. Auriol, "Le problème des médicaments en Indochine de 1940 à 1945," *Produits pharmaceutiques* 2, 3 (1947): 109–19.

who set out on his own in Saigon in the 1930s, developed various procedures to make cholesterol (using beef brains), eucalyptol, lecithin, ben-
zoic acid, and histidine.[107]

Only after 1945, however, did a real pharmaceutical industry emerge in
Vietnam, catalyzed by new political imperatives: at first, to achieve
national self-sufficiency in antibiotics and vaccines, and soon, also, to
renovate a traditional and distinctively Vietnamese therapeutics.[108] Yet
one can locate its precursors in the multiform nascent industrial fabric of
the interwar period, which was fueled by the design and production of,
and the creation of markets for, specialties that circulated in "Asian" and
"Western," as well as "traditional" and "modern," sectors of the drug
business. Both hybrid and Western specialties were given multiple and
dynamic identities that drew on local references while emphasizing innovation. The resulting complexity and confusion in this (or these) eclectic
therapeutic market(s) explains in part why colonial authorities sought to
legislate access to medicines with increasing rigidity, to the extent that
they redefined the field of Vietnamese medicine, a redefinition whose far-
reaching stakes and consequences were as much political and economic
as they were sanitary and commercial.

Private pharmacists who worked in Vietnam, and who greatly out-
numbered pharmacists working for the colonial administration, maintained links with colonial authorities for a variety of reasons – including
but not limited to the search for stable sources of revenue – at least until
the 1910s. On the whole, however, it seems that they kept their distance
from the AMI and its objectives. They had no particular interest in
subscribing to the administration's public health priorities, and so presented themselves as "neutral" health care professionals. They were not
agents of the colonial administration and thus did not necessarily follow
the rules of a "colonial-style" medicalization. While the distribution of
pharmacists matched, to some extent, the density and gaps of the AMI
system, pharmacists did manage to somewhat extend their reach beyond
the largest cities. In addition, qualified pharmacists were far from the only
mediators of access to medicines, including modern medicines, in
Vietnam. Other types of drug traders, including those selling new products labeled as "Sino-Vietnamese," were even more widely spread out.

---

[107] "Les relations nouvelles de l'industrie chimique dans le Sud indochinois," *L'Écho*,
May 11, 1944.
[108] Ayo Wahlberg, "Bio-politics and the Promotion of Traditional Herbal Medicine in
Vietnam," *Health. An Interdisciplinary Journal for the Social Study of Health, Illness and
Medicine* 10, 2 (2006): 123–47. It should be noted that a few French firms continued to
remain active until 1954, and even later in the South of the country, since economic and
commercial links were maintained to some extent between France and the Republic of
Vietnam.

Not only did they draw on a longstanding identity as privileged intermediaries of care and on pre-colonial networks; they also developed new
business practices and new drugs during the first decades of the twentieth
century. In addition to dealing in the ingredients and formulae of a well-
codified pharmacopeia, some of these actors incorporated a variety of new
types of medicines that were at once Asian, traditional, and modern.
Practices, products, and actors constantly crossed the lines between
supposedly separate sectors, becoming entangled in relations of competition, exchange, and mutual influence. Hybrid specialties appear as
a marker of these dynamics. Apparently very similar, the strategies
deployed by both pharmacists and "Sino-Vietnamese druggists" reveal
how these actors identified and leveraged local market opportunities – in
other words, how they sought to adapt to and act on the legal, socioeconomic, and geographic specificities of colonial Vietnam. This, of
course, did not always please the colonial authorities, especially staff of
the Customs Agency and of the AMI. The proliferation of attempts to
tighten legislative control over modes of access to pharmaceuticals and
local responses to these restrictions, both licit and illicit, are in themselves
suggestive of the complexity and dynamism of the Vietnamese drug
market before 1940.

5   Crimes and Misdemeanors: Transactions and Transgressions in the Therapeutic Market

The complexity and creativity of the private trade in medicines in colonial Vietnam manifested itself with particular intensity in the illegal practices reported by French authorities. As seen in Chapter 4, both state-qualified pharmacists and sellers of "traditional" medicines fought, vigorously and with ingenuity, to secure and expand their markets, flexibly adapting to new sources of influence and competition, to changing demand, and to the gaps and shortcomings of the public system. In this, they often tested the limits of legality, sometimes crossing the line into patently illegal practice, for which they were occasionally caught. Laws on the practice of medicine and pharmacy, on the importation and sale of toxic substances, and on trademark registration and infringement defined a number of infractions. Anyone – professional or layperson, public or private, biomedically trained or not – could be accused of these. And, indeed, they were. The colonial and health authorities were apparently much more concerned with controlling the drug market than they were with providing the Vietnamese population with access to efficient and safe drugs. Yet, unsurprisingly, the colonial administration's ability to detect and to prosecute pharmaceutical offenses was limited. The mechanisms created to apply and enforce the increasingly numerous, sometimes redundant, rules of safe therapeutic and commercial practice included the Pharmacy Inspection Service, created in 1908, and the Service de répression des fraudes (Fraud Control Service). Despite their dysfunctions, these two colonial services left precious, although scattered, records of how control measures were enforced (or not), and, especially, on whom and why. The popular press also exposed scandals, reported on trials, and, from time to time, denounced unethical practices, thus providing further information on the contested limits of "proper" drug distribution and on borderline strategies. The focus of this chapter is not on illegal, unethical, or dangerous practices of drug distribution (and possibly consumption) per se. Rather, it seeks, by exploring the margins of legality and appropriateness, to provide an alternative vantage on the extremely dynamic and complex nature of the market for medicines. It pays particular attention to the products traded in this marginal space, from quinine to Dagénan, via anti-opium cures, and to their undeniable power of attraction.

5.1   Regulating Vietnamese Medicine: A Predictable Failure

Illegal and illicit practices – and what they reveal about colonial longings for control as well as about "unruly" commercial and therapeutic impulses – were partly demarcated by the dense legislative framework for the practice of Western and French pharmacy described in Chapter 1. They were further defined by a series of energetic, but ultimately failed, attempts to control non-biomedical actors' involvement in the distribution of remedies, including modern medical and commercial specialties. Indeed, with the exception of the brief and limited case of essential medicines outlets after 1927, traders of the so-called Sino-Vietnamese therapeutic sector were strictly prohibited from the manipulation and sale of "European medicines." This exclusion depended on the ambitious task of defining, at least legally, what the traditional sector actually was, notably, to pin down its practitioners and their therapeutic substances. It was also part of a broader set of attempts – underpinned by a conviction both in biomedicine's superiority and in the dangers of Vietnamese medicine – to use the law in order to marginalize non-biomedical health actors. A vast realm of illegal drug distribution practices was designated by colonial legal attempts to sharply distinguish, and render impermeable, the respective fields of "Western" and "Sino-Vietnamese" medicine and medicines. Yet at the same time, this realm was animated by practices that defied this distinction, playing on the highly flexible cultural and commercial identities of therapeutic products and responding to the demands and desires, opportunities, and accessibility gaps that colonial law failed to address.

Until the late nineteenth century, traditional therapists and druggists were apparently tolerated – and even in some cases employed – by the first colonial hospitals and consultation services.[1] While the professionalization of medical science had already set the scene for a sharper, more hierarchical differentiation between Western and Vietnamese medical systems, their incompatibility was only really established following the advent of synthetic, specific antimicrobial drugs. At the turn

---

[1] Dr. Charles-Édouard Hocquard, *Une campagne au Tonkin*, intro. and ed. by Philippe Papin (Paris: Arléa, 1999 [1892]); "Cochinchine – Cambodge. Statistiques, rapport sur le service sanitaire et les hôpitaux, 1865–1889. Rapport sur l'hôpital de Choquan par le médecin en chef directeur de l'hôpital, 1885," ANOM, AF Indo 323 Y03(1).

of the twentieth century, an increasingly harsh and uncompromising condemnation of Vietnamese medicine emerged in the writings of colonial doctors, as well as of biomedically trained Vietnamese doctors and of some Vietnamese reformist intellectuals and journalists. This intensified contempt was expressed by asserting that its remedies were ineffective and toxic, and that it lacked a scientific basis. Fears of therapeutic as well as commercial competition also, as mentioned previously, played a role. With the declared objective of protecting public health, the project of regulating indigenous medicine essentially took the form of a series of attempted measures to indirectly, yet drastically, restrict its domain of practice, in particular by prohibiting the manipulation and dispensation of toxic substances. These measures were "indirect" because, officially, the control of Vietnamese medicine remained the prerogative of imperial authorities.[2] Thus the main pathway for French colonial regulation was through legislation on toxic substances, buttressed by the law of July 1919, which imposed restrictions handling many substances used in Vietnamese therapeutics. Vietnamese medicine was to be subdued by rendering its remedies inoffensive, thereby relegating its actors to a subordinate status. Without criminalizing it as a whole, the law pushed key areas of therapeutic practice beyond the boundaries of legality.

A first series of bills, remarkably similar in structure and intent, were put on the table between 1913 and 1926. They proposed to impose on non-biomedical therapists and druggists some of the same rules that governed the practice of metropolitan pharmacy, with additional restrictions on the types of medicines they were allowed to manipulate and sell. A first proposal to regulate the "business of Sino-Annamese pharmacies and medicines" in Indochina was put forward in 1913–14. It laid the groundwork for transferring metropolitan requirements for the practice of pharmacy to the sale of Sino-Vietnamese medicines: obligatory "pharmacy" ownership; use of prescriptions for dispensing toxic substances; keeping up-to-date stock inventories, registers of toxic substances, and transcribed prescriptions; and the obligation to submit to regular inspections. It also prohibited the sale of "chemicals and medicines used by the European, American and Japanese pharmacopeias," from which only twenty-two substances, considered to be widely used in Vietnamese therapeutics, were exempt. There is no information in the archives on how this list was established. It included several highly toxic minerals such

---

[2] Some French doctors and administrators were opposed to any attempt to legislate on Vietnamese medicine, on the grounds that this was seen as conceding that it had some value and giving it an officially recognized status.

as yellow arsenic, calomel (mercury chloride), and cinnabar (mercury sulfide).

The 1913 bill was criticized for extending the restrictions but not the protections provided by metropolitan pharmacy legislation. It was quickly rejected by the inspector general of health services, Paul-Louis Simond.[3] While Simond was no fervent advocate of local medical traditions, he firmly believed it would be ill-advised to drastically restrict or to Westernize these, if only because they offered a much-needed source of basic care. At the same time, he warned that the bill did not sufficiently protect consumers from the toxicity of Vietnamese remedies, and suggested instead that a comprehensive list of allowable products, including specified dosage ranges, be drawn up, with the help of local specialists, as a sort of *Codex annamite* (Annamese pharmacopeia).[4] Claiming to revise this and other aborted legislative projects, the 1921 governor general's bill nevertheless again proposed to impose metropolitan rules on the traditional drug sector. In addition, it sought to control therapists and druggists through a licensing system, as mentioned in Chapter 4, which would cap the number of licenses granted per province (determined in proportion to population size) and impose professional taxes.[5]

The law's proposed restrictions on medicines for import and sale by traditional practitioners also went further than the 1913 bill in defining the Sino-Vietnamese therapeutic field by what it should *not* be (i.e., toxic and modern). Prohibited from selling any *produit pharmaceutique* (pharmaceutical product) and foreign specialty, therapists and druggists were left with two (legal) categories: "animal-based medicines" (excluding organotherapeutic drugs and several types of beetles, such as cantharides, mylabris, and meloes) and medicinal plants. There were also proscribed plants, specified in a list of about thirty species. The 1921 list included several substances categorized as "schedule A" by the 1919 law – such as Datura stramonium, aconite, belladonna, and Nux vomica (strychnine) – that were widely and effectively used in Vietnamese therapeutics to treat common afflictions.

This new set of restrictions incensed some traders' associations, who condemned the double standards applied in regulating "Western" and "Asian" pharmacy. They also pointed out that some traditional medicines

---

[3] "Lettre du médecin-principal Dumas, Directeur local de la santé en Cochinchine au Gouverneur de la Cochinchine, Saigon, 5 août 1914," ANOM, Gougal 17172.
[4] "Lettre de l'Inspecteur général de l'hygiène et des services de santé Simond au Gouverneur général de l'Indochine, Hanoi, 6 août 1915," ANOM, Gougal 17172.
[5] Although it lumped potential licensees into the catchall category of "traditional therapists," the 1921 bill at least promised them some advantages by prohibiting the sale of medicines in stalls and public places, with the exception of nontoxic medicinal plants.

were effective, as well as modern, mentioning, in particular, some of the Chinese- and Vietnamese-manufactured products described previously as hybrid.[6] Their anger was also directed at additional taxation: therapists from Tonkin were particularly indignant at being taxed twice, both as "pharmacists" and as "doctors."[7] In the face of these reactions, the 1921 bill was suspended and then abandoned. And yet, the governor general proposed a strikingly similar text in March 1926. Opposition broke out almost instantly, as the new bill coincided with the death and funeral of the popular nationalist leader Phan Châu Trinh, as well as with a major student strike in Saigon Native Girls School.[8] Vietnamese druggists and therapists objected to increased restrictions on substances commonly used in Vietnamese therapeutics, including the elimination of exemptions, notably on mercury sulfide, arsenic sulfide, and strychnine. This again forced the delay, and then the abrogation, of the law.[9]

From the mid-1920s, there was a growing call for gaining better knowledge of the Vietnamese pharmacopeia in which to anchor these proliferating attempts at regulation, as Simond had suggested in 1913. The governor general set up no fewer than three investigative commissions in 1925, 1933, and 1938 to study Vietnamese medicine. At the outset of the first commission, Laurent Gaide, then inspector general of health services, proposed a "systematic study" of the Sino-Vietnamese pharmacopeia.[10] Soon abandoned, this ambitious project was revived as an explicit mandate of the second commission "to study the pharmacopeia in view of elaborating a compendium" as the necessary basis for any regulatory system. The commission generated yet another regulatory proposal – but no compendium.[11] Wisely, the proposal was sounded

---

[6] "Requête adressée par les pharmaciens chinois au Tonkin tendant à obtenir les modifications de la réglementation sur le commerce des médicaments sino-annamites, 1921," VNA, centre no. 1, RST 48343.

[7] Such double taxation was also a legal contradiction, given that, according to metropolitan law, the functions of doctor and pharmacists were strictly exclusive (VNA, centre no. 1, RST 48343; "La médecine sino-annamite dans nos campagnes," *L'Écho*, no. 269, December 1, 1921).

[8] Gail P. Kelly, "Conflict in the Classroom: A Case Study from Vietnam, 1918–1938," *British Journal of Sociology of Education* 8, 2 (1987): 201–2.

[9] VNA, centre no. 1, RST 48079.

[10] Laurent Gaide, "Note sur l'étude de la pharmacopée sino-annamite," BSMI 6, 1 (1928): 13–14.

[11] "Pièces de principe, réponse au vœu 43 tendant au maintien du statu quo pour la réglementation de la vente des médicaments sino-annamites, 1933," ANOM, Gougal 44461. This ambition to elaborate a compendium was never concretized. There are various likely reasons for this, notably its impracticability given that the time and expertise this project would have required, particularly for translations from classical Chinese – the language of the most popular compendia of Vietnamese medicine – to French and then quốc ngữ.

out before the Grand Conseil des intérêts économiques et financiers (Grand Council of Economic and Financial Interests), a mixed assembly of fifty-one French and indigenous members, which gave its advice on economic and financial decision-making pertaining to the colony. Fearing renewed outcry, the counselors advised shelving this project as well. The third commission, which first met in March 1938, concluded with a proposal for a categorical prohibition on the use of any toxic substance by any kind of non-biomedical practitioner.[12] Despite contemporary debates about the utility of Vietnamese therapeutics in the face of the AMI's evident failure to provide universal access to basic care (see Chapter 8), these conclusions were used as the basis for another decree dated October 1939. Its proposed restrictions were protested, even before the law was deposed, under the aegis, in particular, of the Association of Sino-Vietnamese doctors and pharmacists, the Việt nam y dược hội, giving rise to an impressive media campaign. Again, this law was abandoned.[13]

Yet the 1939 decree would rise from the ashes in late 1942 under the Vichy government and wartime conditions.[14] This last regulatory attempt sought in particular to define what should fall under the heading of the *pharmacopée sino-indochinoise traditionnelle* (traditional Sino-Indochinese pharmacopeia). This naming is in itself indicative of the approximations and misjudgments that informed this law – for there is no such thing as a "Sino-Indochinese" pharmacopoeia, given that "Indochina" was a colonial construct and had no shared medical or therapeutic history or culture. Its descriptions of "Sino-Indochinese" therapeutic ingredients, forms, and practices were vague and circular. Essentially, it defined these as being prepared "according to traditional forms," or as "using special traditional means." Its exclusions, however, were extensive and detailed, including any chemical, synthetic, or industrially prepared products; vaccines and serums; mineral waters; and a highly detailed list of pharmaceutical forms, including tablets, capsules, solutions in ampoules or flasks for hypodermic injection, granules, suppositories, and industrially prepared pills, coated pills, or ovules; as well as surgical acts and obstetrical manipulations. It also prohibited medical acts based on Western diagnostic and therapeutic methods and instruments. Not only were practitioners' fields of practice defined increasingly narrowly as "makers of traditional medicines," "traditional therapists," or "merchants of

[12] ANOM, Gougal SE 213.
[13] ANOM, Gougal SE 213.
[14] Although it was ratified in 1943, this text was never really applied. In July of 1942, another decree once again addressed the issue of quotas, per province, for Sino-Vietnamese practitioners.

medicinal plants"; they were also to be subjected to a panoply of authorization, taxation, and other control measures.

The 1942 text tellingly conflates Vietnamese with "traditional" in the
sense of non-modern, non-scientific, and "natural,"[15] reinforcing its
relegation to the status of a second-class and complementary medicine
confined to the treatment of minor ailments. It allowed for no overlap or
similarity between Asian/Vietnamese/indigenous therapies and pharmaceuticals, the latter belonging exclusively to the modern, biomedical
world. This law might be seen as the apogee of colonial desire for
a clear and uncompromising separation between the two medical systems. This separation was incompatible, however, with the dynamic
transformation of the field of Vietnamese medicine during this period,
as well as with the glaring gaps in the accessibility of biomedical care.
Even if they were abandoned, the series of legislative projects proposed
between 1913 and 1942 are a cumulative expression of the deep-seated
and growing conviction of many colonial experts and observers that
Vietnamese medicine was inherently dangerous and devoid of professional or scientific safeguards – ignorance of medicinal dosages, for example, was frequently decried – and thus could not be condoned. Alternating
between a process of biomedicalization and one of disembodiment, in the
sense of severing the connections between the component parts of
a medical system, these legal initiatives heralded the profound ambiguities of later postcolonial and international approaches to so-called alternative medicines and their *domestication*.[16] Pharmacy inspection and
fraud control reports reveal the extent to which this legislation was
impossible to enforce, above all because it failed to grasp the realities of
the "traditional medicines" circulating during this period.

5.2   Pharmacy Inspection and Fraud Control from Discourse to Reality

In 1942, in a letter to the governor general, the inspector general of health
services not only reasserted the necessary distinction between true, well-
trained therapeutic experts and commercially-motivated "pseudo
healers"; he also pointed out that the latter had, among their wares,
"prepared products that have the external appearance of European specialties that are either brought in fraudulently from neighboring countries
or produced in Indochina by firms that would like to avoid any form of

---

[15] "Natural" was meant here as "without any kind of transformation."
[16] Judith Fadlon, "Meridians, Chakras and Psycho-Neuro-Immunology: The Dematerializing Body and the Domestication of Alternative Medicine," *Body & Society* 10, 4 (2004): 69–86.

regulation."[17] This last comment points to the anxiety of colonial authorities in the face of a Vietnamese and traditional therapeutic market that had grown increasingly opaque and complex in its creative responses to the local impact of colonization, including the administration's medicalization policies, as well as to the private market for modern medicines. More obviously, it reveals the existence of fraudulent practices, the attempted control of which, once again, exposes large gaps between colonial discourse and the realities of regulatory practice. Occasionally, the fraud control services did effectively detect, denounce, seize, and pursue cases. These instances provide a glimpse into the drug market in interwar Vietnam, which contributes to a richer, more accurate portrayal of its flexibility and innovative character.

Lacking clear and appropriate legislative texts on Vietnamese medicine, health authorities could fall back on the Pharmacy Inspection Service to police the circulation of all types of therapeutic substances – at least in theory.[18] From 1908, the service was responsible for the annual inspection of every site involved in the sale of medicines, and for official procedures for following up on, and eventually for prosecuting, offenses. Yet the targets of inspection proved elusive – particularly "traditional pharmacies." While itinerant merchants escaped the system altogether, even permanent businesses were numerous, highly diverse, and sometimes very small and discreet. Moreover, the service was never given the means, human or financial, to fulfill its mandate. The result, as each head inspector complained repeatedly to his superiors, was that visits covered only a fraction of existing businesses. For Tonkin, in 1931, the pharmacist in charge of this service, Antonini, calculated that his budget would permit no more than 200 visits.[19] In fact, only 164 sites were inspected that year. This represented slightly fewer than 10 percent of the permanent businesses identified by an official survey.

Of the 157 visits reported for 1934, 124 were to "Sino-Annamese shops," 10 to outlets, and 23 to Western pharmacies – of which 5 were owned by Vietnamese pharmacists. Inspections increased to 191 in 1935, but fell to 171 the following year.[20] The little information available on inspection services in territories other than Tonkin suggests that these

---

[17] "Réglementation de l'exercice de la pharmacopée traditionnelle sino-indochinoise, 1942–1943. Lettre de l'Inspecteur général de l'hygiène et de la santé publique au Gouverneur général de l'Indochine, Hanoi, 16 septembre 1942," ANOM, Gougal SE 213.

[18] The 1908 text specified that the commission would be presided by the highest-ranking military pharmacist of the colony. Its members included another military pharmacist designated by the local administration, a representation of the local health authority, a member of the local hygiene commission, and the regional police commissioner.

[19] ANOM, RST NF 3683.

[20] ANOM, RST NF 3684, 3685, and 3686.

functioned erratically. They were often run by a single pharmacist, or by none at all, since very few pharmacists were employed by the public system: hardly more than forty in 1931. In the 1910s and again in the 1930s, Annam was even absorbed by the Inspection des pharmacies of Tonkin, probably due to lack of money or qualified staff, thus spreading resources very thin on the ground. In 1924, after being ordered by the local director of health to inspect the pharmacies of Annam, Inspector Léon Bloch reported that, in a month, he had managed to visit only a few hospital pharmacies and outlets. Still, he signaled a variety of dangerous and illegal practices in outlets, such as the sale of pharmaceutical specialties and the repackaging, without adequate instructions, of essential medicines for sale in bulk or by the unit. Probably aware of the system's limitations, Bloch merely suggested that outlet managers be chastised . . . by mail.[21] Reports also indicate that the same pharmacies were inspected year after year, chiefly a handful of well-known French pharmacies in Hanoi and Saigon.

As can be expected, there were many obstacles facing coordination between the pharmacy inspection and police services, as well as the judicial system. Another key partner was the fraud control system, but it too was short on staff. In fact, due to the Union-wide shortage of pharmacists, responsibility for the pharmacy inspections and the fraud control service for a given territory was often entrusted to the same person – that is, if the head inspector was not already also in charge of the Central Supply Pharmacy. The TC pharmacists Bloch (in 1915) and Georges Lambert (1926–27) were responsible for both the pharmacy inspection and fraud control services. In 1933, Antonini, another military pharmacist, directed the Central Supply Pharmacy of Tonkin while supervising inspections in both Tonkin and Annam, as had Casimir-Jean Peirier before him.[22] The list of responsibilities given to this handful of pharmacists kept growing. Fraud control entailed the testing of not only medicines but also many other products (primarily foodstuffs, agricultural chemicals, and fertilizers). In the 1920s and 1930s, the fraud control service was asked, in addition, to conduct biological and bacteriological analyses in collaboration with the Instituts Pasteur, as well as tests of food and water composition. It also provided technical supervision for

[21] "Au sujet d'une tournée d'inspection des pharmacies en Annam, 1924. Lettre de M. Bloch, inspecteur des pharmacies du Tonkin et de l'Annam au médecin-inspecteur général des services sanitaires et médicaux de l'Indochine, Hanoi, 31 mars 1924," VNA, centre no. 1, RST 48346.
[22] "Vente et exportation de certains produits toxiques et de leurs dérivés à la colonie, 1915–1917," VNA, centre no. 1, RST 32040; VNA, centre no. 1, RST 32073; "Examen pour la délivrance du certificat d'aptitude à la gérance de dépôt de pharmacie, 1932–1933," VNA, centre no. 1, RST 47835.

disinfection with a Clayton disinfector, investigated Vietnamese remedies and the acclimatization of plants, and prepared therapeutic products for local use, such as chaulmoogric ethers.

The fraudulent contamination, adulteration, and counterfeiting of medicines, along with food, drinks, and agricultural products, was regulated in Indochina by the promulgation, in 1905, of a metropolitan law of 1895. This law defined various types of fraud (against standards of quality and authenticity) and penalties, as well as procedures for seizing and destroying both fraudulent goods and the instruments with which they were manufactured. Its application in Indochina was further detailed in 1914 by a decree that, notably, specified that accused indigenous persons, whether selling European or indigenous products, were to be prosecuted under this colonial law rather than by native tribunals.[23] This provision, which must have favored a high rate of convictions underpinned by questionable judgments, clearly privileged the protection of French rights. The application of the law required laboratory analysis.

From 1915, the Pasteur Institutes, the only facilities in the Union with the required technical and material capacity, were enlisted for this purpose. By decree, the governor of Cochinchina allocated a subsidy of 3,400 piasters to the Institut Pasteur of Saigon for "the establishment and operation, as a trial, within this establishment, of a food fraud control laboratory." Édouard Rose, a TC pharmacist affiliated with the Institut at the time, was put in charge of this laboratory, which was soon named the Laboratoire d'hygiène et de répression des fraudes (Hygiene and Fraud Control Laboratory). In the late 1910s, fraud control services acquired their own, autonomous laboratories placed under the direct authority of the IGHSP. Drug fraud control procedures were initiated by the identification of suspicious products by pharmacy inspectors. The fraud control laboratory was then notified and ordered a seizure. This triggered the transmission of samples and of a report to the Local Directorate of Health, via the head inspector of pharmacies, who again notified the fraud control laboratory, this time to conduct analyses. Test results were reported directly to the Directorate; if fraud was confirmed, the state prosecutor was then notified. Cumbersome and highly centralized, this system was slow and ill-suited to the Vietnamese context.

Inspection reports indeed suggest that administrative delays and difficulties constrained action across all relevant regulatory services, thus

---

[23] In Indochina, at this time, there were French, native, and mixed tribunals. Affairs involving indigenous persons were judged by native tribunals, applying Vietnamese law – except, of course, when cases involved a threat to colonial order. When both indigenous and French persons were involved, the case was referred to a mixed tribunal, which applied French law.

limiting the number of analyses and prosecutions for pharmaceutical fraud. In 1917, only 2 of the 373 analyses conducted by the Hygiene and Fraud Control Laboratory of Cochinchina were of medicines – the rest were biological analyses (295) and food analyses (46).[24] Although inspections and seizures in both "European" and "Sino-Vietnamese" businesses increased in the wake of the 1919 law on toxic substances, very few led to sanctions other than verbal warnings for minor infractions in the registration and stocking of toxic substances. This suggests that, in many cases, suspicious products were not even sent in for analysis, either to avoid paperwork or because test results were expected to lead to no or overly slow action.[25] By 1919, medicines were the target of nearly 13 percent of the analyses conducted by the Laboratory of Cochinchina, and of none in Annam due to the lack of a pharmacist.[26] In 1923, out of 227 tests conducted in Tonkin, 26 were of medicines, while more than half were of nước mắm, the local fish sauce. Two years later, medicines accounted for 38 out of 289 analyses.[27] The Tonkin laboratory was the only one with a steady increase in analyses performed on medicines and medicinal substances in the 1930s. In 1934, it tested 59 samples of French and Sino-Vietnamese specialties and therapeutic products labeled as "other," of which 14 medicines of the "Hindu pharmacopeia," as well as several products suspected of containing quinine (but which were not QE tablets), krabao oils, and an injectable solution of methylene blue.[28] By 1935, 20 percent of the laboratory's analyses were of therapeutic products. The reason for this seems to be that more institutions were now requesting analyses, such as the Hygiene Office of Hanoi, AMI hospitals, the police, the Customs Agency, and even private individuals, including pharmacists.[29] The proportion of products found to be fraudulent by this laboratory remained, however, very low.

Why was this? Is it possible that compliance with the law increased over time? Given, on the one hand, the increasing rigidity of the legislative corpus and, on the other hand, the dynamism and hybridity of the Vietnamese medicines marketplace, this seems highly unlikely.[30] It is much more plausible that the cumbersome and inadequately-resourced

---

[24] ANOM, Gougal 65327.

[25] VNA, centre no. 1, RST 32073.

[26] ANOM, Gougal 65329. Someone would finally be appointed in 1921 (ANOM, Gougal 65331).

[27] "Détail des analyses effectuées au Laboratoire d'hygiène et de répression des fraudes du Tonkin en 1923," ANOM, RST NF 4012.

[28] ANOM, RST NF 3684.

[29] ANOM, RST NF 3683.

[30] In an article on fraudulent quinine in British India, Patricia Barton puts forward a different hypothesis, according to which the British authorities were much too preoccupied by opium trafficking to pay any serious attention to a traffic in medicines: Patricia Barton, "Powders, Potions and Tablets: The 'Quinine Fraud' in British India,

regulatory system failed to capture infringements, either because the inspection services failed to visit the "right" businesses, or because inadequate staff and equipment were unable to detect new and creative means of counterfeiting and adulteration. Although these colonial labs contributed to the rise of modern toxicological knowledge and expertise, including in the field of legal medicine, they do not seem to have significantly increased public protection from risky medicines.[31]

5.3   Crosscutting (Clever) Crimes, (False) Accusations

Unlike the French "charlatans" of the nineteenth century, druggists and merchants of medicines in Vietnam were not marginal actors heading toward obsolescence; they were numerous and well-organized. Like qualified pharmacists, they had to adjust their practice to comply with the law but also, at the same time, survive commercially and professionally. Some seem to have been ill-equipped to ward off the constant legal threats thrown at them, or even to fully comprehend the rules they were meant to obey. Others, however, demonstrated a formidable resourcefulness and capacity to retaliate, whether by opposing restrictions, as described previously, or by maneuvering around the law, often in ever more clever and innovative ways.[32] It must also be emphasized that breaking and bending the law was not the preserve of "Sino-Vietnamese empiricists"; nor were indigenous and traditional actors necessarily more closely controlled than biomedical ones. However, they were constantly under suspicion, and therefore more often accused and punished for illegal drug trading than their French counterparts. That being said, illegal practices were widely shared across these two sets of actors.

In fact, the popular press often denounced AMI staff for trafficking medicines, or for failing, more generally, to respect professional codes of conduct. Colonial functionaries and health professionals, as well as French private pharmacists, were also known to commit offences, knowingly or not. The most frequent illegal practices pertained to the illegal importation of certain types of medicines, notably narcotics and products not listed in authorized pharmacopeias; the sale of toxic substances by an

---

1890–1939," in Mills and Barton, *Drugs and Empire,* 144. Yet the two are not mutually exclusive, especially if defined as matters of regulating the circulation of toxic substances.

[31] Arnold, *Toxic Histories*; Monnais and Tousignant, "The Values of Versatility." See also Noémi Tousignant, *Edges of Exposure: Toxicology and the Problem of Capacity in Postcolonial Senegal* (Durham: Duke University Press, 2018).

[32] In some cases, it is possible that laws were broken in ignorance rather than intentionally. Legal texts, prolifically promulgated, were not well publicized, while French (and legislative) language was not necessarily clear to everyone ("Au sujet de la traduction de la nouvelle réglementation sur le commerce des médicaments de la pharmacopée indigène, 1921," VNA, centre no. 1, RST 48344).

unauthorized person; the sale of medicines without a prescription (or with a fake one); and the production and sale of counterfeit, stolen, or contraband medicines. They involved a wide range of medicines other than narcotic and psychotropic drugs, such as QE, Dagénan, arsenobenzols, and various commercial specialties. This illicit market for medicines turns out to have been extremely dense, revealing much about diverse responses to new therapeutic possibilities and constraints under colonial rule.

By law, as mentioned previously, the only Asian medicines that could be legally imported and sold in Vietnam were those identified as "Sino-Vietnamese." Yet French traders and pharmacists, as much as Asian and Vietnamese actors, seemed eager to sell, alongside Western pharmaceuticals, medicines produced in Asian countries that they identified as modern medicines. This eagerness, along with perceptions of potential local demand for these products, are expressed in official requests to colonial authorities for authorization to import specialties from non-Western pharmacopeias. For example, in 1901–2, the firm Bourgouin-Meiffre unsuccessfully applied to the Customs Agency for authorization to import stocks of Wonderful Specific, a specialty produced in Shanghai that was reputed to effectively cure dysentery.[33] In 1907, a certain Mr. Yokohama applied to the superior resident of Tonkin for permission to sell pharmaceutical products. He countered, as Maire would later, that laboratory tests and reputable Japanese clinicians had validated these.[34] This kind of request was systematically refused. While there is no indication, in this particular case, that the decision was not complied with, official paper trails do contain hints and traces of the importation and sale of Asian pharmaceuticals, especially of Japanese pharmaceuticals, in Vietnam.

Attempts by Japanese pharmaceutical firms to seek a stable market for their products in Indochina, and a widespread acceptance, including among some French pharmacists and Vietnamese businessmen, of the scientific validity and marketability of these products, created a fertile terrain for illegal practices. In August 1908, a month after the Maire scandal, a Vietnamese-owned drug shop in Ha Dong City was shut down for selling Japanese medicines imported by the Haiphong-based

---

[33] "Pharmacie B. Au sujet de l'importation d'un des médicaments ne figurant pas à la pharmacopée officielle, 1901," ANOM, Gougal 17156; "Introduction au Tonkin du Wonderful Specific par MM. Meiffre et Bourgouin, 1902," ANOM, RST NF 3710.

[34] "Demande formulée par M. Yokohama en vue d'être autorisé à vendre des produits pharmaceutiques, 1907," ANOM, Gougal 17162; "Interdiction prononcée contre Yokohama, sujet japonais, de vendre des produits pharmaceutiques japonais, 1907," ANOM, Gougal 9967; ANOM, RST 894.

firm Société Bao Dien.[35] Both cases suggest that intermediaries for the trade of Japanese drugs were already well established in Vietnam. These must also, however, be situated in a context of particularly tense relations with Japan. Combined with the anxiety arising from the poisoning of military personnel (see Chapter 1), this political tension may have favored such crackdowns. Yet there is evidence that Japanese pharmaceutical firms maintained a foothold in Vietnam – through direct product distribution using Japanese representatives or Vietnamese businesspersons – throughout the colonial period. For example, in 1917–18, the pharmacist Edmond Chassagne mentioned, in his correspondence with the Local Directorate of Health on the topics of import difficulties and shortages, that he had long-standing relations with Japanese firms.[36] Similarly, in 1939, a certain Bùi Duy Dan pointed out – to support his own request to import specialties from Japan – that two Hanoi-based firms were openly selling, in the city and via outlets, several well-known Japanese specialties such as Kobeol, an anti-syphilitic drug.[37]

To facilitate the entry of specialties from Japan as well as from continental China, Hong Kong, and Singapore, many were falsely labeled as "products of Sino-Vietnamese medicine." In 1940, for example, the Customs seized stocks of two medicines: Chekouchoi, for intestinal parasites in children, and Chaplintan, for fever and headache in children. These had been imported as Sino-Vietnamese products by a Mr. Ma Hoa Huu, who claimed to be a representative for two Hong Kong–based pharmacies, Wang Hing and Ling Chi. Analysis revealed that their contents corresponded with compositions listed in the French pharmacopeia.[38] The products of the famous entrepreneur Aw Boon Haw, maker of Tiger Balm, were particular targets for this type of seizure.[39] Many foreign specialties, including hybrid specialties, must have nevertheless slipped through the customs net by claiming to be traditional Vietnamese remedies, a category that was defined only vaguely, at least until the law of 1942. French pharmacists, as much as Asian drug traders, appear to have been willing to defy the boundaries dividing markets for Western and Asian medicines in order to broaden their product range, to obtain cheaper or more readily available Asian products, and to push sales of their merchandise.

[35] "Fermeture de l'officine de Le Duc Diu, marchand de médicaments japonais, 1908," ANOM, RST NF 895.
[36] "Lettre d'Edmond Chassagne, pharmacien de 1ère classe, au Directeur local de la santé, Hanoi, 14 février 1918," ANOM, Gougal 33693.
[37] ANOM, RST NF 3710.
[38] "Droguistes. Mise en vente de médicaments dits chinois mais qui relèvent en réalité de la pharmacopée occidentale, 1940," ANOM, Gougal SE 219.
[39] Cochran, *Chinese Medicine Men*, 118–50.

In addition to selling Japanese specialties in his own pharmacy, Maire had, as the 1908 investigation revealed, opened a well-advertised "traditional pharmacy" in Bac Ninh in the name of his Japanese partner Shigetaro Kuroshima. Maire could defend himself neither by claiming it to be a Western-style pharmacy, since he could not by law own two businesses and his accomplice was not a qualified pharmacist, nor by claiming it to be a Sino-Vietnamese business, since the sale of traditional remedies was forbidden to French citizens. In the end, the stocks of both businesses, defined as both secret and Sino-Vietnamese remedies by the local director of health, were confiscated.[40] Other French pharmacists sought to sell Asian specialties, or to have indigenous traders sell French specialties, under specific conditions and under their supervision.[41] Thus, in 1920, the pharmacist Trombetta was denounced for supplying a Cholon-based pharmacy whose owner was found guilty and fined one hundred piasters for selling the French pharmacists' brand of anti-opium pills.[42] The subsequent investigation by the Pharmacy Inspection Service revealed that Trombetta had imported ten kilograms of morphine hydrochloride through a British wholesaler, which he then resold under various forms, including his famous pills, to several Cholon-based business associates – acts that could be prosecuted as both the illegal practice of pharmacy and the illegal sale of toxic substances.[43] Attempts to import products from illegal sources were particular numerous during times of crisis, particularly of war, due to shortages combined with the temporary tightening of drug import regulations. In 1941, some Tonkin-based pharmacists even attempted to purchase quinine from "Chinese clandestines," who disposed of large stocks of unknown origin.[44]

Before the 1919 application in Indochina of the 1916 metropolitan law, it appears that the distribution of toxic products to unauthorized persons, or without a prescription, was generally tolerated. However, vigilance had grown over the previous years as narcotics control took

[40] "Circulaire du médecin-principal Collomb, Directeur local de la santé du Tonkin, au maire de Hanoi, Hanoi, 15 juillet 1908," ANOM, Gougal 17166.
[41] "Lettre de L. Sarreau, pharmacien à Phnom Penh au Résident supérieur du Cambodge, Phnom Penh, 25 mars 1916," ANOM, Gougal 17172; "Vente de médicaments européens par des indigènes, 1912," VNA, centre no. 1 RST 48337.
[42] "Police de l'Indochine, Cholon, 1er juin 1920, note," VNA, centre no. 2, Goucoch IA-8/237(4); ANOM, Gougal 17174.
[43] "Demande d'autorisation d'importation de stupéfiants, 1919–1920," ANOM, Indo AF 326 Y51(1).
[44] The Sûreté générale investigated the case in March to April of 1941, only to conclude, a month later, that instead of tracking down traffickers and sellers, it would have been more productive for the AMI to turn a blind eye to certain practices and thus obtain high quality medicines ("Contrebande de quinine, 1941," ANOM, RST NF 4181).

a prominent place on the international agenda. By the beginning of World War I, the Cochinchina Pharmacy Inspection Service was keeping an eye on the pharmacists Dourdou and Renoux. This was for good reason: by late 1915, they had each imported up to several hundred kilograms of morphine for resale to unauthorized persons in Vietnam and China.[45] Investigative documents reveal that, between 1912 and 1915, Dourdou sold his stocks to doctors ("Dr. Levier" and "El Kantara"), AMI facilities, pharmacists (including Brousmiche, who was based on the other side of the country), and, in significant quantities, non–health care professionals, in particular to Chinese individuals – a certain "Lam" in My Tho, a "Chinese from Cholon," and an "unknown Chinese." Renoux's morphine buyers were equally diverse: the rather long list of clients included a "Chinese pharmacist," who was said to have purchased nine kilograms, and Thieu Pham, identified as a Chinese druggist, who received five.[46]

Around this time, debates arose within the colonial health administration on the circulation of opium cures, and particularly on their OTC sale. Renoux and Dourdou argued, in 1916, that non-prescription sales of Solution Holbé, then owned by Renoux, should remain legal on the basis of its value as a cure for addiction problems in the local population. The pharmacists also mentioned their efforts to make this "marvelous specific" more widely available through the use of indigenous intermediaries, namely Chinese and Vietnamese druggists who also sold similar preparations from China.[47] Renoux and Dourdou's petition was firmly denied with reference to the law, requiring prescription-only sale by a qualified pharmacist for any remedy containing a higher than 1 percent concentration of a poisonous substance.[48] The 1917 creation of a governor general's commission to examine the possibility of stricter surveillance of morphine, which was likely motivated by the prevalence of these remedies, followed by the promulgation of the law of 1919, seems to have curbed the sale of anti-opium cures. Dourdou modified his formula in order to avoid prescription requirements, while most other products ceased to be advertised in Vietnamese newspapers from 1920. Private pharmacists nonetheless continued to discretely sell other products defined by law as toxic. Soon, preparations containing cocaine were seized during routine inspections, while Chassagne was found guilty of both storing toxic substances in an unlocked cupboard, and of selling

[45] "Requêtes formulées par MM. Dourdou et Renoux, pharmaciens à Saigon, 1916–1917," ANOM, Amiraux, Box 189, Folder 279.

[46] ANOM, Gougal 17174.

[47] VNA, centre no. 2, Goucoch IA-8/237(4).

[48] "Lettre de l'Inspecteur général de l'hygiène et des services de santé au Gouverneur général de l'Indochine, Hanoi, 18 mars 1916," ANOM, Amiraux, Box 189, Folder 279.

dangerous medicines, including an ergotin lotion, OTC in 1920.[49] The same year, Montès was found to have dispensed an impressive list of schedule A and schedule B substances (mercury, codeine, Fowler's Liquor, Nux vomica, digitalis, etc.) without requiring prescriptions, as well as his Vin Tonique Tonkinois, which contained Arrhenal, an arsenical compound.[50]

From the interwar years, reports of infringements of toxic substance laws by pharmacists decreased, probably under the influence of an increasingly radical narcotics control movement, as well as the threat of frequent inspections.[51] By this time, the majority of seizures occurred in "traditional" businesses. Substances commonly used in Vietnamese therapeutics were among those most frequently confiscated, such as strychnine, mercury (as calomel or cinnabar), and arsenic (as arsenic sulphide).[52] In 1935, the local director of health for Tonkin, Dr. de Raymond, deplored that he lacked the means to contain the circulation of large quantities of strychnine, of which he was informed by military intelligence.[53] Also in the 1930s, Hanoi's Laboratoire de répression des fraudes analyzed a variety of "red pills," an inexpensive treatment often imported from China that contained Heroin, and was used to treat opium addiction and anxiety.[54] Chinese businesses were also found to sell the latest synthetic drugs, including arsenicals such as Compound 914, Treparsol, and Stovarsol, under their trademark or false names.[55] Illegal sales of toxic substances were also reported in some essential medicines outlets, including of mercury-based syphilis medicines

[49] Laurent Gaide, "Notes sur les médications anti-opium et sur le traitement de l'opiomanie," BSMI 8 (1930): 963–64.
[50] "Police urbaine de Hanoi, 1er arrondissement, 24 avril 1920, objet: infraction au décret du 16 juillet, nr 259. Procès-verbal, 23 avril 1920 du commissaire de police Lecoeur," VNA, centre no. 1, RST 38306.
[51] "Police de l'Indochine, Sûreté de Cochinchine, commissaire spécial à l'administrateur chef de la Sûreté, Saigon, 18 mars 1920," VNA, centre no. 2, Goucoch IA.8/237(4).
[52] ANOM, RST NF 3684; "Vente par certains pharmaciens annamites de Nam Dinh de médicaments chinois à base de strychnine, 1935," VNA, centre 1, RST 48079. Recall that, according to the first two study commissions on the Sino-Vietnamese pharmacopeia, many of these substances should have been included in the list of "traditional substances" exempt from the law on toxic substances.
[53] VNA, centre no. 1, RST 48079.
[54] These pills contained a rather volatile combination of Heroin, sometimes with morphine, and caffeine, quinine, or even strychnine (ANOM, RST NF 3683). Predating the era of combination drugs, these famous red pills were also quite prevalent in the Western world in the 1930s: Dikötter, Laaman, and Zhou, Narcotic Culture, 156–60.
[55] VNA, centre no. 1, RST 32073; "Rapport d'inspection des pharmacies de Hanoi, les 27 et 28 décembre 1927 faites par l'Inspecteur des pharmacies du Tonkin, VNA, centre no. 1, RST 32116; "Vente de Stovarsol et Tréparsol par un commerçant chinois à Phan Rang, 1936," VNA, centre no. 2, 3715. RSA/HC.

(Pilules de Ricord and Hectargyre), and of paregoric, a camphorated tincture of opium used to treat diarrhea.[56]

5.4   Fine Imitations: The Colonial Genesis of Pharmaceutical Counterfeiting

In 1931, the inspector of pharmacies for Tonkin identified several French specialties on sale in a shop in Hanoi, on Hué Street. Two of these were trademarked specialties, Oléo Résine and Kalmine, the first being indicated for the treatment of gonorrhea and the second for fever, fatigue, and anxiety. These were not listed as toxic substances, and were not confiscated. The "tonic wines with French presentations," however, while apparently no less harmless than the other medicines, raised a red flag – for the inspector suspected counterfeiting.[57]

The sale of nontoxic Western specialties by unauthorized persons (anyone other than a licensed pharmacist or outlet manager) was very rarely mentioned in inspection reports. This suggests that the practice was rare, very well hidden, or simply tolerated. Inconsistencies in the law may have encouraged the latter. Indeed, legislative measures combined extreme rigidity (totally prohibiting the sale of any "Western medicine" by Asian traders)[58] with flexibility (authorizing laypersons to distribute quinine and nontoxic medicines in various types of outlets). Furthermore, the law tended to define the category of *spécialité européenne* (European specialty) in vague terms, which varied from one text to another. It seems, in the end, that most commercial specialties circulated relatively freely, making it possible for French pharmacists to do business with Chinese or Vietnamese drug traders, or with public and private outlets. When these otherwise innocuous medicines were suspected of being counterfeit, however, the law bared its teeth.

While the imitation of pharmaceutical forms was not in itself condemned by colonial law, other types of plagiarism were. These included, from 1909, the use of registered trademarks, and, following a 1915 governor general's decree, the falsification and alteration of pharmaceutical specialties (by reducing, omitting, or substituting active ingredients); the copying of specialties (in terms of the ingredients and formula or in the

---

[56] "Le médecin principal de 1ère classe Gaide, Directeur local de la santé en Cochinchine à M. le Gouverneur de la Cochinchine, au sujet de la visite des dépôts de produits pharmaceutiques faite à Vinh Long," VNA, centre no. 2, Goucoch IA-8/237(4); "Rapport de gendarmerie sur une saisie de médicaments français chez un Chinois à That Khé, septembre 1930," VNA, centre no. 1, RST 48024.
[57] ANOM, RST NF 3683; VNA, centre no. 1, RST 32073 and RST 47835.
[58] "Rapport de la commission d'inspection des pharmacies, 1913. Cholon (extrait)," ANOM, Gougal 17172.

presentation of the product); and false representations (of contents, of therapeutic indications, or of claims concerning efficacy or toxicity). One can imagine that these laws provided ammunition for zealous colonial authorities to "punish" indigenous traders suspected of counterfeiting for their "incompetence" and "greed."[59] Pharmaceutical firms, French and foreign, also filed complaints for brand theft, as did the Hong Kong–based British firm Watson and Co. in 1915.[60] In 1931, an inspector seized "176 boxes of Pastilles Valda labeled in Annamese" from a shop in Haiphong: the harmless but counterfeit throat lozenges were found to be sold by several shops.[61] Some products were confiscated because they were found to contain compositions listed in the French pharmacopeia, as mentioned previously, with the 1940 seizure of Chekouchoi and Chaplintan. The law on trademarks was also deployed to seize and destroy several local hybrid specialties in the 1910s. In fact, pharmacy inspectors, upon coming across hybrid products, generally defined them as illegal, calling them either counterfeit French specialties or traditional medicines prohibited by the law on the sale of toxic substances. The majority of confiscations, however, were for products that were falsified, altered, or falsely represented, sometimes in combination with brand theft.

These products were viewed as public health risks, given that their composition and concentrations in active substances were unknown (and thus might be overly active, leading to toxic side effects or drug interactions, or too weak, resulting in failed treatments) and/or were not accompanied by appropriate therapeutic instructions. Reports of quinine counterfeiting were particularly numerous. In 1926, the inspector of pharmacies for Tonkin, Georges Lambert, sounded the alarm upon finding that several shops were selling quinine that had been cut with starch. He reported that "a native" was being prosecuted for acting "as the middle-man in the supply of the shops" in his neighborhood.[62] A few months later, Lambert mentioned that large quantities of so-called QE, which were entirely devoid of quinine, were in circulation.[63] In 1934, the Grand Council of Economic and Financial Interests received reports of cases involving the distribution of quinine with a lower than 25 percent

[59] Some pharmacy inspection reports indeed hint that inspectors used these aspects of the law to intensify their repression of Sino-Vietnamese traders.

[60] "Au sujet du dépôt de marques de fabrique en Indochine, 1915," ANOM, Gougal 18773.

[61] ANOM, RST NF 3683. Pastilles Valda, a menthol and eucalyptol–based green lozenge, was invented by the French pharmacist Henri-Edmond Canonne in 1904 and became extremely popular worldwide in the 1930s.

[62] VNA, centre no. 1, RST 32073.

[63] VNA, centre no. 1, RST 32073.

concentration in alkaloids.[64] In late 1938, the sale of inexpensive quinine tablets by "Chinese shopkeepers of Cholon and inland" was brought to the attention of the Cochinchina fraud control service. An investigation located the sellers and determined the tablets were not QE; genuine tablets were rose-tinted and stamped with "QE." The following year, the TC pharmacist Marcel Autret reported that nine antimalarial products analyzed by the Fraud Control Laboratory were found to contain lactose or starch or both; he believed these were made locally using genuine QE tablets. In Hanoi, Franck Guichard, also a military pharmacist, came across "very well-made" tablets of starch and lactose that he thought had been locally manufactured with a tablet press.[65] Over the years, reports indicate, quinine fraud not only continued; it also became increasingly sophisticated.

Indeed, the skill of drug fraudsters, which some colonial doctors and administrators would call "deviousness," was noted as early as the 1920s. Lambert, in 1926, remarked on the "cleverness" of Sino-Vietnamese drug traders. The individual from whom he had confiscated starch-cut quinine also carried "a large supply of santonin admirably falsified with pulverized gypsum." He also gave another illustrative example of ingenuity, involving "a Hanoi merchant" who was being prosecuted at the time: having been first found guilty of selling "fever pills" containing quinine, the merchant had eliminated the active substance. However, when his clients had likely found these "no longer had the same taste and effect," the merchant substituted quinine with a similarly bitter ingredient: powdered false angostura bark (the bark of the Nux vomica tree), a "violent poison."[66] As in many other cases, this "cleverness" was equaled only by the tenacity of some officials in cracking down on such illegal pursuits.

5.5   Black Market Medicines

When the head doctor for Lai Chau, in Upper Tonkin, noted the presence of very cheap quinine tablets sold by Chinese merchants in 1919, at a time of severe shortages in the QE service, he suspected these were either falsified or stolen.[67] Drug theft and trafficking – including but not only of opium, which often made the news in Indochina and neighboring colonies – was also on colonial authorities' radar.[68] There is also evidence

---

[64] "Grand conseil des intérêts économiques et financiers de l'Indochine, Procès-verbal des séances plénières de la session ordinaire de 1934," ANOM, NF Indo 2298.
[65] Marcel Autret, "La fraude sur la quinine en Indochine," RMFEO 17, 1 (1939): 925–28.
[66] VNA, centre no. 1, RST 32073.
[67] "Rapport sanitaire annuel de la province de Lai Chau, 1920," ANOM, RST NF 4011.
[68] Tagliacozzo, Secret Trades, 187–207.

of black markets for other colonial medicines, including cutting-edge medical specialties (arsenobenzols such as 914 and Stovarsol, and sulfonamides such as Dagénan) and toxic substances stolen from pharmacies.[69] Black market activity increased sharply (or perhaps was more closely monitored) with the outbreak of World War II, as drug shortages in the public system became more acute. In November 1940, two women were arrested in the colonial capital for possession of seven hundred piasters' worth of medicines, apparently stolen from an army infirmary. A few months earlier, the Institut Pasteur in Hanoi was robbed.[70] In 1943, Dr. Vũ Ngọc Anh, an AMI doctor posted in Thai Binh, reported that, upon his request, the police services confiscated more than two hundred ampoules and syringes, most of which had been diverted from AMI facilities. He explained that this trafficking was orchestrated by "a band of charlatans, former nurses who had been fired, coolies with long-standing urban clienteles and who, no longer able to obtain pharmaceutical products, attempt to corrupt our subordinate personnel to get [what] they need."[71] The same year, Soludagénan, an injectable form of Dagénan, could only be found in Cochinchina on the black market, or so the Directeur local de la santé confided to the director of Specia-Rhône-Poulenc. The official further hinted that a few private pharmacies, having sold their stocks illicitly, were partly responsible for this shortage.[72]

AMI staff members were often accused of being involved in the illicit trading of Western drugs. From at least the late 1910s, official documents and newspaper articles frequently exposed unlawful transactions between patients and health care workers, as well as the existence of larger, better organized trafficking operations. Vietnamese public sector nurses were castigated in a circular letter dated June 1921, signed by the governor of Cochinchina, for reselling "medicines that are extremely difficult to handle, such as intravenous injections of arsenical salts (606, 914, etc.)."[73] Reprinting an excerpt of this letter a few days later in L'Écho, the journalist Nguyễn Hữu Ích depicted such activities, which

[69] L'Écho, no. 97, September 28–29, 1924.

[70] "Note de l'administrateur résident de France à Yen Bay au Résident supérieur du Tonkin, Yenbay, 20 novembre 1940" and "Note postale 26-S du 25 juillet 1940 du pharmacien gestionnaire de la pharmacie centrale au sujet d'un vol de médicaments au pavillon Pasteur," ANOM, RST NF 3710.

[71] "Vol de produits pharmaceutiques à Thai Binh, mais 1943" and "Note postale, Thai Binh, le 16 mars 1943, le médecin de l'Assistance médicale à M. le Résident de France à Thai Binh," ANOM, RST NF 6440.

[72] "Note confidentielle du Directeur local de la santé (Dr Simon) au Directeur de la Maison Specia (Saigon), Hanoi, 29 juin 1943," ANOM, RST NF 3710.

[73] L'Écho, no. 215, July 21, 1921.

combined the illegal practice of medicine with counterfeit prescriptions and the diversion of public medicines, as widespread, pointing out that several nurses had already been suspended.[74] Clearly, public health care workers had good reasons for participating in such activities, for they worked under difficult conditions and had easy access to pharmaceuticals, in particular the latest medical specialties and hypodermic syringes. Still, these accusations must also be seen as part of a broader stigmatization of the AMI and of its indigenous subordinate staff. While colonial reports convey particular mistrust of nurses and midwives, the editorial press condemned nurses' illicit practices as part of a general diatribe on the failures of the public health care system. This critique ranged from minor failings such as hospital dirtiness to the incompetence or greediness of its personnel (who, for example, were said to make patients pay for free public services).[75]

Such accusations, which were prevalent into the 1920s, also point to a real phenomenon, which often featured improper dealings in some of the most expensive medicines, such as sulfa drugs.[76] In June 1925, a Vietnamese nurse by the name of Le Van Con was arrested for selling six ampoules of 914 (for the price of eighteen piasters, quite a lot of money at the time) and injecting it into a patient of the Hôpital indigène in Phan Rang City. The client, an "Asian doctor," had denounced Con after experiencing "unexpected side effects" and attempting, unsuccessfully, to get his money back.[77] In an article published in 1926, Dr. Coppin reports the case of another patient who, consulting for a motor impairment, admitted to having similarly purchased and received injections of 914 from a nurse acquaintance.[78] By 1942, AMI authorities were alert to the risk of diversion by subordinate agents, as "ha[d] already happened on a large scale with Dagénan," wrote Tonkin's local director of health.[79] AMI nurses were also accused of taking advantage of the opportunity, offered by firms based in France, to place direct mail orders, a system that sometimes allowed even prescription-only medicines to reach buyers

[74] Nguyễn Hữu Ích, "L'exercice illégal de la médecine," *L'Écho*, no. 217, July 26, 1921.
[75] "A l'hôpital municipal de Cholon," *La tribune indigène*, no. 218, October 25, 1919; "La déchéance de la médecine française," *La tribune indigène*, no. 307, June 17, 1920.
[76] "Nouvelles d'Annam, Phanrang, exercice illégal de la médecine," *L'Écho*, no. 323, July 4, 1925; A. Le Roy des Barres and Henri Marcel, "Infirmiers et infirmières indigènes de l'Assistance médicale au Tonkin," BSMI 5, 1 (1927): 1–6.
[77] Dong Chau, "L'exercice de la médecine par les infirmiers," *La tribune indigène*, no. 310, June 24, 1920.
[78] Henri Coppin, "Un syndrome rare chez l'Annamite: signes de la série tabétique, alcoolisme, hypertension artérielle," BSMI 4 (1926): 611.
[79] "Lettre du Dr Simon au président de la Chambre, Hanoi, 25 août 1942," ANOM, RST NF 6264.

without inspection. They thus obtained products they were not authorized to manipulate or dispense, and resold them at a profit.[80]

If the doubly subaltern AMI nurses were most often and most vehemently accused, other actors were occasionally exposed for trafficking in medicines. In 1911, there was a final-year Vietnamese medical student said to have diverted public hospital stocks for sale to private clients. In 1920, similar acts were committed, claimed *La tribune indigène*, by a "Mr. officier de santé, resident in Saigon."[81] Non–health care professionals who had connections to the public or private medical world, such as domestic employees or colonial agents, were also sometimes implicated. In July 1942, *La dépêche d'Indochine* reported that Võ Văn Tam, a "boy"[82] employed by an unnamed doctor, was being convicted for having written a Dagénan prescription for a friend on his boss's letterhead paper.[83] Police documents from the early 1940s describe illicit networks that were directed by former indigenous managers of big commercial firms, such as Descours & Cabaud, which, as we have seen, also imported medicines in bulk.[84]

The motivations of those who engaged in illicit drug markets were probably very diverse. For many subordinate AMI employees, this was a way of supplementing low salaries, but also of responding to patient requests, which were often both very specific and insistent – especially, some said, in hospital settings.[85] Such requests were not only likely to kindle empathy among health care providers. They might also make them feel useful and needed, while generally, they worked for long hours, routinely performing tasks that were unrewarding, even unbefitting of their training, often under the scornful gaze of their French or Vietnamese superiors.[86] When no doctors were available to dispense, they may have felt especially compelled to satisfy requests for prescribed medicines and injections. Indeed, several nurses defended themselves by explaining that,

---

[80] Nguyễn Hữu Ích, "L'exercice illégal"; "Lettre de Thanh Van," *L'Écho*, no. 220, August 2, 1921.
[81] Tu Do, "Dix ans après," *La tribune indigène*, no. 491, October 4, 1921; "Exercice illégal de la médecine," *La tribune indigène*, no. 496, October 15, 1921.
[82] Boy meant "houseboy," or domestic servant, in the context of French Indochina.
[83] The prescription had then been passed on to another friend to make the purchase in a pharmacy. The pharmacy detected the falsification, then called the doctor. The domestic employee and his friend were each condemned to a four months conditional jail sentence: "Le boy docteur," *La dépêche d'Indochine*, July 2, 1942.
[84] "Détention de stocks de médicaments par le Chinois Lyao-A à Haiphong, 1942," ANOM, RST NF 6440.
[85] It is true that AMI nurses were poorly paid. In 1928, their starting salary was of 360 piasters. After 30 years, it might increase up to 1,150, while, at the time, auxiliary doctors were paid between 1,200 and 3,600.
[86] Dong Chau, "L'exercice de la médecine"; Nguyễn Hữu Ích, "L'exercice illégal."

given the scarcity of doctors, they were justified in stepping in to take care of patients, even if that meant stepping outside the law. From the perspective of buyers and consumers, this was one, sometimes the only, if often expensive, route for accessing sought-after therapeutic tools to take care of oneself or of kin.[87]

Some of the motivations behind informal and illicit exchanges of medicines can be glimpsed in the following excerpt of an intercepted letter, dated December 1942, written by "Ngô," employee of the Residence of Nam Dinh, to a Mr. Nguyễn Đăng, lieutenant at Saigon's military hospital, the Grall Hospital:

My wife had a miscarriage [. . .] Now she is weak [. . .] To give her relief, she must be given laminaria sticks. For now, I am not worried, as my wife does not have fever. Each laminaria stick cost only one piaster at the time, but now I am forced to pay twenty for an injection given to my wife because this product can no longer be found in [. . .] pharmacies [. . .] My wife also needs to take Dagénan pills, but the supply of this medicine is completely finished here, so I have to give her Septoplix instead [. . .] I have already received the Solucalcium you sent me, and I express my sincere gratitude for it.[88]

The two protagonists of this letter lived more than one thousand kilometers apart, yet they maintained a relationship based on familiarity and mutual trust (Ngô's letter also offered financial advice), the similarity of their positions (both were employed by the colonial administration), as well as the exchange of medicines. Their correspondence proves the existence of a black market for pharmaceuticals in a context of shortages and rising costs. It also paints a picture of growing demand for, and familiarity with, Western pharmaceuticals, which some were willing to risk breaking the law, and to trust friends and accomplices, to get their hands on.

By 1940, colonial authorities clearly believed that the illegal practice of medicine and pharmacy, and illicit markets for counterfeit, toxic, and diverted public medicines, were pervasive across the Vietnamese territory.[89] It was also clear that this parallel economy was not only a product of minor traders' attempts to survive, but was made up of powerful and well-known actors whose networks and influence reached

---

[87] Although in some cases, illegally traded medicines were less expensive than legal ones, as seen above in the case of quinine.

[88] "Fiche de renseignements des commissions C et K du contrôle postal et de contrôle télégraphique et téléphonique de Saigon issue d'une interception postale. Expéditeur: Ngo, résidence de Nam Dinh; destinataire: Nguyen Dang, lieutenant, Hôpital Grall; date de la communication: 1er décembre 1942 (langue: annamite)," ANOM, RST NF 3710.

[89] ANOM, Gougal 44461.

beyond the borders of the Indochinese Union. This suggests that medicines circulated more widely, or at least with greater ease, outside the
AMI than within it. And yet, there seems to have been no real reflection,
at the time, on the roots and determinants of these transactions. While
their logics and stakes were surely heterogeneous, and despite uncertainty
about their true extent, the existence of these practices at the very least
indicates an insistent and enthusiastic demand for remedies in general,
and colonial medicines in particular, from within the Vietnamese population. There are clear, cumulative indicators of this demand in evidence of
how it was kindled and catered to, from the imitation of Western pharmaceutical labels or products to the marketing hybrid specialties, as well
as the trafficking of syringes, Dagénan, and QE. At the same time, this
demand, which defined modern medicines as commodities, as the objects
of potentially thwarted consumer desire, was marginalized, even
criminalized.

Other examples of transgressive imitation included the use of the title of
"Doctor" by Sino-Vietnamese therapists in the 1930s (for which they
were reprimanded), and the display, by druggist shops, of the Red Cross
insignia to attract clients.[90] French food products were also frequent
targets for counterfeiting. For example, the newspaper *L'Opinion*
reported the sentencing of a certain Trần Gia Dat to three months of
imprisonment and a huge fine in compensation to the Nestlé Company
for the fraudulent use of its labels to pass off milk tins as authentic
products.[91] Such signs of the popularity of French products and of
modern pharmaceuticals contradict AMI professionals' complaints of
"native mistrust" toward biomedicine, suggesting, once again, that
other reasons were at the root of Vietnamese under- or non-
consumption of medicines.

By the interwar years, colonial medicines, in the expansive sense
defined in this book's introduction, were being given an increasingly
central role in changing practices and perceptions of health within some
segments of the Vietnamese population. This is perceptible in the busy,
eclectic, and rapidly changing market for medicines in Vietnam, in the
wide variety of products that circulated within the colony and in the
proliferation and intensification of legal measures to control this circulation. The pharmacy inspection and fraud control services were challenged
not only by lack of means, but also by the moving target of rapidly
evolving practices of pharmaceutical production and distribution, behind

---

[90] "Lettre de Tissot président de la Croix-Rouge au Résident supérieur du Tonkin, Hanoi,
20 août 1938," ANOM, RST NF 3656.
[91] Cited in VSB, no. 62, March 1931.

which they always seemed to lag, struggling to police the boundary between legal and illegal practice. At the same time, the range of reported offences, and hints that reported cases were only the tip of an iceberg of illegal practice, are indicative of growth in the offer and demand for "modern" – whether "Western," "Asian," or "hybrid" – pharmaceuticals, and of a willingness to defy the legal boundaries drawn around biomedicine and the public health care system, as well as between hierarchical levels of health work. Additional problems, from rigid systems of supply and recurring shortages to the high cost of medical specialties, as well as the lack of financial and human means to strictly and thoroughly implement the system of pharmacy inspection, left the door open to a wide range of adjustments, compromises, elusions, as well as innovations by a variety of actors. Colonial authorities were seemingly wary of the popularity of medicines and of their transformative potential. Drug sellers of all sorts, however, seized it as an opportunity, presenting themselves as accessible pathways to desirable therapies, at least for (peri-)urban populations who could pay for medicines. But who were these consumers and how did they make their therapeutic choices? Why did Ngô specifically request Dagénan from his business partner? How did this low-level clerk come to discriminate between brands of sulfonamides according to their therapeutic efficacy, given that these products had only just been introduced to the colony, and that their official distribution was likely limited to a handful of carefully selected hospital patients? The rest of this book addresses the difficult task of deciphering the consumption of colonial medicines through the eyes of those who sought them out.

6 Learning Effects: Lived Experiences, Pharmaceutical Publicity, and the Roots of Selective Demand

The very existence of a private market for medicines, in all its density, diversity, and creativity, testifies to the popular success of colonial medicines in Vietnam. The three final chapters further probe the roots, vehicles, characteristics, and consequences of Vietnamese pharmaceutical consumption, examining, in particular, the patterns and underlying rationalities of what emerged, over the first decades of the twentieth century, especially during the interwar period, as both a highly selective and persistently plural demand for medicines. The information we have already seen on QE, illicit practices, and commercial strategies indicates that the Vietnamese attraction to colonial medicines was both partial and differentiated. It was anchored in a rational and experiential process of selection oriented by both attraction and skepticism, shaped by highly uneven access to information and care, and integrated into therapeutic geographies and itineraries that continued to include non-biomedical substances and representations. In this first chapter on patterns of Vietnamese therapeutic demands and consumption, I examine how these were profoundly transformed by the increasingly tangible presence of pharmaceuticals. Representations and expectations were far from static, and they evolved in response to the embodied effects of colonial medicines – whether these were experienced personally, witnessed, or spoken about – and to publicity representations of relief and cure that took up an increasing amount of space in the popular press. While emphasizing a capacity to learn about and to adopt new therapeutic representations, as evidenced in the popular press (including several health magazines), I also draw attention to how these dynamic processes may have been facilitated by points of intersection between colonial medicines (and the ways in which they were diffused) and preexisting therapeutic practices and expectations.

6.1 Efficacy versus Toxicity: An Embodied Calculus

Colonial doctors often blamed their patients' fear of toxicity as the main reason for rejecting medication or for failing to take it properly. In some cases, they associated this refusal with distinctive representations of the Vietnamese body and of its response to foreign medicines.[1] An AMI doctor reported in 1913 that sellers of Vietnamese medicines in the Haiphong area had supposedly attempted to discourage individuals from attending consultation services by spreading the following message: "French medicines are very good for French temperaments but they are dangerous for Vietnamese constitutions."[2] Fear of toxicity remains, across very different contexts, one of the main factors for non-adherence to therapy.[3] In the first half of the twentieth century, this fear was not unfounded. As discussed previously, a growing number of pro-ducts circulating in Vietnam, as well as elsewhere, were defined as toxic by biomedical practitioners and laws. In Vietnam, such substances were often used on an experimental or even on a trial-and-error basis. This seems to have given rise to multiple local experiences of reactions and side effects.

Some of the unpleasant, in some cases even deadly, effects of Western pharmaceuticals are documented in medical publications and AMI reports. For Vietnamese patients, these effects were often unexpected and inexplicable, which would explain why some medicines were unpop-ular. Medical specialties such as arsenical drugs, sometimes used in excessive doses and durations, frequently caused "accidents," as unplea-sant and dangerous effects were called, and even death.[4] The risk of adverse effects was more likely in patients who were already vulnerable due to advanced disease, malnutrition, and comorbidity – this is another likely factor for the persisting therapeutic skepticism of AMI doctors described in Chapter 2. Intramuscular injections of chaulmoogra oil were also widely agreed, even by colonial doctors, to be quite painful; they often provoked fever, nausea, rashes, and skin discoloration. This, among other factors, might explain the frequency of attempts to escape from leprosaria before the 1930s. Some commonly used products also caused side effects. Quinine, especially when used intravenously in ser-ious cases of malaria, could provoke fever spikes, violent chills, and aches that some found unbearable. The regular consumption of preventive quinine was also associated with intense fatigue, tinnitus (and even

[1] As we will see, toxicity was associated, by some Vietnamese, not only with "Western" drugs but also with Chinese medicines.
[2] "Rapport sanitaire de Haiphong, 1913," ANOM, RST NF 4014.
[3] Pandora Pound et al., "Resisting Medicines: A Synthesis of Qualitative Studies of Medicine Taking," *Social Science & Medicine* 61, 1 (2005): 133–55.
[4] Dupuy, "Accidents mortels"; Séverin Abbatucci, "Accidents convulsifs mortels survenus au cours d'un traitement antisyphilitique par des injections intraveineuses de Néo-Salvarsan," AMPC 19 (1921): 210–14.

temporary deafness), heartburn, vertigo, local inflammation, and vomiting.[5] Copper sulphate eye drops caused intense pain and conjunctival reactions, which, AMI doctors wrote, drove some patients away. Others complained about the unpleasant effects of taking Pyramidon, such as perspiration.[6] And yet there is also evidence of rapid and enthusiastic acceptance of some medicines despite their (potentially) aggressive effects.

Vietnamese patients' appreciation of santonin, for example, was mentioned frequently, from very early on, in health reports. Apparently, the medicine was widely seen as highly effective in eliminating various common parasites such as roundworms and pinworms. Already in 1897, Dr. Gouzien reported that, in Tonkin, it had been renamed *thuốc giun*, literally "medicine-worm."[7] Many AMI reports from the 1910s to 1920s concurred. The 1923 report for Ninh Binh states: "At the consultation we see at least twenty [Vietnamese children] who come each day with a big belly and cramps and who say they have found worms. Having taken it or seen it given out, they are now very familiar with the specific remedy santonin; with quinine, it is one of only two Western medicines with the rare quality of being popular."[8] Santonin was also seized a few times by the pharmacy inspectors in druggists' shops in Saigon in 1913. It was among the medicines that Chassagne sought to import from Japan in 1918, which he justified in terms of AMI's supply needs.[9] Santonin was not, however, an innocuous medicine. Its effects could be drastic and occasionally caused the death of children; some doctors recommended semen contra as a safer alternative.[10] Yet these effects were also visible and striking. As the medical officer for Phu To Province wrote in 1921, "santonin is certainly [. . .] the therapeutic agent most highly appreciated by the masses due to its tangible and striking results. The absorption by their children, on the night before, of a powder, which to mothers seems to be insignificant, is followed on the morrow by the unfailing expulsion of bunches of worms. The family finds itself wonderstruck."[11] Another

---

[5] Pierre Millous, "Les injections intraveineuses de quinine comme traitement du paludisme chronique," *Paris médical* (July 26, 1924), cited in AMPC 22 (1924): 282–83.

[6] ANOM, RST NF 4007; Readers' correspondence, BAYB, no. 21, March 1936, 25.

[7] Paul Gouzien, *Manuel franco-tonkinois de conversation spécialement à l'usage des médecins* (Paris: Challamel, 1897), 95–96. Other medicines were also listed in the manual as having become part of Vietnamese life by this time: Antipyrin, cocaine, iodoform, Laudanum, and Helmerich's ointment.

[8] ANOM, RST NF 4021.

[9] "Pharmacie. Réglementation de la pharmacie indigène en Indochine. Correspondance, 1914–1918," ANOM, Gougal 17172; "Importation de produits chimiques et pharmaceutiques en Indochine, 1918," ANOM, Gougal 33693.

[10] "Causerie médicale. Le parasitisme intestinal," *L'Écho*, no. 271, April 30, 1925.

[11] ANOM, RST NF 4019.

medicine said to be popular due to strong and immediately perceptible bodily effects was Quinobleu, a drug used to amplify the effects of quinine in malaria treatment, which produced "a certain euphoria felt from the outset of treatment."[12] Quinobleu was, like santonin, a risky medicine (it contained an arsenical salt) that was nevertheless appreciated for its perceptible effects.

Over time, comments on toxicity as a reason for Vietnamese refusals of treatment grew fewer and far between in doctors' reports. Gradually, the factor of efficacy instead took center stage in explanations of why medicines were accepted or rejected. The arsenical compounds 606 and 914 sometimes caused adverse effects, which were occasionally identified as causes of therapeutic non-adherence and abandonment. And yet, they were said to be the object of a nearly instant and highly enthusiastic demand. Already in 1912, doctors at the Hôpital du protectorat in Hanoi reported that their syphilis patients had a "tendency [. . .] to ask for [606] instead of mercury," a demand which they "fought firmly" when it seemed inappropriate.[13] In Nam Dinh, a local dignitary had, in 1913, proposed before his peers of the Council of Notables that a ton of 606 be imported for the treatment of syphilis and relapsing fever. Dr. Paucot took this as a sign of the "natives'" appreciation of its "rapid action."[14] During an epidemic of relapsing fever in 1913, Dr. Mouzels reported, "patients were coming to the doctor of their own will to demand" the injection of Salvarsan.[15] In 1915, the annual health report for Phu Ly Province remarked that 606 was widely known for "its effectiveness against syphilis," especially among educated people but also even "deep in the countryside"; it was a topic of everyday conversation and had been nicknamed "the sainted remedy." This was only five years after the drug was introduced to Vietnam.[16] As mentioned in the introduction, Compound 914 (under its various brand names) was, in the late 1930s, the most frequently mentioned product in the readers' correspondence of the Hanoi-based health magazine BAYB.[17]

This does not imply universal acceptance of these drugs. Yet it makes clear that knowledge and appreciation of the action of arsenical compounds quickly spread beyond the initial confines of hospital-based trials.

---

[12] H. Chabaud, "Quelques considérations sur l'emploi du Quinobleu dans les hôpitaux d'Assistance," RMFEO 14, 6 (1938): 820.

[13] Roux and Tardieu, "Ulcérations balaniques," 38.

[14] Paucot, "Emploi du Salvarsan," 240. The Council of Notables retained control over day to day matters at the village level within the structure of the Union Indochinoise; it was also in charge of raising direct taxes for the colonial administration.

[15] Mouzels, "La fièvre récurrente," 281.

[16] ANOM, RST NF 4015.

[17] Acétylarsan is mentioned forty-three times in the BAYB readers' correspondence, Sulfarsénol is mentioned twenty-three times, and Stovarsol is mentioned eighteen times.

And this popularity lasted. As seen in Chapter 5, these drugs were often
the objects of illegal transactions by AMI nurses or drug traders. Indeed,
beginning in the 1920s, AMI doctors denounced their overconsumption.
In 1926, for example, Drs. Sambuc and Ha Văn Sua blamed a rash of
accidents on the overuse of injections of arsenicals for the treatment of
syphilis, thus linking this problem to the huge popularity of 914.[18] Also
recall that in the early 1930s, there were intense debates within the
international and colonial medical communities about arsenobenzols in
the treatment of syphilis, and in particular about the connection between
inadequate use and the development of neuro-syphilis.[19] In Vietnam, at
a conference of the Société médico-chirurgicale de l'Indochine (Medico-
surgical Society of Indochina) in 1926, Dr. H. G. S. Morin clearly
associated "the increasingly marked zeal of the Annamites for injections
of Novarsénobenzol" with the "frequency of neurological syndromes
[. . .] observed among them."[20]

I am suggesting here that lived experiences of therapeutic efficacy
shifted perspectives on colonial medicines, and reconfigured individual
and collective treatment priorities. Especially in cases of serious, life-
threatening conditions, apprehensions of toxicity were displaced by
quests for efficacy. This implies a potential pathway of familiarization
with colonial medicines – especially those which produced clearly perceptible and repeated displays of therapeutic efficacy – through an accu-
mulation of experiences. These experiences might have been felt within
one's own body, but also witnessed in others or conveyed by word of
mouth (for example, in the transmission of stories about the cure of
a village dignitary), or they were disseminated by the press, which
reported the results of successful trials and reproduced open letters
describing spectacular cures.[21] Such accrual of therapeutic proof, of
efficacy outweighing toxicity, might help explain why sulfonamides were
adopted with such alacrity and enthusiasm when they were introduced to
Vietnam, so much so that they almost immediately made their way onto
the black market. In other words, the prior success of arsenical drugs,

---

[18] Sambuc and Hà Văn Sua, "Note sur les accidents," 409–12.
[19] M. L. R. Montel, Trần Văn An, and Dan Van Cuong, "Adénopathies iliaques primitives
chez les Annamites de Cochinchine," BSPE 17 (1924): 75.
[20] Cited in: Nguyễn Văn Tùng, "Note sur la syphilis," 129.
[21] ANOM, RST NF 4014; Drs. Reboul and Ung Tong, "Notes sur les cures d'opiomisme
faites à l'Hôpital central de l'Annam," AHMC, 16 (1913): 756–65, "Rapport sanitaire
annuel de la province de Ha Dong, 1926," ANOM, RST NF 4024. Remarkable cures
were also mentioned in letters published in *L'Écho* and *La tribune indigène*, especially in
the 1920s; these often named and praised specific doctors. Conversely, toxic effects could
also be perceived indirectly, witnessed in a family member or a hospital roommate, for
example, or even read about in the press, thus arousing fear and non-compliance.

which had built up a reputation for efficacy despite their tightly controlled distribution within the AMI, seems to have facilitated the acceptance of sulfa drugs.[22]

Exchanges between the readers and editor of the BAYB also reveal emerging expectations of pharmaceutical efficacy. Dr. Nguyễn Văn Luyện and his editorial team were often asked to confirm that a particular medicine, which had been recommended, prescribed, or heard about, was truly effective. Also striking, however, are frequent complaints about a medicine's lack of efficacy. The tone of many complaints was not merely disappointed; it was also angry, suggesting a betrayal of therapeutic promise. This is indicative of the strength of readers' expectations that pharmaceuticals should obtain rapid and specific effects. Many types of medicines were accused of coming up short of such expectations, including elite medicines such as the arsenical drug Acétylarsan, essential medicines such as Aspirin and sodium bicarbonate, as well as other medical and commercial specialties, and even vaccines and serums.

Some readers, as we will see in more detail when we examine their therapeutic itineraries in Chapter 8, described desperate attempts to find efficacy. While these quests sometimes led to prolific and potentially risky self-medication, they could also motivate the use of biomedical channels of diagnosis and prescription. For example, the Grand Council of Economic and Financial Interests commented, in 1930, on high levels of adherence to treatment in a specialized STI service, the Institut prophylactique de Saigon (Saigon Prophylactic Institute). This was supported by figures suggesting that patients returned for follow-up treatment (an average of 5 consultations per patient, calculated on the basis of 6,072 patients for 39,574 consultations) and received multiple injections (31,747 in total, of which 14,654 were bismuth salts and 11,824 were arsenical compounds). Hospitalization rates for STIs were also increasing across the Union, with as high as a 35 percent rise in Cochinchina in a single year.[23]

Concerns about drug toxicity did not vanish. In the late 1930s, many Vietnamese patients still complained of intolerance to 914; others abandoned treatment or requested safer substitutes. There was collective anxiety about the addictiveness of some medicines, and the risk in others of causing sterility or potential harm for babies and children, provoking

---

[22] A. Seyberlich and Lê Thị Văn, "Action véritablement merveilleuse d'un pansement annamite à base de plantes," RMFEO 17 (1939): 909.
[23] ANOM, Gougal 47474.

persistent rumors about the colonizers' "real" intentions.[24] Yet not only
did quests for efficacy temper worries about adverse effects; the expansion
of pharmaceutical research and development also put safer products on
the market. For example, some of the synthetic antimalarial drugs introduced to Vietnam in the 1930s were known and preferred for having
significantly fewer side effects than quinine.[25]

6.2   The Appeal of Injections

Another sign of change in lay calculations of efficacy versus toxicity was
the growing demand for injections. In contrast with other drug forms,
notably pills, injection techniques had no precedents in local practices
and were thus a novelty when introduced by the French to Indochina.[26]
Needles are also invasive, while their coercive use in mass vaccination
campaigns or in the closed spaces of hospitals and leprosaria made them
easy to interpret as symbols of colonial and biomedical control. Injection
techniques also require an expert mediator – someone able to prepare the
product (which usually requires some mixing, sometimes dosing as well)
and to insert and depress the needle in the right position to ensure efficacy
and limit the risk of adverse effects. There were thus good reasons for
injections to appear as unfamiliar, inaccessible, risky, and even violent to
the Vietnamese. Yet many seem instead to have perceived the advantages
of the technique, which allows substances to enter organisms faster than
oral administration, and to act in a quicker and more targeted way, thus
limiting, for example, reactions such as stomach irritation.

Hypodermic syringes were used in Vietnam from the end of the nineteenth century.[27] By the early years of the AMI system, injections of
quinine, caffeine, camphorated oil, mercury, and artificial serum seem
to have been rather common in hospitals.[28] As I mentioned earlier, some
types of injection and injectable products were quite painful and thus
unpopular. For Dr. Mouzels, "horribly painful" intramuscular injections
of 606 were the obvious reason some of his patients had abandoned

[24] Readers' correspondence, BAYB, no. 15, September 1935, 34; no. 19, January 1936, 33;
no. 24, June 1936, 29.
[25] BAYB editorials, no. 5, October 1934, 28; no. 33, March 1937, 27.
[26] Since acupuncture was not common in Vietnam at the time, it is unlikely that the practice
facilitated the adoption of injections as has been hypothesized for China: Dikotter,
Laaman, and Zhou, Narcotic Culture, 175.
[27] Gouzien, Manuel franco-tonkinois, 130–31.
[28] Dr. Renault, "Fonctionnement du premier service de l'Hôpital de Hué pendant l'année
1911," AHMC 16 (1913): 401; Dr. Koun, "Fonctionnement du deuxième service de
l'Hôpital de Hué pendant l'année 1911," AHMC 16 (1913): 421.

treatment in 1913.[29] Injections also caused adverse reactions. These were sometimes reported in the popular press, such as the case of a woman who developed "two formidable abscesses" after being injected with Tonikeine, a tonic, by an auxiliary doctor, for the treatment of puerperal fever at the hospital of Bac Lieu, which had caused an "alarmed" family to transfer her to the hospital of Soc Trang.[30] By the interwar period, however, many Vietnamese were becoming familiar with highly effective therapies that were administered by injection.

News of the curative effects of arsenical therapies, such as 606 in the treatment of syphilis and epidemics of relapsing fever, spread quickly and widely. From 1912, injections of emetine were used to treat amoebic dysentery, significantly reducing morbidity, notably by lowering the risk of developing life-threatening liver abscess.[31] Some may have learned of the rapid relief from pain and cough obtained by injections of opiate analgesics.[32] Over time, patients might also have learned about differences between types of injections, allowing them to distinguish often-painful intramuscular and especially subcutaneous injections from usually painless intravenous shots.[33] Displays of rapid, dramatic efficacy prompted a reevaluation of the risks and pain associated with the technique. As early as 1915, the head doctor of Binh Dinh Province reported that more and more malaria sufferers sought out injections of quinine and sodium cacodylate, despite the length of treatment (daily injections for up to ten days) and the sting of the needle.[34] Residents of Lao Kay reportedly believed that quinine was active only when administered by hypodermic injection. Blaming this conviction as an obstacle to treatment, the AMI doctor labeled it "a regrettable local tradition."[35] His report was written in 1919. That a demand for injections was already being called a "local tradition" is, in itself, quite telling.

Familiarization with, and perhaps demand for, injection techniques was also likely to have been stimulated by the large number of injectable products in circulation in Vietnam during this period. Up to 12 percent (136 products) of all the medicines I identified were chiefly or exclusively distributed in injectable form; for specialties, this figure was nearly

---

[29] Mouzels, "La fièvre récurrente."
[30] Tu Do, "Dans l'Assistance . . . règnerait aussi le régime du bon plaisir?," *La tribune indigène*, no. 577, May 13, 1922.
[31] C. Coste and R. Deschiens, "Données relatives à l'histoire médicale des dysenteries avant la découverte de l'amibe dysentérique," BSPE, 38 (1945): 15–27.
[32] Dikötter, Laaman, and Zhou, *Narcotic Culture*, 174–75.
[33] Pierre Millous and Phạm Văn Chi, "Essai de médication stibiée dans le traitement des lépreux," BSMI 4, 6 (1926): 305–8; Guillon and Keruzore, "Quelques précisions," 526; Nguyễn Văn Luyện, "Tiêm thuốc phải cần thận," VSB, no. 62, March 1931, 1–3.
[34] ANOM, RST NF 4003.
[35] ANOM, RST NF 4011.

16 percent (107 products). The arsenical compounds so often mentioned by BAYB readers were available only in injectable form. By the late 1930s, many sulfonamides were also available for injection, as were several antiseptics and other antibacterials.[36] A few anesthetics were also stocked by public facilities. The therapeutic indications of injectable products were diverse, but four general categories of therapeutic activity may have created an association between injectability and specific types of effect. Most obviously, injections cured serious and highly prevalent infectious diseases, notably STIs. All active therapies for syphilis were administered by injection, including not only arsenical compounds but also bismuth- and mercury-based medicines (branded Bismuthoidol, Bivatol, Muthanol, Olbia, Quinby, Collobiase, Hectargyre, and Hermophényl). Injections could also act rapidly and powerfully on acute conditions such as hemorrhage, asthma attacks, intense pain, epilepsy, heart problems, malarial fever, poisoning, infected wounds, and septicemia. A few medicines for chronic conditions were injected, notably insulin, available in Vietnam from the Byla and Roussel firms as early as 1935, while other injectable organotherapeutic and hormone therapy products were indicated for various women's health issues (such as Agomensine, Angioxyl, Endocrisine, Hormocrine, Hormovarine, and Crinex).[37]

Injections did not just deliver highly effective cutting-edge medical specialties: a wide range of tonics and restoratives were also sold as injectable products, including medicines containing calcium, vitamins, and kola. Thus a positive association, almost a metonymic one, developed between the technique and tonic drugs. Organ- or hormone-based substances (Colloidogénine, Hépacrine, Hépatrol, Pancrinol, Syncrines Choay) were often injected to "boost" one's system. Readers of BAYB were apparently avid consumers of stimulant specialties sold as injectable ampoules, which they sought out to treat anemia, exhaustion, lack of energy, as well as "debilitating" diseases such as tuberculosis.[38] Strychnine injections were mentioned on several occasions as a treatment for nervous problems or spermatorrhea.

---

[36] The world production of syringes increased exponentially in the interwar period: from about 100,000 in 1920 to 2 million in 1940 and 7.5 million in 1952. This was partly due to advances in manufacturing (the cost per unit dropped 80 percent during this period), but also to the popularity of some injectable drugs: Ernest Drucker, Philipp G. Alcabes, and Preston A. Marx, "The Injection Century: Massive Unsterile Injections and the Emergence of Human Pathogens," *The Lancet* 358 (2001): 1989.

[37] ANOM, Gougal SE 2920. Insulin was used not only to treat diabetes but also morning sickness, undernutrition, and some skin conditions at the time.

[38] Several injectable specialties mentioned in the BAYB (Cinnozyl, Colloidogénine, Panxylon, Nucléarsitol, Francalcium, Vitadone) are listed in Vidal's repertory, as both indicated for the treatment of tuberculosis and for the relief of conditions often associated with the disease, such as asthenia, anemia, weakness, and rickets.

Those who wrote about injectable products to health magazine editors in the 1930s expressed particularly high expectations of efficacy.[39] The editor-in-chief of the BAYB, in turn, warned that, without proper guidance, this enthusiasm for injectable products could lead to risky practices, particularly when toxic products were involved, such as Sérum-neurotrope, Strychnarsitol, strychnine phosphate, and, of course, arsenobenzols.[40] Dr. Nguyễn Văn Tùng also noted in the BSMI in 1931 that AMI patients "very often get injected with Novarsénobenzol unnecessarily, if only as a fortifying remedy, for problems that have no relation to syphilis or other affections for which arsenical medication is indicated. They consider Novarsénobenzol as a veritable panacea, of which some go as far as to request a prescription from their doctors."[41]

Yet French and Vietnamese health care professionals, in both the public and private sectors, also seem to have become more inclined to give injections over time, as the efficacy and popularity of the technique grew. This inclination could have been transmitted to patients, as is suggested in this excerpt of an article published the same year in the health magazine *Vệ sinh báo. Journal de vulgarisation d'hygiène* (VSB):

When a case of flu has more serious symptoms, a doctor must be consulted. He may need to administer injections of ether, camphorated oil, strychnine and sometimes of Electrargol or of Septicémine. If the flu is severe and has spread to the lungs, a flu vaccination is needed [. . .] If one cannot eat, it is possible to be given, by injection, fortifying substances such as sodium cacodylate or sodium glycerophosphate. If there is hypotension, one can take Hépatrol, Pancrinol or Hémostyl or even iron supplements [. . .] If one is very weak, it is a good idea to get an injection of strychnine of half to ten milligrams.[42]

Injectable medicines also had their disadvantages. For example, ampoules were fragile, difficult to transport, and hard to preserve. Indeed, orally administered alternatives, including for the treatment of syphilis, were advertised for their practicality. For example, Comprimés de Gibert (Gibert tablets) were advertised in the Vietnamese popular press as being as effective as arsenical drugs, but much more discrete and easy to use, especially when traveling, while Sigmargyl was not only "scientific" but practical: "tablets replacing needles."[43] Overall, however,

---

[39] Readers thus felt particularly let down when injected medicines failed to produce desired effects. Among the medicines that disappointed them were Olbia Moyneyrat, a syphilis treatment (BAYB, no. 5, November 1934, 29); Laroscorbine Roche, a vitamin C–based product (BAYB, no. 40, October 1937, 27); Panxylon, a remedy for anemia (no. 40, November 1937, 28); and Natibaine, for hypertension (no. 42, December 1937, 24).

[40] Nguyễn Văn Luyện, "Tiêm thuốc."

[41] Nguyễn Văn Tùng, "Note sur la syphilis," 127.

[42] "Khi có người cảm thì chữa thê nào?," VSB, no. 67, October–December 1931, 13–14.

[43] Advertisement, *La dépêche d'Indochine*, March 30, 1938.

there are clear signs of a growing appreciation for the curative and adjuvant effects of injections, which may have paved the way for an acceptance of preventive products such as vaccines and serums, thus facilitating the application of key public health measures.

6.3   Promoting Efficacy

In addition to embodied experiences of efficacy, direct or mediated, another mode of familiarization with pharmaceutical (good) effects was through the editorial content and publicity of the print media. In other words, knowledge about medicines was obtained from a variety of sources that transmitted "messages" about therapeutic effects, indications, risks, and value.

Both the general editorial press and health magazines disseminated various types of health education and advice, in which promotional messages were often subtly embedded. Explicit direct-to-consumer advertising was, by the 1920s, however, the most abundant and visible source of printed information about medicines. It told readers which products were available and where, what they were for, and what they should be expected to do. By then, publicity was occupying an increasing amount of space in the press, and was displayed more prominently. Advertisements for medicines, as well as for other health products and services, accounted for a significant part of this increase, especially in Vietnamese-language publications.[44] Medicines, modern but also traditional and hybrid, were most often advertised in quốc ngữ script, either alone or as part of bilingual (with French) or even trilingual (with both French and Chinese) inserts. It is difficult to determine how the language of advertising was selected. While hybrid specialties and traditional medicines were always advertised in quốc ngữ, many European specialties, such as Aspirin, could be advertised in different languages, even within the same publication. It is also unclear how advertisers chose publications: the previously mentioned Sygmargyl advertisement appeared in the Vietnamese papers BDP, *Lục tỉnh tân văn*, and VSB, but also in the colonial forum *La dépêche d'Indochine*.

The proliferation of pharmaceutical advertising suggests that it became, or at least that it was seen as, an important site for fashioning Vietnamese expectations of new kinds of drugs. At the same time, advertisers surely sought to speak to, and make a profit from, what they saw as the existing or potential demand for medicines. To "sell," publicity must

---

[44] *L'Écho* and *L'Annam nouveau* carried fairly little advertisement, while publicity was increasingly present at the time in the BDP and the *Lục tỉnh tân văn*.

identify and integrate readers' references to capture their attention, inform them, and attempt to alter their behavior.[45] For historian Peter Zinoman, publicity in Vietnam was, by the interwar years, already part of a "supra discourse" that was marked by significant transformations in perceptions of language, interpersonal relations, and representations of progress. For George Dutton, the prominence of publicity reflects the centrality of the press in Vietnam's effervescent commercial life during this period.[46] As both a site for representing of modernity and an object of market relations, publicity opens onto a dynamic and emergent culture of health at the intersection of professional and lay, as well as Western and Asian, references, representations, and practices. It both reflects and was a source of transformations in consumer demands for therapeutic effect.

While the general press carried direct publicity for medicines, it rarely published substantive textual content on the topic. Only a few articles in the 1930s addressed wartime shortages, the QE service, recent European drug discoveries, and problems of access to essential products. The health magazines that proliferated from the 1920s, however, were saturated with content on medicines, both as direct advertisement and as informative texts, although many of these are also identifiable as indirect publicity. This is not surprising, given that several of these publications were created, financed, and even edited by locally established pharmacists, both French and Vietnamese. Indeed, magazines seem to have been one of these pharmacists' main marketing strategies. While it is sometimes difficult to trace the precise nature of their involvement in these publications, it is easy to imagine their motivations: by "helping" readers to manage their health, they sought to diffuse information about their own products and to attract and stabilize an indigenous clientele. Almanacs and catalogues, which also provided routine health advice alongside product information, played a similar role. It is telling that those I was able to locate were all published in quốc ngữ. These specialized publications also represented a considerable enterprise. Given the linguistic, technical, and scientific complexities and cost of running these publications, as well as

[45] Judith Williamson, *Decoding Advertisements. Ideology and Meaning in Advertisement* (London: Marion Boyars, 1978), 99. T. J. Jackson Lears emphasizes the importance of a "fertile soil" (made up of suitable institutional, economic, and "moral" environments) for a consumer culture to "take": T. J. Jackson Lears, "From Salvation to Self-realization: Advertising and the Therapeutic Roots of the Consumer Culture, 1880–1930," in *The Culture of Consumerism. Critical Essays in American History, 1880–1980*, ed. Richard Wightman Fox and T. J. Jackson Lears (New York: Pantheon Books, 1983), 1–38.

[46] Peter Zinoman, "Introduction," in Vũ Trọng Phụng, *Dumb Luck. A Novel*, trans. and intro. Peter Zinoman (Ann Harbor: University of Michigan Press, 2002 [1936]), 14–15; Georges Dutton, "Advertising, Modernity, and Consumer Culture in Colonial Vietnam," in Nguyen-Marshall, Drummond Welch, and Bélanger, *The Reinvention of Tradition*, 21–42.

the time, energy, and staff they required, it is remarkable, and again revealing, that they were run at all – some from quite early on and some for many years. These publications illustrate the dynamism and eclecticism of the colony's mediascape; they are also an additional expression of the growing weight of qualified pharmacists in the drug market, and of their marketing skills and creative competition strategies. On a more general level, they show the importance given by health care professionals, especially pharmacists but also doctors, to educating the general population in biomedical ways, teaching them about health and about *informed* health care practices.

The *Nam trung nhút báo. Le courier de la Cochinchine*, owned by the pharmacist Gabriel Renoux and published in Saigon from April 1917 to the end of 1921, appears to be one of the earliest initiatives, although it is not a health magazine per se.[47] Described as a vehicle for the "popularization of French thought," this weekly had an average length of eighteen pages and cost 0.15 piasters per issue. Publicity for drugs soon occupied a significant amount of space, advertising Renoux's pharmacy along with its merchandise. Other than explicit publicity, the content of the newspaper ranged from a literary column, which occasionally reprinted poems, to news features, and included articles on health broadly defined. Many of these articles, behind a veneer of scientific authority, were in fact thinly veiled advertisements for products sold by Renoux. The address of Pharmacie Chassagne is listed as the editorial office of another periodical, the VSB, which was, from February 1926, published monthly (ranging from ten to twenty pages in length), then, from mid-1931 to late 1933, every three months (with an average length of thirty pages). Its title, the "popular health journal," announced its intentions more explicitly than the *Nam trung nhút báo*. It was also cheaper: 0.10 piasters per issue and 1 piaster for a yearly subscription; for a short time, it was even distributed for free.

Like the latter, the VSB's pages were filled, increasingly in its later years, with explicit publicity for its sponsor, and repeated advertisements, sometimes more than once per issue, for a limited range of ten to twenty products. It also published, alongside humorous features, articles containing scientific descriptions of disease and practical advice on the identification of symptoms, as well as on the principles of hygiene and treatment. While even the most serious and scientific of these articles contained discrete references to products that happened to be sold at 59

---

[47] Renoux remained its owner even after he sold his pharmacy to Solirène in 1919. The magazine was integrated into the *Lực tình tân văn* in October 1921. I have not found information about how or why this merge happened.

Paul Bert Street, the newspapers' owners – Chassagne, then Lafon and Lacaze – insisted that its primary motivation was not to serve their commercial interests but instead to serve the population by disseminating the "rich knowledge" of Western science and therapeutics and helping the Vietnamese people benefit from Western medicine. While this effort to distinguish their publication from similar initiatives must be taken with a grain of salt, the VSB's editorial board did enlist health care professionals, including Drs. Petitjean and Nguyễn Văn Luyện, who took an active role in it before founding and running his own, the BAYB. Still the VSB's contents, while avoiding explicit support for self-medication, often minimized or at least did not insist on the importance of medical diagnosis, prescription, and follow-up. Instead, it put forward an image of the accessible pharmacist, who was competent to provide health advice, in particular for the treatment of common conditions, in articles with titles such as "What to Do while Waiting for the Doctor?"[48] This type of publication marketed not only the efficacy of drugs, but also the availability and expertise of health care professionals other than doctors.

Other health magazines run by pharmacists seem to have been less successful, as suggested by their less frequent and durable publication. The TKVSCN, for instance, was published monthly in 1930–31 by the Pharmacie Imbert of Hué. It was filled with publicity and sparse in original content, although several articles were written by local AMI doctors. It also published a "formulary" feature that provided instructions on how to prepare some common remedies at home. Established in Tourane, the pharmacist Phạm Đoàn Điễm published only two issues of the *Vệ sinh y báo. Revue mensuelle de vulgarisation d'hygiène et de médecine*, in 1928. Yet the very existence of these publications in the late 1920s and early 1930s, even beyond Hanoi and Saigon, shows that pharmacists aspired to this type of strategy, through which they might play multiple roles in their clients' health management strategies.[49] This kind of advertising was legal in Indochina and was still common in the metropole;[50] so was the collusion between doctors and pharmacists, as is suggested by the sustained presence of Nguyễn Văn Luyện on the editorial board of the VSB. At the same time, the language and style of these periodicals, and the pragmatism of their content, also characterize them as profoundly local initiatives.

These publications can also be seen as a response to the commercial aggressiveness of local druggists and merchants of "Asian medicines,"

---

[48] "Khi đợi thấy thuốc phải làm thế nào?," VSB, no. 56, September 15, 1930, 1–3.
[49] The *Vệ sinh y báo* content was strikingly similar to the VSB. It was probably among the "pale copies" VSB editors complained of in several editorials of their own magazine.
[50] Blondeau, *Histoire des laboratoires*, vol. 3, 12–13.

who also filled the press with publicity. Indeed, the frequent use of Vietnamese-language periodicals for advertising Western, mainly French, pharmaceuticals is indicative of a demand from the colonized population. This demand was perceived as expansible and exploitable, not only by direct publicity, but also through the cultivation of "educated" health practices and attitudes, as was the objective of publications like the BAYB (see the Introduction and Chapter 7).

6.4   Selling Relief and "Pep"

What did this publicity seek to sell? A systematic scan of a broad sample of printed media, both general and specifically health-related, turned up direct advertisement for about 350 products – this excludes medicines identifiable or advertised as traditional products, but includes hybrid specialties. Presumably, these products were sold in Indochina, in at least one location. This number seems low relative to the quantity of products that were probably advertised in the metropole during this period, but the overall composition of product types is similar. As in France, advertised products included both older types of medicines and the most recent specialties, and their therapeutic indications were very diverse, confirming this to be a period of therapeutic transition in Vietnam. Most medicines originated in the metropole, but some were from other European countries, as well as from North America, Vietnam, China, and elsewhere in Asia. The vast majority of directly advertised medicines were commercial specialties authorized for OTC sale.[51] These were mostly mass-produced, as indicated by standardized forms and packaging: pills, tablets, and granules that were sold in tubes and boxes.

Of these 350, about 50 specialties were advertised more heavily, with greater frequency, and for longer periods of time than the rest. In health magazines, an even narrower range of products was aggressively promoted. The *Nam trung nhút báo* advertised only a few products: a mint extract, Pâte du Dr. Zed (a medicated cream containing codeine and tolu balsam), a guaiacol expectorant syrup, Thomas brand sandalwood oil capsules, Dépuratif Richelet (a plant-based tonic syrup with added B vitamins), Dragées Ferrugineuses du Dr. Rabuteau (iron-supplement pills), and a few personal toiletries including, unsurprisingly, Renoux-brand soaps. The VSB carried advertisements for forty-nine different products and the BAYB for thirty-one. Some of these products appeared issue after issue, or even several times in a single issue, such as the Collyre

---

[51] I did, however, find publicity for a few toxic and injectable products and even for vaccines.

Jaune in the VSB. Inserts were also increasingly big and bold, taking up half and even full pages. In both publications, thirteen to twenty inserts were published in a single issue, adding up to between a third and half of overall content. While some medicines were advertised persistently across different titles (including the famous Canadian Pink Pills for Pale People, as well as Dépuratif Richelet, Grains de Santé du Dr. Franck, and Neurotrophol Byla), others were more aggressively advertised in one or the other, resulting in little overlap between the ten most advertised specialties by title (Table 6.1). Each magazine, however, typically promoted both cutting-edge medicines launched only recently in France and locally produced specialties, such as Collyre Jaune, Sirop Iodotannique Imbert, and Poudre Saint André.

What were these heavily advertised medicines meant or said to be able to do to the body, to symptoms, and to pathological processes? While a few products' contents and indications were unidentifiable, I was able to draw a general portrait on the basis of clearly advertised effects and indications and/or on listings in Vidal's repertory. The strong predominance of medicines with stimulating or restorative properties (130, or 37 percent of the 350 advertised products) is the most striking trend echoing the growing "taste" for injectable tonics I mentioned earlier. Stimulation and regeneration, particularly of the blood, were often advertised in tandem, such as in publicity for Phoscao ("to regenerate [one's] blood and fortify [one's] nerves"), while Pink Pills would "enrich, purify and regenerate the blood," and Deschiens hemoglobin syrup was called a "blood regenerator." The active ingredients in tonic specialties included phosphorus, kola, cinchona, calcium, and magnesium; all of these substances were widely known at the time for their stimulating and regenerative properties. Many also contained iron or iron-rich hemoglobin. Tonics promised to treat a wide range of "weaknesses," including anemia, fatigue, "chlorosis," "asthenia," and several "nervous" conditions.

After tonics, the most prevalent class of medicines is anti-infectious agents (34 percent). This is consonant with the dominance of infectious disease, and especially STIs, as a therapeutic indication in the full set of medicines I identified as being in circulation in Vietnam. Medicines with purifying properties, including laxatives, purgatives, and some diuretics, come third. They account for about seventy of all advertised medicines. These drugs typically promised to return sufferers to a "happy disposition." If we combine products with stimulating and regenerative properties with those promising to help eliminate toxins and waste, more than half (57 percent) of all advertised products were meant to procure a general effect in the organism.

Table 6.1 *Top Ten Most Widely Advertised Specialties in Vietnamese Health Magazines (in Decreasing Order)*

	VSB	BAYB	TKVSCN
1	Collyre Jaune	Collyre Jaune	Sigmargyl
2	Vin J. K. Watson	Tricalcine	Diéménal
3	Sirop Roche au Thiocol	Vin 33.500	Panbiline
4	Poudre Saint André	Sirop Roche au Thiocol	Junase
5	Vin 33.500	Choléopeptine Logeais	Lipocire
6	Sirop Delabarre	Quinimax	Delbiase
7	Pangaduine	Kalmine	Sirop Iodotannique Imbert
8	Injection Strychnophospharsinée	Fer de Quévenne	Pastilles Tussis
9	Élixir Déret	Pilules Robur	Grains de Vals
10	Inotyol	Grains Miraton	Vernine

Likewise, a clear majority was indicated for the treatment not of a specific disease but rather of symptoms such as fatigue, digestion problems, pain, and other discomforts. These medicines relieved the discomfort of hemorrhoids, as well as coughing and wheezing with diverse etiologies: the well-advertised Sirop André, for example, relieved the coughing associated with whooping cough, colds, and flus, while codeine tablets were said to help control tuberculosis symptoms and asthma attacks. Other medicines were indicated for sore throat, gout, rheumatism, arthritis, fever, skin rashes, and back pain. Furthermore, many of these products were presented as having multiple indications and/or general constitutional effects. Indeed, two-thirds of the most advertised specialties were promoted as panaceas, whether explicitly, such as Alcool de Menthe Ricqlès (a "supreme panacea: excellent for dysentery, stomachache, nausea or headache"),[52] or by promising to relieve (nearly) everything. Regularly advertised in the TKVSCN, tablets of halogenated magnesium Delbiase (Laboratoire Grimault, Vial & Cie) were said to "fortify the individual for better digestion; for those who [have] pain in the liver, the eyes, the brain, the muscles; itching and skin conditions." Lê Văn Minh's Kola Stabilisée was sold for its preventive virtues, but was also described as an effective treatment for the flu and as able to fortify the organism and protect it from measles, smallpox, scarlet fever, and even

[52] Advertisement, *La Cochinchine française*, no. 40, November 18, 1907.

typhoid. And if one had already caught one of these diseases, one could still take the kola for strength and faster recovery.[53]

Among the tonic and purifying medicines on the Vietnamese market were a significant number of organotherapeutic products, many of which were similarly promoted for their multiple or general effects. They accounted for about 10 percent of drugs circulating in Vietnam in the 1920s and 1930s, and included products recently launched in France by leading firms such as Byla, Choay, Roussel, Scientia, and Lumière. This suggests that they were in high demand in Vietnam, as they were in Europe at the time. Tricalcine and Peptalmine, produced by Scientia, were particularly well-advertised in both general and specialized periodicals. The first was to be taken for weakness of many origins (breastfeeding, tuberculosis, or convalescence); the second was for various pains and types of discomfort. These medicines were also regularly mentioned in correspondence with the editor of the BAYB: Peptalmine (eleven times) for digestive problems, itching, and eczema, and Tricalcine (six times) as a good tonic for whooping cough, breathing difficulties, pregnancy, and rickets. Opocalcium was the "nutritional supplement" most recommended by the TKVSCN; the product was also mentioned regularly (thirteen times) by readers writing to the BAYB, for a variety of indications, notably for the treatment of rickets as well as flu and weakness in children.

Cutting across the wide range of indications and effects that featured in publicity was a widely shared emphasis on the qualities of efficacy (the gonorrhea cure Santal Midy was proclaimed to be "marvelously effective"[54]) and of being "scientific." The scientific nature of medicines was alluded to in different ways: by referring to a product's laboratory origins and modern production (Lê Văn Minh's Purgose was a "synthetic purgative" sold as "effective [. . .] tablets");[55] by using adjectives such as "rational" ("Pierrol: a rational remedy for constipation");[56] or through the Pastorian metaphor of battle against pathogens. Even mere throat lozenges like Pastilles Valda were described as "an antiseptic respiratory remedy" that could "armor [one's] throat, bronchi, lungs, defending and preserving them by volatile antisepsis."[57] And while many medicines promised global or multiple effects, a subset of drugs was promoted as "specific" – a term that was used very loosely and could refer, simultaneously, to curative efficacy, scientific validation, and basis in modern

[53] Advertisement, La tribune indigène, no. 294, May 11, 1920.
[54] Advertisement, L'Écho, no. 390, October 7, 1922.
[55] Advertisement, La tribune indigène, no. 294, May 11, 1920.
[56] Advertisement, Le progrès annamite, no. 269, January 4, 1927.
[57] Advertisement, BDP, no. 26, March 10, 1925.

therapeutic principles. Boldo Verne was promoted as a "specific of liver diseases," while Entericine, Lactobacilline, and Elkossam tablets were boasted as "specifics of enteritis and dysentery." Borostyrol promised "specific healing of skin inflammations" and was used successfully to treat tropical ulcer and "bourbouille," prickly heat – an itchy rash caused by heat and humidity, particularly common in children. Others claimed to be specific cures for syphilis, such as Sigmargyl, or tuberculosis, including medicines that were probably just cough suppressants.

The safety or harmlessness of commercial specialties was also frequently highlighted. While scientific origins were put forward as a guarantee of quality, many products, including local and "house" products, were also further characterized as gentle, nontoxic, and devoid of side effects. Lê Văn Minh Purgose was not only effective; it was also "gentle" and "pleasant."[58] Gonoryl, a local gonorrhea medicine produced and marketed by the pharmacist Barberousse, was advertised in *L'Écho* in 1931 as fast acting yet safe.[59] Élixir Déret, a tonic, and Sigmargyl were presented as "mild" syphilis cures, suitable for those unable to tolerate mercury or arsenic-based treatments, including children. Épicral made by the Laboratoires G. Lambert was also said to be valuable as a mild tonic medicine for syphilitics. Such characterizations may have been meant to emphasize the product's suitability for Vietnamese bodies and tastes. They clearly picked up on a strong demand for both tonics and treatments for STIs. Whereas most advertisements for French products were simply reproductions or translations of metropolitan versions, in a few cases, this suitability was quite explicitly put forward: "Neurotrophol. From the Byla firm in Paris. Medicine for the liver (gout). The taste is sweet, which is why it suits people from Annam."[60]

Although pharmaceutical publicity rarely contained images, these were occasionally also used to illustrate this local suitability, by representing tropical environments and pathologies, or Asian features. Sudol, a powder for skin infections, was advertised by an image of children scratching furiously, sweating under a scorching sun amidst palm trees (Figure 6.1). In another case, a shirtless man, who also complained of itchiness, was apparently being given a recommendation for Inotyol salve by an Asian-looking man behind a desk, presumably a doctor. This unusual image was probably meant to express that the product was recommended by doctors, rather than as a message to seek professional

[58] Advertisement, *La tribune indigène*, no. 294, May 11, 1920.
[59] Advertisement, *L'Écho*, no. 1, March 15–16, 1939.
[60] This advertisement was published in the PNTV from June to December 1930.

medical advice for using a harmless product. Most (of the few) images, however, conveyed more general impressions of discomfort in need of alleviation (suffering, coughing, and itching bodies that would find relief in Sirop André, Fer de Quévenne, Kalmine, Foster Pills, or Sirop Nofal) or of therapeutic efficacy (the radiant, restored faces of those who had taken Pink Pills).

6.5   Learning at the Intersection: Tradition for Change

This proliferation of pharmaceutical advertising, along with comments in AMI reports on the growing popularity of injections and of effective medicines, suggests that Vietnamese perspectives on colonial medicines were far from static. On the contrary, the demand for therapy they reveal was highly responsive to new sources of information on the indications and effects of new types of medicines. Still, this emerging demand was selective, privileging some types of medicines and modes of administration – such as arsenical compounds, santonin, injections, and tonics – above others. What we have seen so far suggests that the popularity of medicines in Vietnam was correlated with how well their efficacy was "demonstrated," whether through highly perceptible bioactivity, widespread availability, and a prominent as well as persuasive presence in publicity.

While arguing that these factors played a major role, I also want to point out that information about colonial medicines circulated within a *space of inter-comprehension*. By this, I mean that medicines – their effects and efficacy, as well as their availability and publicity, and advice on how to obtain and to use them – interacted with prior expectations of how therapy should modulate the body; of what conditions were most important to seek treatment for; of how information and expert advice about therapy should be obtained; and even, more broadly, of the meaning of therapy. In other words, processes of learning and developing expectations about colonial medicines may have been facilitated by prior, pre-colonial therapeutic concerns and understandings. This draws attention to the *cultural accessibility* of at least some colonial medicines.[61]

---

[61] The concept of cultural accessibility is used in migrant and minority health studies to draw attention to the fact that the geographical and economic availability of public health services does not guarantee their accessibility: they must also be "culturally sensitive" – that is, compatible with users' sociocultural understanding, their prior experiences of care, and their life trajectories – in order to become acceptable (and be used) among such communities.

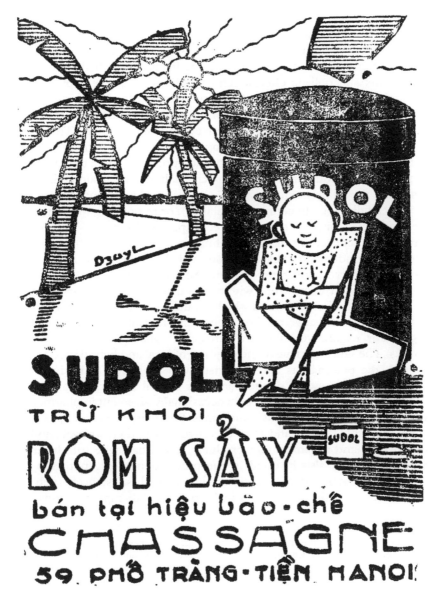

Figure 6.1 Advertisement for Sudol, 1928 (*Vệ sinh báo* [VSB], no. 28, May 1928)

The emphasis on symptomatic relief and global effect on the body in pharmaceutical publicity in Vietnam is, on the one hand, very similar to contemporary trends in the metropole.[62] On the other hand, the striking predominance of tonic and purifying medicines, with highly versatile indications and holistic effects, echoes older Vietnamese expectations about the functions and goals of therapy. Images of unbalancing excess or deficiency in the body, with commercial specialties presented as sources of counter-effect, were often evoked in the press. Thus, the body appeared as a whole, made up of interactions with the mind, between the micro- and the macrocosmic, functioning in a binary mode (equilibrium/disequilibrium, harmony/chaos, hot/cold). Maintaining and restoring the body's equilibrium – by controlling emotions, eating a balanced diet (i.e., to counter imbalance), or responding to changes in weather – was likely a constant preoccupation for most Vietnamese. Traditional conceptions of vital equilibrium in the East Asian region are generally considered to be based on four main bodily functions: digestion, circulation, nerves, and reproduction. An attack on one of these functions, which can come from within or outside the body, first causes weakness, then disequilibrium, which, in turn, can lead to disease.[63]

Some of the best-advertised medicines in Vietnam promised stimulating and/or restorative effects, which acted against such unbalancing attacks. The same was true of the majority of local and hybrid specialties. Indeed, the pharmacists and druggists who produced and advertised these were likely aware of the particular appeal and marketability of these effects. The promotional gifts occasionally given out in pharmacies were usually tonics, especially tonic wines. Pharmacists including Lê Văn Minh (who sold Gaduol and a "tri-digestive"), Montès (owner of another tri-digestive and a hemoglobin product), and Chassagne (producer of a peptone elixir) also invested in the production of organotherapy.[64] Organotherapeutic products, containing animal substances such as blood, were already widely used in Vietnam as "therapeutic foods" to

---

[62] In France, the most prevalently advertised therapeutic indications remained stable from the late nineteenth to the early twentieth centuries. These included digestive problems, fatigue, rheumatism and gout, arthritis and sciatica, heart and circulatory problems, allergies, colds, and women's health issues. Fortifying medicines, especially tonic wines, were still sold as remedies for those with "languishing constitutions," stomach pain, intestinal troubles, diabetes, or excessive nervousness: Myriam Tsikounas, "Quand l'alcool fait sa pub. Les publicités en faveur de l'alcool dans la presse française, de la loi Roussel à la loi Evin (1873–1998)," *Le temps des médias* 1, 2 (2004): 99–101.

[63] David Craig, *Familiar Medicine. Everyday Health Knowledge and Practice in Today's Vietnam* (Honolulu: University of Hawai'i Press, 2002), 67–87.

[64] Pepsin and peptone-based products were quite numerous. Pepsin is an enzyme that was extracted from pig stomachs; peptone was obtained from the artificial digestion of meat by pepsin and/or pancreatin.

prevent disease or boost the organism.[65] Similarly, hormone-based specialties were presented as compensating deficiencies and restoring equilibrium at the level of the organism.

These were also promoted as being good for women's health problems. The instant and enthusiastic demand expressed by BAYB readers for Roussel's Folliculine to treat dysmenorrhea and fatigue might be explained as a product both of preexisting understandings of disease and therapy, which seems to have stimulated a demand for colonial medicines offering holistic, re-equilibrating effects on the body, and of a particular societal preoccupation with treating "female" and reproductive issues. Indeed, conditions affecting both men and women's reproductive capacities (menstrual irregularities, problems of male genitals, and sperm production and infertility) were frequently addressed. In other words, afflictions seen as posing a particular threat to both the individual and the social body may have kindled more determined quests for new, more effective therapies.

This preoccupation is another reason that accounts for the popularity of medicines for the treatment of STIs. Many of the highly popular arsenical drugs were indicated, some exclusively so, for the treatment of syphilis. Other medicines for STIs, especially syphilis and gonorrhea, also seem to have been in high demand: Pilules de Ricord and Hectargyre were seized in an outlet in Vinh Long in 1919, while a large cache of potassium iodide was stolen from the Pharmacie Sarreau in 1924. Many commercial and hybrid specialties as well as traditional remedies were also indicated for these two infections, such as sandalwood-based remedies, La Rose du Dr. Aboud, and Ablennol. Bismuth-based products were the third most frequently mentioned medicines in the BAYB. In addition, magazine readers often expressed anxiety about STIs, or sought advice for symptoms associated with such infections, such as itching, rashes, and lesions in the genital area, as well as signs of inflammation of the urinary tract or testicles. Readers were particularly worried about the threat these conditions posed to reproduction, including mother-to-child transmission of the disease, its hereditary consequences, and the risk of sterility following infection.[66] Furthermore, syphilis was highly prevalent in Vietnam, with infections rates in 1930 estimated (probably underestimated) at 4 to 10 percent in rural Tonkin, and 9 to 16 percent in Hanoi.[67]

---

[65] Du'o'ng Bá Bành, *Histoire de la médecine au Việt nam* (Hanoi: École française d'Extrême-Orient [EFEO], 1947–50), 68.

[66] 914 was also used at the time to protect children of syphilis infected mothers (BAYB no. 18, December 1935, 29).

[67] Exposition coloniale internationale, Laurent Gaide and Paul Campunaud, *Le péril vénérien en Indochine* (Hanoi: IDEO, 1930).

The rapid, enthusiastic adoption of arsenical compounds could thus be explained in terms of a pragmatic acceptance of proof of efficacy in the treatment of fatal afflictions that were widespread and potentially fatal, and which also affected reproductive health and were not effectively cured by traditional therapeutics.

BAYB readers also frequently mentioned children's health problems, including acute diseases, such as whooping cough, chickenpox, measles, and developmental problems, such as stunting and rickets.[68] Similarly, the top problems mentioned in the *savoir-vivre* (lifestyle) column in the women's magazine PNTV were menstrual problems, syphilis, and childhood diseases. These recurring concerns with producing and protecting future generations also echo a more general preoccupation with strength, vitality, and equilibrium. BAYB readers often complained of various minor but painful or bothersome conditions (hemorrhoids, rheumatism and arthritis, headache, cough, sore throat, runny nose, especially from seasonal allergies, rashes, itching), as well as asthma and hypertension, and a range of "stomach" problems (diarrhea, constipation, dyspepsia, and "trouble eating"). They generally associated these conditions either with a general state of weakness or with "stress" (discussed further in Chapter 7), while gastrointestinal conditions can be seen in terms of flows and blockages. This constellation of concerns correlates with the most prevalent indications among the best-advertised specialties in Vietnam. In other words, the therapeutic offer in Vietnam matched up with – and probably cultivated, but must also have picked up on – the potential demand for medicines arising from dominant preoccupations relating to health, specifically with threats to equilibrium and reproduction. By contrast, such preoccupations do not seem to have been shared by health authorities, or to have ranked high among the AMI's priorities and actions.

Pre-colonial understandings of the body and longstanding worries intersected with some colonial medicines' modes of action and indications, stimulating a demand for some types of pharmaceutical efficacy. Shared ingredients, common to both Western and Asian therapeutic arsenals, form another type of intersection that may have facilitated Vietnamese familiarization with biomedical therapies. Despite colonial lawmakers' recurring attempts to detoxify Vietnamese medicine and the growing, and increasingly emphasized, differences between biomedicine and Vietnamese medicine, some therapeutic overlap persisted.

---

[68] The importance given by readers to children diseases in the BAYB can also be explained, at least in part, by the fact that the magazine's owner, Dr. Nguyễn Văn Luyện, was a respected pediatrician.

Both therapeutic systems, for example, used mercury, arsenic, camphor, copper sulphate, and zinc. Some substances were even used for similar purposes in both medical systems, such as mercury to treat syphilis, ergot to stop bleeding, castor oil as a laxative, iron for anemia, and camphor to relieve rheumatism and nerve pains. Both systems recognized the digestive properties of menthol, which was the main ingredient in several well-advertised local specialties such as Holbé-Renoux and Lê Văn Minh brands of peppermint oil. Zinc and copper sulphate were used in Vietnamese remedies for several eye diseases; they were also the active ingredients of most eye drops distributed in public facilities and private pharmacies, including Collyre Jaune and Dr. Motais' Collyre Vert.[69] Moreover, the use of similar material forms probably contributed to some drugs' popular success: as mentioned previously, the pill form was widely used to prepare Chinese and Vietnamese medicines, which may explain why pills and tablets were quickly accepted.[70]

Traditional healers and druggists drew on biomedical references and techniques, encouraging further therapeutic entanglement. There are reports of therapists who prescribed sulfonamides for their "magical" properties, and of others who administered their own products by injection in order to speed up and magnify their action. Another way of enhancing medicines was to combine traditional ingredients with Western substances, a strategy that seems to have become popular by the mid-1930s, as this passage published in L'Annam nouveau indicates:

The Sino-Annamese pharmacy Tham Thiên Duong was brought before justice several times for contravening a law prohibiting the mixing of local and European remedies. Despite several trials, [the pharmacy] remains alive and well. Maybe the judge also thought that this mixing was essential to treatment [. . .] given that curative virtues are better guaranteed in mixed remedies composed of Annamese and Chinese materia medica, or Annamese and French, than in simple and pure remedies. M. Hoang Hy Tuân, a qualified

---

[69] If intersections between therapeutic systems explain the adoption of some medicines, then the converse also seems to be true. The "milk diets" that colonial doctors sought, usually in vain, to impose in the treatment of dysentery in the 1910s must have struck patients as particularly bizarre and probably also literally sickening, given a widespread lack of familiarity with milk and high prevalence of lactose intolerance (up to 75 percent of the Asian population is estimated to be lactose intolerant): "Rapport sanitaire annuel de la province de Haiphong, 1913," ANOM, RST NF 4014, "Rapport sanitaire annuel de la province de Ninh Binh, 1917," ANOM, RST NF 4007.

[70] Vietnamese consumers were also reported to have a particular appreciation for red- and blue-colored remedies (both had positive associations in the Confucian tradition, the first symbolizing good fortune and the second vitality). This appreciation perhaps contributed to the success of Pharmacie Chassagne's Pilules Bleues Antiblennorragiques.

pharmacist in Vinh, has also observed this curious property of remedies: Annamese [medicines for fever and worms], he says, have a faster and surer effect when mixed with European remedies.[71]

Indeed, there was a long history of using ingredients or medicines of Chinese origin to "boost" Vietnamese remedies.[72] Existing modes of hybridization were thus adapted in response to new influences and substances, and were thus diversified, modernized, and Westernized. Sherman Cochran and Perry Link have suggested that early-twentieth-century urban Chinese already made a clear distinction between "ancient" and "modern" medicines. The latter category encompassed not only Western products but also a complex, ill-defined range of neo-traditional, or hybrid, specialties.[73] The same hypothesis can be made for Vietnam, at least for late-colonial urban Vietnam.

Given the marginalization of medicines from official initiatives of health education and care, how did a Vietnamese demand for pharmaceutical specialties emerge and grow? Part of the answer is in the innovative and competitive private market described by the last two chapters, as well as in the efforts made by private pharmacists and doctors, both French and Vietnamese, to publicize therapies through direct advertising, educational texts, and readers' correspondence columns. Publicity displaying the indications and effects of new, practical, convenient, efficient drugs surely had a major impact on readers. Embodied experiences of drug effects, whether felt directly, witnessed, or heard of by word of mouth, may have reached an even broader audience. This clearly contradicts colonial sources that denounced the Vietnamese population's collective ignorance and "resistance to change." Familiarization with colonial medicines was nevertheless a complex learning process that shows continuities – which were skillfully and innovatively exploited – with older therapeutic and health practices that AMI agents could not see, or did not want to acknowledge. This leads to the broader question of whether colonial medicines acted as vectors of social change. Was the emerging demand "merely" a pragmatic search for relief and cure? Or did other values – associated with modernity, science, social status, consumption, individual rights – also enhance, and perhaps arise from, the popularity of medicines? What role were medicines given in a dynamic, modern Vietnamese interwar urban culture? Were quests for medicines

[71] L'Annam nouveau, no. 491, October 27, 1935.
[72] Albert Sallet, "Les vers intestinaux et leurs traitements dans les thérapeutiques annamite et sino-annamite," BSMI 6, 1 (1928): 15–90.
[73] Cochran, Chinese Medicine Men, 159–61; Perry E. Link, Mandarin Ducks and Butterflies: Popular Fiction in Early Twentieth-Century Chinese Cities (Berkeley: University of California Press, 1981), 204.

an indication of, or steps toward, a growing acceptance of biomedical principles, institutions, and practitioners? In other words, to what extent were colonial medicines vectors of modernization and of medicalization? The answer, of course, is multifaceted, differentiated along social and geographical lines that are not always easy to delimit with precision, and many of the clues are difficult to validate or interpret. Yet it is worthwhile to situate the consumption, and non-consumption, of medicines both in the health care field as a whole (public and private) and in relation to the major changes, from nationalist activism to urbanization via consumer commodities, that transformed Vietnamese interwar social and political worlds.

7 Medicines as Vectors of Modernization and Medicalization

To explore the question of whether, and how, the popularity of (some) colonial medicines participated in the modernization and medicalization of Vietnamese society, we first turn to the media. Interwar Vietnam's prolific and vibrant popular press both reflected and shaped a self-conscious quest for modernity. It described, and stimulated, the role of medicines in this quest. Indeed, the media was not simply an arena for marketing pharmaceutical efficacy; it also presented health as modern, as an individual right and responsibility, as well as a consumer good. Yet modernity brought both new imperatives and new obstacles – through overwork, stress, and lack of time – to the management of one's health. Medicines offered solutions. Modernity and medicines thus converged in several ways. We then return to colonial sources. While dominant discourse posited an incompatibility between Vietnamese demand for drugs and a "proper" process of medicalization, I examine how data on medical consultations and private doctors suggest a different story. This demand may have constituted an alternative pathway for medicalizing the colonized. Vietnamese therapeutic practices may not have wholly conformed to the prescriptions and expectations of colonial agents, yet they did not inasmuch systematically contradict them. Medicines thus, in the end, may have created a productive yet unexpected and unintended meeting point between the AMI's objectives and Vietnamese quests for health.

7.1 Media and Social Change

In the 1920s and 1930s, projects of colonial modernization, stemming from the dual logics of "mise en valeur" and of the "civilizing mission," were pursued with greater intensity in Vietnam. As the colonial provision of both basic and higher education expanded, new socio-professional categories (workers, civil servants, liberal professionals) as well as new tensions emerged. In Hanoi and Saigon, modernity was made increasingly tangible in public architecture, electrification, public transportation, new sites of leisure, sociability, and consumption, as well as the growing availability of consumer products. It was adopted by segments of the urban population as a Vietnamese value and goal, driving both the personal cultivation of new dispositions and forms of individuation, and a collective movement for the development of a new civilized (*văn minh*) society. Carried by the Vietnamese intellectual and professional elite, this movement advocated modernization as a tool for strengthening the nation. It was pitted against a colonizers' modernity to which the colonized had little access and which was used to exploit their labor and resources.[1] The interwar years are thus a critical period in the history of Vietnam, with still untapped potential for studying the profound and ambiguous impact of colonial encounters on the emergence of distinctive understandings, experiences, and practices of modernity, particularly in relation to health. Studies in other locations of European influence and domination, particularly in British India and China, have described how such *medical modernities* were actively driven by subalterns, and were highly differentiated by location, social status, as well as political and cultural context.[2] Analogous processes of rational, active, yet selective and modulated appropriations of "modern/Western" norms, values, and technologies of health, including medicines, have been little studied in Vietnam.

There is no better source for capturing such processes than the popular press. Following David Marr, Shawn McHale, and George Dutton, I argue that these publications' content both shaped and responded to readers' expectations, concerns, and values. The press promoted modern ideals and forms of emancipation, but also provided an arena for open discussion and debate about key issues and ideas – for instance, the status of women, the future of Confucianism, and filial piety. Interactive columns and letter-to-the-editor sections were particularly explicit spaces of exchange between editors, contributors, and readers. In these discussions, we can see the emergence of a novel public space, formed around the discussion and adoption of new norms. Christopher Goscha has called this a "cultural revolution," from which could be constituted new "imagined communities," as Benedict Anderson has so elegantly described.[3] It is important to again emphasize that no other French

---

[1] Brocheux and Hémery, *Indochine*, 212–44.

[2] See, in particular, Bhattacharya, "Between the Bazaar and the Bench"; Hodges, *Contraception*; Sivaramakrishnan, *Old Potions*; Bridie Andrews, "Tuberculosis and the Assimilation of Germ Theory in China, 1895–1937," *Journal of the History of Medicine and Allied Sciences* 52, 1 (1997): 114–57.

[3] Christopher Goscha, "'Le barbare moderne': Nguyen Van Vinh et la complexité de la modernisation coloniale au Viêt nam," *Outre-mers. Revue d'histoire*, 88, 2 (2001): 328–32; Benedict Anderson, *Imagined Communities. Reflections on the Origins and Spread of Nationalism* (New York and London: Verso, 1983).

colony had such a prolific popular written press in the interwar years as in Vietnam, where hundreds of titles were published. While this profusion was certainly stimulated by the power attributed to writing in a Confucian society, colonial literacy efforts also played a role. It is estimated that around 1930, at least 20 percent (and perhaps up to 30 percent) of the male adult population could read a newspaper in quốc ngữ.[4]

Print-run figures provide an indication of the rapid rise in popularity of some of these publications.[5] *L'Écho*, created in 1920, had a stable official print run of 3,000 to 4,000 copies per issue from the outset, while *La tribune indigène* quickly jumped from 900 to 2,000 copies. The main women's magazine, the PNTV, could print up to 8,500 copies in the early 1930s. Popular health and science serials had lower but still substantial print runs. The *Nam trung nhứt báo*, owned by the pharmacist Gabriel Renoux, had a print run of 750 copies in 1921 – a modest, but not negligible, circulation for the time. In late 1923, 2,000 copies of each issue of the *Khoa học tạp chí. Revue de vulgarisation scientifique*, the main science magazine, were printed. At the turn of the 1930s, 1,300 copies of the VSB were distributed; 1,500 of the BAYB in 1935.[6]

Editorial statements and letters to columnists and editors provide a glimpse of readership profiles. Some BAYB readers came from far outside Hanoi, including smaller Vietnamese cities (Hué, Tourane, Phan Rang, Pleiku, Ben Tre) as well as Cambodia, Laos, and even southern China and Siam. They were almost exclusively male.[7] Readers of the PNTV were similarly far-flung, but most were educated women, although the column also elicited questions from men. Of the few who revealed more about themselves in their letters to the BAYB, most identified as intellectuals, civil servants, and students. Yet some content may have reached audiences wider than direct readerships, making it difficult to determine exactly who was exposed to their messages. There is evidence that some articles, probably because they struck readers as interesting or important, were read aloud, discussed, reproduced, and sometimes translated from French to Vietnamese.[8] These modes of diffusion, which may have

---

[4] Marr, *Vietnamese Traditions*, 44–50; McHale, *Print and Power*, 28.

[5] Periodical publications varied widely in size and circulation: some were run with very minimal staff and resources, and were forced to slow, suspend, or stop publication in situations of war, economic crisis, or the loss of a journalist.

[6] Subscriptions to *L'Écho* cost 20 piasters per year, and only 1.50 for civil servants and company clerks residing in Saigon-Cholon and Gia Dinh. Yearly subscriptions to VSB and BAYB were 1 and 1.50 piasters, respectively. The health serials were generally cheaper than editorial publications, surely due to their promotional nature.

[7] Men often wrote on behalf of women, on rare occasions they wrote for themselves on gynecological problems and once even on contraception (BAYB, no. 15, September 1935, 29).

[8] McHale, *Print and Power*, 134; Marr, *Vietnamese Traditions*, 140.

reached beyond educated urban circles, seem to have been particularly suited to the content of health magazines. Simple recipes for remedies (a few magazines even had specific formulary sections) could easily be memorized, copied, and passed on; letters sent to the BAYB sometimes requested information about medicines the writer "had been told about," or "shown an advertisement for," by a reader of the magazine.

Health and science–related content was prominent in both the general and specialized press; it played a central role in the articulation and promotion of modern values. This was also the case in early twentieth century Europe and North America, where the mass media played a key role in shaping lay health conceptions and practices under the influence of increasingly close ties with medical institutions and professionals, as well as an explosion in advertising.[9] I estimated that health-themed articles, sections, publicity, and letters to the editor made up nearly 20 percent in the PNTV and up to 60 percent of the BDP in the late 1920s. About one out of every three issues of *L'Écho* featured an in-depth article on health and well-being, often on the first page, adding up to about 520 health-related articles over its publication span from 1920 to 1944. In the 1930s, the impact of these articles would have been boosted by the expansion in direct-to-consumer advertisement. In fact, the advertising sector as a whole was dominated, from the 1920s, by publicity for health products and services, which included medicines but also hygiene and cosmetic products, private clinics and professional services from private doctors and midwives, dentists, and even dental technicians.

From the 1910s, several editorial journals also featured health-related columns, such as the "doctor's corner" in *Le progrès annamite*, the "doctor's opinion" in *L'Écho*, and the "medicine discussion corner" in *La tribune indigène*. The PNTV's "lifestyle" rubric often offered health advice. Health care professionals, especially Vietnamese doctors, wrote, advised, or edited much of this content in both general and specialized publications. *Le progrès annamite* was even founded by a doctor: Jean-Marie Lê Quang Trịnh. Lê Quang Trịnh was the first Vietnamese to obtain, as a French citizen, a doctorate in medicine in Montpellier in 1911. A decade later, in 1922, he opened a private clinic in Cholon and, two years afterward, became a member of the Colonial Council. Dr. Trần Văn Đôn, another key figure in the Vietnamese medical elite, owned the scientific magazine *Khoa học tạp chí* from 1923 to 1926, then became the first Vietnamese vice-president of the Société médico-chirurgicale de

---

[9] Claire Hooker and Hans Pols, "Introduction. Health Medicine and the Media," *Health & History* 8, 1 (2006): 6–7. These two sources of influence, professional and commercial, are not necessarily contradictory: publicity helped promote new ideals of health through images of cleanliness, beauty, youth, and healthiness.

l'Indochine (in 1934) and later wrote dozens of articles for other journals, including the PNTV.[10] I mentioned previously the role played by Nguyễn Văn Luyện in both the VSB and the BAYB. A private general practitioner and pediatrician, Nguyễn Văn Luyện was committed to popular health education (he also wrote manuals on childcare and STIs[11]) and was apparently convinced that such media were a particularly good, cheap, and accessible vehicle for information about medicines and health, and to educate the public for the sake of future generations.

These publications diffused heterogeneous, even at times contradictory, messages about health and care. Their tone ranged from didactic and laudatory to more openly informative, leaving room for interpretation, and perhaps also, at times, room for confusion. Yet across diverse editorial positions and policies, there was a deep and widely shared conviction of the value, even the superiority, of science and biomedicine. By contrast, Vietnamese medicine was frequently a topic of criticism and ridicule; articles denounced, in particular, the abuses and incompetence of "imposters" as well as the use of toxic or unscientific remedies, and thus called for stricter regulation.[12] This promedicalization position was part of the promotion, by the Vietnamese elite, of Westernization more broadly, as civilizing by virtue of its universal scientism. For example, the liberal newspaper L'Écho, headed by the constitutionalist Nguyễn Phan Long, was particularly in favor of Westernization for Vietnam, but also demanded reforms to colonial rule as a beneficial yet transitory source of "progress." In the late 1910s and 1920s, the constitutionalist movement advocated for greater Vietnamese participation in colonial modernization under the banner of Sarraut's Franco-Vietnamese collaboration. It attracted landowners and liberal professionals, including doctors, who were convinced that colonialism could be reformed, and that collaboration with the colonial authorities might lead toward building a Vietnamese nation capable of taking its future into its own hands.[13]

L'Écho was central to the emergence and development of this nationalist movement in Cochinchina from 1917. The newspaper often supported colonial health policy, praising the AMI and its "heroes," including its Vietnamese staff, giving frequent and positive coverage to

[10] Marr, *Vietnamese Traditions*, 54–100.
[11] *Sản dục chỉ nam*, a vademecum to help mothers taking care of their babies, was published in 1925; *Phong tình y an*, a manual to prevent STIs, in 1932.
[12] Un nhà quê, "Nécessité de réglementer la vente de strychnine," *L'Écho*, no. 196, June 4, 1921; "Serait-ce un phénomène"; "Une pratique dangereuse de la médecine annamite," *L'Écho* no. 1256, July 27, 1929.
[13] Peycam, *The Birth of Vietnamese Political Journalism*.

the feats and success of biomedically trained Vietnamese doctors.[14] In parallel, it promoted Pastorian principles of mass prevention through didactic advice addressed to a population considered to be "ignorant and gullible." In 1926, for example, it published a multi-issue article under the title "Germs That Think," to provide, in a playful manner, scientific information on microbes. It also regularly announced public vaccination sessions and published the number of stray dogs "eliminated" in Saigon in the fight against rabies. Yet as defenders of a "real" medical modernization of Vietnam, both newspapers did not hesitate to point out the failures of the colonial administration to deliver it, thus fueling criticism of the AMI's gaps and shortcomings.

7.2   Criticizing the AMI, Advising on Therapy

Such criticism occupied a surprisingly high number of articles in *L'Écho* and other progressive publications, such as *La tribune indigène* and its successor *La tribune indochinoise*. Subaltern AMI staff, as pointed out previously, was regularly accused of incompetence, corruption, and immoral conduct. Some articles also warned readers about doctors who, although qualified, cheated their patients and abused their power. Poorly managed AMI facilities made headlines as well: they were described as dirty, decrepit, and lacking in equipment and staff. There were even exposés on the mistreatment of patients.[15] More general problems of inaccessibility were also denounced and blamed for allowing the population to be exploited by unqualified therapists and unscrupulous traders, especially in rural areas. Such critiques and calls for reform conveyed a distinction between the ideal of biomedicine, assumed to be superior, and its imperfect, even inadequate, implementation in colonial health care, which likely both shaped and was informed by readers' concerns. In other words, they articulated the expectation of a *right to health* as an intrinsic dimension of modernity, while denouncing its denial to the Vietnamese. By the 1930s, many journalists, especially those who were doctors, made explicit claims to this right on behalf of a profoundly disappointed public. AMI doctors' responses to a questionnaire item

---

[14] It published detailed administrative information on doctors' graduations and changes in rank and position.

[15] Among the most virulent articles are "A l'hôpital municipal"; Lê Trung Nghĩa, "La bagarre de Cholon et les infirmiers de l'Hôpital indigène," *La tribune indigène*, no. 59, December 24, 1926; Thọc Mạch, "Le gâchis dans les hôpitaux de Hué," *La tribune indigène*, no. 783, January 18, 1927; Linh Vê, "Les malades indigènes. Dédié à la direction de l'Hôpital indigène de Cholon," *La tribune indigène*, no. 1104, February 24, 1928, and no. 1110, March 2, 1928; "Un peu d'humanité à défaut d'égards pour les malades, s'il vous plaît!," *La tribune indochinoise*, no. 614, September 29, 1930.

asking about "indigenous aspirations in matters of health" in 1937–38 provide a glimpse of these expectations and their betrayal. The majority answered: "free medicines and hospitals."[16] "Free," of course, is the keyword here; yet it is also significant that what the population, according to doctors, most wanted were medicines. Their lack was identified as a core element of the AMI's failings.

At the same time, the local media articulated and promoted a modern, and modernizing, *responsibility for health* that entailed obligations on the part of the general public. These obligations were to oneself, but also toward others: to maintain personal hygiene as well as public order and cleanliness; to prevent disease transmission; to engage in physical activity; and to commit to attentive mothering.[17] Calls to take on this responsibility were, once again, increasingly relayed through advertising. Articles on topics such as vitamin deficiency in the 1930s stressed the importance of good diets and strong, healthy children. These more or less explicitly linked to publicity for products that blurred the distinction between food and medicine.[18] Nestlé products, especially its range of baby formulas and condensed milk, were advertised ubiquitously. These and enriched foods (like Blédine, Phosphatine Fallière, Banania, and Ovomaltine, the latter marketed as sources of strength for children and parents alike)[19] were promoted with messages about the crucial role of early dietary supplementation. Publicity for soaps, toothpaste, detergent, and other personal and household hygiene products also emphasized the obligations of those hoping to participate in the biomedical citizenship promised by colonization. There was, at the time, a flourishing local soap industry that included brand names such as Dragon d'Annam, Ng Huu, and Đại Quang, named after the famous Cholon "traditional" drugstore. It was implied that the fulfillment of these obligations would contribute to the making of a new, and newly vigorous, social body that might, one day, be the body of the nation.

This call to take responsibility for one's health and others' was also conveyed, more or less directly, in educational content and in the advice

---

[16] The question was from a questionnaire on Indochinese health, nutrition, and housing distributed for the purposes of the Commission Guernut, French Front Populaire commission of inquiry in 1937 that was mandated to gather and review information about the "needs and aspirations" of the colonized population in order to make some appropriate reforms in the empire (ANOM, CG, Box 107, Folder 18).

[17] Eugenia Lean describes similar trends in the contemporary Chinese popular press: Eugenia Lean, "The Modern Elixir: Medicine as a Consumer Item in the Early Twentieth-century Chinese Press," *UCLA Historical Journal* 15 (1995): 65–92.

[18] The 1930s were a time of growing alarm among the colonial administration about malnutrition, whereas several regions of Vietnam were facing an expansion of poverty, overpopulation, and even famine: Brocheux and Hémery, *Indochine*, 252–70.

[19] *L'Écho*, no. 795, February 7, 1927.

provided by columnists and editors. Health magazines, in particular, provided, alongside explicit and embedded promotional messages, information ranging from straightforward advice on simple, practical measures for preventing infection and treating illness to highly technical explanations of the etiology, transmission, and Vietnamese epidemiology of infectious diseases.[20] Many articles described hygienic measures for protecting pregnant women and newborns. There were also passionate pleas for vaccination, sometimes alongside information meant to reassure readers about the procedure; many reminders of the importance of a healthy diet and of safe or moderate sexual and other lifestyle habits; and the occasional article about the dangers of addiction to opium (and to anti-opium medicines), alcohol, and tobacco.[21] These publications also offered guidance for *rational self-medication*. This was particularly explicit in the VSB and in the BAYB, in which Nguyễn Văn Luyện provided instructions on how to manage minor health problems. He also gave detailed therapeutic advice for preventing adverse effects and for determining dosages, including on how to adjust posology to an individual's condition, age, sex, intolerance, and so on.[22]

Doctors often offered medical advice, and even remote consultations, through the press. VSB and BAYB editors did not present all self-medication as suitable or safe. They warned readers that some health conditions and therapies called for a medical consultation, and that some medicines, particularly if used outside validated therapeutic indications, could be dangerous. If direct-to-consumer publicity quite obviously encouraged its audience to make choices about which medicines to take, some inserts also offered guidance for avoiding therapeutic misuses. For example, some advertisements for Collyre Jaune warned that using the eye drops for the wrong conditions could lead to blindness. The BAYB editor also cautioned readers about drug risks. For example, in March 1936, he responded to one reader's letter with a reminder that the arsenobenzol Acétylarsan should only be taken by prescription and under medical surveillance.[23] A few months later, another reader asked for

---

[20] Some articles used a vocabulary so specialized that I suppose most readers were unlikely to fully comprehend. Yet some publications also offered French-Vietnamese lexicons of scientific, including medical, terms, surely in order to increase the accessibility and familiarity of biomedical information.

[21] On vaccination promotion, see for instance several articles published in *L'Écho* in 1928: "Faites-vous vacciner!," no. 1144, April 12; "Le vaccin BCG," no. 1302, October 19; "Le vaccin tuberculeux. Peut-il être nocif? Une controverse intéressante," no. 1343, December 10.

[22] Nguyễn Văn Luyện, "Khi ngộ độc phải làm thế nào?," VSB, no. 69, April–June 1932, 1–4, and no. 70, July–September 1932, 1–4; "Tiêm thuốc."

[23] Readers' correspondence, BAYB no. 21, March 1936, 24.

information on how to use Plasma de Quinton, which he had purchased, but for which he had no instructions. Nguyễn Văn Luyện responded with precise information about dosage depending on age, the length of treatment, and therapeutic indications and contraindications.[24] While the PNTV's "savoir-vivre" column regularly provided information and advice on health, the editors grew worried about the difficulty of validating the quality of its information, and announced, in 1931, that they were stopping its publication. In the future, they promised, the magazine would avoid providing any information on "unscientific" (ngoài khoa) remedies unless verified by recognized professionals.[25]

Editors and advertisers thus recognized, if implicitly, that readers were likely to obtain and to take medicines without consulting a doctor, providing tools for making informed choices about self-medication. This willingness to accept and strengthen patients' aptitude to manage their own medication contrasted with contemporary dominant biomedical discourse, especially with the official position of colonial doctors. And while the proliferation of drug publicity and medical advice was driven by commercial interests, it was also compatible with Confucian principles of self-education and responsible management of health. Deeply-rooted values were thus adapted to new scientific, technical and material realities. And despite representations of "quality of life" as emblematic of the cultivation of the modern self, advice on how to maintain this quality did not always point toward biomedical solutions. Even in the 1930s, the PNTV and health magazines often provided simple recipes for traditional remedies, either for minor health problems or as a solution to the problem of unavailable or unaffordable biomedical doctors and medicines. These were pragmatic suggestions, for recipes sometimes included plants used in the Sino-Vietnamese pharmacopeia that were readily and often cheaply available. Yet they invite us to consider how longer-standing Confucian traditions of care, as much as a quest for modern values and technologies of health, might account for the popularity of the Vietnamese press and its success in instilling a sense of obligation to "live healthily." Indeed, its advice may have improved everybody's quality of life: this is what the government official in charge of the Binh Dinh Province affirmed in an open letter sent to the VSB in 1929, in which he thanked its editorial team for the precious contribution they had made to the well-being of the Vietnamese population.[26]

[24] Readers' correspondence, BAYB no. 29, November 1936, 31. It is not impossible that the magazine editor-in-chief fabricated some of the correspondence published in the BAYB, for educational purposes – that is, to raise readers' awareness of a particular treatment or issue.
[25] PNTV, no. 98, September 1931, 18.
[26] VSB, no. 43, August 1929.

Health was clearly central to the self-conscious cultivation of modernity advocated by the press and its readership, which challenged colonial authorities to deliver on their promises of medicalization, while also calling on the lay public to take responsibility for their own health. From this perspective, modern medicines were both a right to which colonial authorities should ensure access, and a privileged tool of self-care. But beyond this, to what extent were medicines perceived by the Vietnamese as emblematic modern technologies of care and, more generally, as essential tools of modern life? We saw in Chapter 6 that medicines were increasingly visible in the pages of the popular press via the modern medium of advertising that, despite a continued emphasis on holistic and symptomatic effects, also mobilized images of modern science, specificity, and efficacy. For many Vietnamese, even in rural areas, the material and visual presence of medicines increasingly took the shape of mass-produced forms and packaging. While many highly effective and popular medicines came in injectable forms, the majority of commercial specialties and rural essential medicines were presented as tablets, granules, sugarcoated pills, capsules, and so on. Ready for sale and consumption, easy to ingest, stock, and carry, as well as to protect from the effects of time, heat, and humidity, these forms were appreciated by consumers and distributors alike. Pills in particular were now increasingly numerous, well-displayed, and well-advertised as products of scientific innovation, industrial production, and commercial consumption. Mass-produced forms conveyed distinctly modern therapeutic principles – shifting the locus of specificity from the patient to the treatment – as well as more abstract representations of modern identities and forms of belonging.

Observers remarked that medicines, like other consumer goods including toiletries and cosmetics, as well as clothes, perfume, jewelry, and cars, were consumed not only because of an "attraction" to Western ideals, but also as a marker of social distinction. In the mid-1930s, the journalist, novelist, and satirist Vũ Trọng Phụng openly mocked members of Hanoi's fashionable society who took Western medicines because it was the "done thing," through his comic antihero the "king of venereal disease."[27] Even earlier, in 1923, Vong Buc denounced, in L'Écho, such "trend effects" as being superficial and out of place in Vietnamese society, hinting at their potentially harmful impact on health:

Now that we have given up our civilization, we have given up the books that guided us for so long. And we have imported science, industry, champagne, silver cutlery [. . .] the pornographic postcard, and the impudence of women [. . .] [Thrown into] the heap there is [also] Pastorian medicine and pharmacy, fresh

---

[27] Vũ Trọng Phụng, Dumb Luck.

out of the laboratory. And all this, indiscriminately, helter-skelter. So that the grimiest nhà quê wears patent leather booties and limps, and the most worn-out ba già drinks a Chinese decoction with conviction yet superstitiously asks for some "[intra]venous shot." Anyhow, Annamites have shown themselves to be infinitely permeable to ideas from the outside and to passing fashion.[28]

Three editorials published by the BAYB in 1936–37 also warned of the potentially dangerous influence of drug advertisements. Noting how fast the messages in health publicity circulated, the first article warned that the content of this information was guided by "vogues" rather than a concern for safety. The two other articles similarly attacked "dangerous" and "misleading" publicity: one pointing to the specific case of "pseudo-specialties" promising cures for syphilis and gonorrhea, and the second calling more broadly for tighter regulation of health advertisement, concluding that only "a few really useful medicines" were worth promoting to the public.[29] Yet these warnings indicated that, by then, advertising was surely seen as an influential, if not necessarily reliable, source of information about the value and effects of medicines in Vietnam.

7.3   Modern Medicines for a New Society: Lack of Time, Neurasthenia, and Consumerism[30]

Publicity for toiletries and cosmetics played on the association between consumption, health, and modern belonging. They offered an entry into a state of modernity that manifested as visible and desirable, if superficial, signs of health. Toothpastes (Obanil and Dentol brands), soaps (Cadum), antiseptic or beauty creams and powders (Satine, Tokalon, Helena Rubinstein, Reina), and hair products (Petrole Hanh dandruff lotion or pharmacist Lê Văn Minh's Venusol) promised consumers, especially women, an attractive (i.e., healthy and youthful) physical appearance. This promise put forward new aesthetic standards influenced by Western ideals of beauty: wrinkles vanished in an advertisement for Crème Parisienne Keva, while Pilules Orientales were recommended "for firmer breasts," and Crème Siamoise was "whitening." Notably, however, publicity also emphasized these products' scientific qualities and curative efficacy – that is, their medicine-like qualities. Obanil

---

[28] Vong Buc, "Lettres d'un villageois. Pour l'expansion de la pharmacie française," *L'Écho*, no. 442, February 22, 1923. *Nhà quê* means "peasant" and *bà già* "old lady." Vong Buc uses both terms in a derogatory manner purposefully, as some French colonials would do, to emphasize the ridicule of these so-called civilized practices.

[29] Editorials, BAYB, no. 25, July 1936, no. 39, October 1937, and no. 40, November 1937.

[30] The arguments in this section were inspired by Nancy Vuckovic's, "Fast Relief: Buying Time with Medications," *Medical Anthropology Quarterly* 13, 1 (1999): 51–68.

toothpaste was marketed as a "scientific toothpaste that whitens the teeth."[31] The text of a 1934 advertisement for Crème Tho-Radia, containing radium and thorium "according to the formula of Dr. Alfred Curie," provides an even more striking illustration of this promotional strategy:

What makes a pharmacist particularly competent for the preparation and sale of a beauty cream? Because a beauty cream, to be beautifying, must not only be safe but also have truly curative virtues [. . .] The signature of a pharmacist on a cosmetic product is a sure guarantee of respect for the formula and of the therapeutic value of the ingredients used. In addition, only the pharmacist is allowed to sell a beauty cream of which the medical properties make it a true pharmaceutical specialty.[32]

These marketing strategies extended the reach of scientific medicine and modern ideals of health into new realms of everyday life, an extension that resulted from, but also actively drove, the adoption of new practices of prevention, care, and consumption. Modern consumption was promoted by appealing to science – as proof of efficacy as well as guarantee of quality and the competence of experts – and the promise of improved quality of life. As a 1930 advertisement for a digestive aid powder, Poudre Maubar, proclaimed pithily: "Western quality, benefits: digestion, joie de vivre."[33] The consumption of medicines was surely stimulated, in part, by the broader, and aggressively promoted, appeal of Western goods and lifestyles, as well as by more insidious pressures to assimilate to the norms of French colonial society.

Yet as material substances that enter and transform bodies, medicines cannot merely be seen as symbols of membership in modernity. One must also ask how their transformative potential was represented and harnessed in terms of capacity to function, to work, to enjoy life, and to have children in a rapidly changing world – that is, as practical and powerful tools for modern living. Time, or rather lack of time, was a growing concern in interwar urban society, as much for traders and workers as for colonial clerks and liberal professionals. Problems, especially those impinging on the capacity to work, required quick solutions. The price of medicines from a nearby private pharmacy or shop was offset, at least in part, by savings in time and cost (of transportation, lost working hours, and fees) of not having to consult a clinician.[34]

[31] Advertisement, BDP, no. 156, January 19, 1926.
[32] Advertisement, PNTV, no. 237, April 12, 1934.
[33] Advertised regularly in the PNTV, *Le progrès annamite* and *La tribune indochinoise*.
[34] There are several mentions of access problems posed by transportation and lost work time for both urban clinics and rural settings, where the sparsity of facilities forced patients and kin to abandon their fields for up to several days to visit a consultation or

If self-medication was thus already a shortcut, publicity further fueled the expectation that medicines should be easy to administer and deliver swift and powerful, sometimes even instant, effects. Indeed, speed was central to the promotion of Baume Tue-Nerf Miriga for toothache, Nobial pills for head colds, and Amibiasine for diarrhea, the latter described as "easy to administer, with immediate and durable efficacy."[35] Dépuratif Richelet would fix circulatory problems and relieve the pain of arthritis and rheumatism in only a few days. Its publicity often featured the image of a well-dressed man who was clearly suffering, holding his head or back or walking with difficulty. Thus fast effects were associated with therapeutic versatility and with the restoration of functionality for people with fast-paced lives. Even Banania, a simple cocoa-based drink powder, was sometimes marketed as "food for busy people."[36]

Publicity for Poudre Saint André featured a distinguished-looking man, writhing with pain in his stomach, who was unable to function (Figure 7.1). Foster Pills were often advertised in the BDP as a remedy for all kinds of pains, especially back pain, which was widely seen as an ill of modern society. Back pain was only one of the symptoms and pathologies that were widely associated with the pressures of work in Vietnam's large urban centers.

Other modern afflictions included fatigue, anxiety, insomnia, and other nervous problems, such as stress and especially neurasthenia, for which dozens of products promised relief.[37] Among these were well-advertised commercial specialties, many of which had a wide range of indications, often including the treatment of spermatorrhea and anemia.[38] Pink Pills, for example, were said to prevent the escalation of "weariness,"

---

medicines outlet, while the common rule of dispensing only twenty-four hours' worth of treatment entailed additional transportation and/or time away from work.

[35] Advertisement, BDP, no. 76, July 16, 1925.

[36] Advertisement, *La tribune indochinoise*, no. 548, April 19, 1930, and no. 562, May 23, 1930.

[37] Neurasthenia was defined in 1868 by the American neurologist George Miller Beard as "a chronic, functional disease of the nervous system" or a state of "nervous exhaustion," associated with the pressures of urban life and modern work. In the 1910s, it was still a "fashionable" diagnosis in the West. It was linked to a wide range of symptoms, including headache, various pains, irritability, loss of appetite, insomnia, dizziness, dyspepsia, extreme fatigue, loss of sensation, palpitations, and impotence: Laurence Monnais, "Colonised and Neurasthenic: From the Appropriation of a Word to the Reality of a Malaise de Civilisation in Urban French Vietnam," *Health & History* 14, 1 (2012): 121–42.

[38] Spermatorrhea was greatly feared in East Asia both as a result of broader anxieties about modernization and long-standing associations of sperm loss, STIs, impotence, and the risk of sterility: Hugh Shapiro, "The Puzzle of Spermatorrhea in Republic China," *Positions. East Asia Cultures Critique* 6, 3 (1998): 571–81.

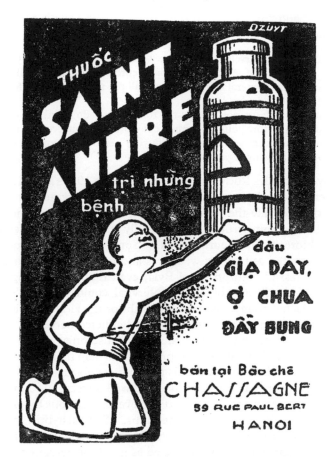

Figure 7.1 Advertisement for Poudre Saint André, 1932 (VSB, no. 70, July–September 1932)

"depression," and "overwork" into full-blown neurasthenia by restoring physical and nervous strength:

Don't put off treating yourself [. . .] You are weary, weak, depressed by work, by worries, by overwork. Be aware that [this] depression of yours will soon be anemia, neurasthenia, general exhaustion and all the troubles and suffering that comes with these.

Don't put off until later, don't wait until tomorrow to do a Pink Pill cure [. . .] Pink Pills will soon restore your strength because they will give you richer, purer, more vibrant blood, because they will fortify your nervous system and will energetically stimulate all your organic functions[39]

Similarly, Ampoules Rudy were advertised in the 1920s as indicated for "neurasthenia, convalescence, overwork," as well as in the treatment of infectious diseases like the flu and malaria. By regenerating the blood, Deschiens hemoglobin syrup would allegedly increase one's resistance to weakness, chlorosis, and neurasthenia.[40] Some cutting-edge specialties were also promoted as treating weakness and nervousness. "No state of fatigue could resist" Neurotrophol Byla, even though the drug's main indication was for liver problems.[41] Nervital could control "sadness, anguish, headache, cramps, pain in the limbs or the kidneys [which] are some of the symptoms of neurasthenia; [. . .] afflicted nerves."[42] Billonal would allow one to get rid of "dark thoughts," insomnia, and all kinds of nervous symptoms. Céphalose even promised to help manage "timidity" as well as "cerebral fatigue," and thus to eliminate obstacles to social and professional success.[43] The well-named and well-advertised Kalmine was to be taken for anxiety and was seized on several occasions by pharmacy inspection services in Sino-Vietnamese shops.[44] Several hybrid specialties and Vietnamese remedies, such as several Đâu Rông and Lu'o'ng Minh Ký brand products, were also publicized as good for nervous problems, stress, as well as overwork and competition, also identified as conditions of modern life.

Readers regularly mentioned such medicines and nervous afflictions in their correspondence with BAYB's editor; they were worried about

[39] Advertisement, BDP, no. 1, January 12, 1925. This issue contains no fewer than five publicity inserts for Pink Pills.
[40] This product was regularly advertised in the BDP in the 1920s.
[41] Advertisement, L'Écho, no. 442, November 26, 1925.
[42] The two products were advertised side by side in La tribune indochinoise, no. 562, May 23, 1930.
[43] Advertisement, La tribune indochinoise, no. 562, May 23, 1930.
[44] VNA, centre no. 1, RST 32073 and 47825; ANOM, RST NF 3683. Kalmine, in French also, evokes "calming" or "to calm." Introduced in 1914, the product sold well internationally during the interwar period: Michèle Ruffat, 175 ans d'industrie pharmaceutique française. Histoire de Synthélabo (Paris: La Découverte, 1996), 47.

conditions such as insomnia, irritability, exhaustion, and hypertension, often in conjunction with nervousness or heart problems or both, which they explicitly attributed to modern work environments.[45] Brought up on eighteen occasions, the medical specialty Geneserine was indicated for the treatment of indigestion, but it was also used in subcutaneous injections to treat the "painful crises" and "anxiety and insomnia" suffered by dyspeptics.[46] A certain L. N. L., from Haiphong, said to perform "intense intellectual work," wondered in 1936 whether his symptoms (pressure in the chest, loss of appetite and weight, irritability and trouble sleeping) were signs of neurasthenia.[47] In 1937, a student complained of weakness, insomnia, and depression.[48] Another, an AMI nurse, blamed his suffering (he had trouble eating and sleeping, and was so exhausted that he could not perform routine activities) on five years of exposure to a harmful work environment.[49] For these afflictions, which threatened their ability to function and manage their lives, readers expected readymade pharmaceutical solutions, asking the editor-in-chief to recommend a "miracle cure."

This quest to treat emerging pathologies of modern life, particularly nervous problems, coincided, in the 1930s, with a growing consumption of recently introduced hypnotics, sedatives, and barbiturates. Among the products mentioned in the BAYB are Gardénal (Rhône-Poulenc),[50] Allonal (Roche), Vérogénol (Laboratoire Veinot), Neurinase (Genevrier), and Spasmine (Jolly). Soon, doctors began to worry about abusive usage of these "overly soothing" medicines in Vietnam, which were also distributed in growing volume within AMI facilities.[51] This (over)consumption of tranquilizers was linked, as it was in European and North American debates, to the harmful effects of industrialization and urbanization. In 1939, L'Écho complained that noise pollution in Saigon plagued a population already in the throes of "a feverish existence, so hectic, so irritating in so many ways in this

---

[45] Among the products mentioned for treating hypertension were Passiflorine, a plant-based product, Angioxyl (Roussel), and Spasmosédine (Laboratoires Deglaude), which were also used in the West to treat neurasthenia.
[46] Vidal, Dictionnaire, 745.
[47] Readers' correspondence, BAYB, no. 19, January 1936, 32–33.
[48] Readers' correspondence, BAYB, no. 31, January 1937, 27.
[49] Readers' correspondence, BAYB, no. 40, April 1938, 23.
[50] Gardénal (phenobarbital, previously called Veronal) was the most frequently mentioned barbiturate in the Vietnamese press.
[51] "Lúc ngộ độc phải làm thế nào? Ngộ độc bởi thuốc ngủ," VSB, no. 72, January–March 1933, 6–8; Massias, "Intoxication volontaire." In the late 1930s, some AMI hospitals stocked also Prominal, Phanodorme, Ruthonal, Sonéryl, Adaline, Somnifène, Evipan, and Sédol (ANOM, Gougal SE 217 and 2921).

century of mechanics, of speed [. . .] and of frenzied work."[52] Yet it should not be forgotten that, in Vietnam, this change occurred under and was driven by an extractive colonial enterprise that made heavy demands on the time, energy, and health of its agents and workers. Some suggested that colonial rule was directly responsible for the cumulative assaults on the health and well-being of urban dwellers and might lead to a desperate search for relief, any kind of relief. Barbiturates, Nguyễn Văn Luyện wrote in 1933, were already seen by some as a source of ultimate relief – in other words, as a means of committing suicide. In May 1934, the PNTV published a long article, which was immediately censored, on suicide as a "new social problem," describing it as the conclusion of a downward spiral, progressing from depression and stigmatization to death, caused by the aggravation of economic conditions and poverty.[53]

If many well-advertised and best-selling medicines addressed long-standing Vietnamese concerns about health – to maintain equilibrium through stimulation and elimination, and to protect reproductive and children's health – at least a portion of Vietnamese consumers turned to medicines to solve new kinds of problems, including troubled nerves, stunted growth, and hypertension, that were at once medical and social, somatic, and psychic, thus shifting the boundary between the normal and the pathological. This extended the range of conditions identified as treatable – that is, as falling within the reach of biomedicine and perhaps also as requiring treatment, signaling lowered thresholds of tolerance to suffering and dysfunction. Was this expansion of medicalization a sign of modernity, of Westernization, of an imminent health consumerism?[54] Whatever we call it, by the late 1930s, AMI doctors clearly complained much less than they had in the early 1910s of their patients' stoicism and tendency to delay seeking treatment. Growing (learned) hope of relief and cure, perhaps even new aspirations to well-being, might be supposed to have shifted lay perceptions over these two to three decades, at least among those in closest contact with new therapeutic possibilities, toward greater convergence with expert biomedical perspectives on medicalization.

---

[52] E. A., "Contre le tapage nocturne. Trop de bruit à Saigon aux heures indues: la sieste et la nuit," *L'Écho*, no. 17, April 24–25, 1939.

[53] "Nạn tự tử! Dịch tự sát!," BDP, no. 423–24, October 18 and 20, 1927; "Sự tự tữ," PNTV no. 241, May 10, 1934.

[54] Health or medical consumerism is usually defined in terms of linking health with the pleasure, uncontrolled desire, and individualization of the consumption process: Arthur W. Frank, "What's Wrong with Medical Consumerism?," in *Consuming Health, the Commodification of Healthcare*, ed. Sara Henderson and Alan Petersen (New York and London: Routledge, 2002), 18–19. Thus it is probably an anachronistic term with which to describe the situation in Vietnam, where the accessibility of medicines and of health care was still very limited, and pharmaceutical products were not yet considered to be banal and necessary commodities.

7.4   (In)compatible Representations (Part I): Disciplining the Demand for Medicine

This being said, to what extent and by what channels did demands for medicines lead to a medicalization of Vietnamese lives, bodies, and health practices within and beyond the urban male elite? What forms did these processes of medicalization take? I have already suggested some of the ways in which the advertising and consumption of medicines mutually interacted with new, modern ideas and values of health. Beyond this, however, available sources do not allow for the elaboration of direct and detailed answers to these questions. I now offer two indirect routes for exploring whether and how an emerging selective Vietnamese demand for medicines converged, or not, with the broader colonial project of medicalization.

I first revisit biomedical portrayals of Vietnamese demands for medicines as excessive, irrational, and undisciplined. Even if they were often pejorative, doctors' comments on lay demands and refusals of treatment also contain hints about the nature of their underlying logics and motivations. It is thus possible to identify some points of convergence or compatibility between colonized representations of medicine(s) and colonial medicalization policies – as well as points of divergence and misunderstanding. I then return to the question of how medications were obtained in French Indochina, and particularly to the refusal or acceptance of clinical consultations as gateways to free and effective medicines. Biomedical and colonial rules placed the doctor-patient encounter at the heart of a proper therapeutic process. Of course, it was often bypassed. While the practical problems of access to consultations was a major reason for this (see Chapters 2 and 3), we must also consider that potential patients also, in some cases, chose to engage with consultation services as a pathway for obtaining therapy, and wonder why. The rise of private medical consultation services in the 1930s suggests that a demand for medicines could indeed be a vector of medicalization. These two "diagonal" readings of sources – for reasons behind Vietnamese acceptance and refusal of biomedicine, colonial services, and their therapies – show how medicines both revealed and bridged a cultural gap in colonial Vietnam.

Early French observers had seen an opportunity to "convert the natives" in the Vietnamese "ancestral taste" for medicines, which they attributed to the central and long-standing role of remedies in Vietnamese health practices. For missionaries such as Father Cadière, offering medicines could ease relations and create opportunities to speak about God.[55] The first military doctors and explorers also provided medicines as gifts to demonstrate the benevolence and benefits of French presence, even if the therapeutic results were not always persuasive in themselves.[56] With the official creation of the AMI system, the indigenous demand for medicines was increasingly described in dismissive terms. The Vietnamese liked medicines "too much"; they were "pharmacophages" (eaters of medicines) by taste and by education.[57] In the late nineteenth century, colonial medicines were still similar in many ways to Sino-Vietnamese remedies. In the first decades of the twentieth century, however, modern pharmaceuticals were increasingly set apart from traditional therapeutic forms by new modes of production, regulation, commercialization, and administration, as well as by changes in understanding of etiology and treatment of disease. These growing differences between the two types of medicines, from their material appearance to their underlying rationales, were emphasized by an increasingly assertive colonial medicalization project.

AMI doctors often suggested that their patients' failure to take adequate preventive measures, as well as their tendency to delay seeking treatment and to abandon it too early, was due to their poor grasp of disease etiology. This made them ignorant or indifferent to underlying pathology, and led them to focus exclusively on superficial symptoms and discomfort. Given as an explanation for Vietnamese resistance to (proper) medicalization, this emphasis on an inability or unwillingness to adhere to Pastorian understandings of disease was certainly exaggerated. Indeed, we have seen that drug advertising used images of battle and resistance against microbes. Still, references to the persistence of Vietnamese beliefs in the supernatural origins of some diseases were widespread. In 1932, for example, the VSB noted that "many people" did not seek vaccination or hospitalization for cholera because they believed the disease was "brought by genies," and instead "pray[ed] to Quan ôn."[58] This suggests that, even as biomedical models of etiology became more familiar, they continued to coexist, sometimes in tension or conflict, with local explanatory models for some diseases, leading to selective appropriations and variable interpretations. Leprosy, for example, continued to be seen by many as a karmic illness, suffered in

[55] Léopold Cadière, *Croyances et pratiques religieuses des Vietnamiens* (Saigon: EFEO, 1955), 211.
[56] Foiret, "Topographie médicale"; Dr. Mougeot, "Un rapide voyage chez les Mois," *Bulletin de la Société des études indochinoises* 5 (1887): 29–44.
[57] Sarrailhé, "Extraits du rapport annuel," 309–10.
[58] "Cái thiên tai hàng năm. Bệnh dịch tả," VSB, no. 69, April–June 1932, 4–9.

retribution for grave sins committed in a previous life.[59] Some conditions were also identified as "Vietnamese diseases," against which biomedicine was expected to be powerless. Dr. Massias, working in Soc Trang in the early 1930s, suggested that this was why typhoid fever patients were brought to him only as a last resort.[60] A few years earlier, the same Massias had asked the Byla firm to create a treatment for beriberi that would appeal to "indigenous tastes," in order to convince the population that this condition was, contrary to "local belief," a treatable entity.[61]

Other diseases, however, prompted recourse to biomedical care. Tuberculosis was widely recognized to be contagious and fatal, and its symptoms were well known. The expression then used for the disease, *bệnh ho lao*, referred to its wasting cough. The press reported that specialized consultation services created in the late 1920s and new treatments – such as the subcutaneous beeswax injections proposed by Dr. Normet at the Hôpital indigène of Hué –attracted patients in droves.[62] Young people, from Hanoi and the provinces, suffering from persistent cough were said to have immediately flocked to the new tuberculosis dispensary established in the early 1930s in the city's Richaud Street.[63] Yet even when they did seek biomedical treatment, the Vietnamese were said by colonial doctors to be overly or exclusively preoccupied with symptoms (pain, tiredness, itching, coughing) rather than with identifying and treating an underlying cause.[64] This tendency was mobilized as an argument against the use of medicines as tools of medicalization. A particularly clear example of this can be found in debates about the (mis)use of arsenical compounds in syphilis control that arose in the BSPE, then in the BSMI, in the 1930s.

These debates, described in Chapter 2, centered on the erratic therapeutic behavior of Vietnamese patients (and the impossibility, in a thinly spread and understaffed colonial health care system, of keeping a close eye on them) as a cause of complications – namely neuro-syphilis, a condition associated with incomplete courses of therapy. They provide a striking illustration of the clear, persistent rift between the AMI's

---

[59] Monnais, "Lepers and Leprosy," 133.

[60] Charles Massias, "La fièvre typhoïde en Cochinchine. Étude de 89 cas à l'hôpital de Soc Trang," BSPE 27 (1934): 406–13.

[61] The resulting product – tablets of B1 vitamins, brewers' yeast, and amino acids – was later trademarked as Vitaminol: Charles Massias, "Le traitement du béribéri par une préparation contenant vitamine B et acides aminés (Vitaminol)," BSMI 11 (1933): 389–91.

[62] Linh Vê, "La lutte contre la tuberculose pulmonaire en Annam," L'Écho, no. 1088, February 6, 1928.

[63] "Pour les tuberculeux," L'Annam nouveau, no. 1102, February 25, 1932.

[64] VSB and BAYB editors also often insisted on the importance of going beyond visible symptoms and seeking a doctor's diagnosis.

objectives and the goals of potential patients. On the one hand, colonial doctors and health policies prioritized prevention-based public health measures that implied tight control over potential or declared disease carriers. On the other hand, potential patients sought treatment for an affliction that threatened their lives and the future of their families. An example of how AMI professionals sought to undermine drug treatment in favor of preventive measures is the fact, reported by Vũ Trọng Phụng in the late 1930s, that prostitutes in Hanoi were taught in a public specialized dispensary to practice good hygiene to prevent venereal disease so that they might avoid the need for "painful" arsenical injections and pills that were "difficult to swallow."[65] The alternative, therapy-centered routes to health traced by astutely advertised commercial specialties and the advice of health magazine editors, may have better responded to potential consumers' expectations and preoccupations.

In the case of syphilis, Vietnamese preoccupations seem to have intersected with health authorities' concerns. By contrast, other infectious diseases – notably malaria, but also dysentery, smallpox, cholera, plague – were priority targets for the IGHSP but were rarely mentioned and never discussed in readers' correspondence and had little presence in pharmaceutical publicity. When these diseases did appear in the press, it was as part of educational articles on disease prevention or in announcements of official colonial actions. There are other explanations for this silence: for one, several of these conditions, being acute, fatal, and having no effective drug treatment, were unlikely to prompt written requests for advice or treatment recommendations. Still, this mismatch in apparent priorities draws attention to possible divergence between popular and colonial interpretations not only of disease etiology but also of the severity and preventability, or curability, of specific afflictions. From a broader perspective, this also calls attention to the gap between individuals' quest for personalized therapeutic solutions and the public system's persistent emphasis on collective prevention.

Such tensions also manifested as contradictory representations of the goals and functions of therapy. Quinine provides an interesting case. The drug, as we saw in Chapter 3, was invested in by the colonial government as a tool of mass prevention and became the cornerstone of its malaria control policy. At the same time, the State Quinine Service prioritized broad distribution outside the AMI facilities, putting the circulation of quinine largely in the hands of lay distributors and consumers. While there is little information on the consumption or refusal of quinine – and

---

[65] Vũ Trọng Phụng, *Lục Xì. Prostitution and Venereal Disease in Colonial Hanoi*, trans. and intro. by Shaun K. Malarney (Honolulu: University of Hawai'i Press, 2011), 103.

what little that exists is indirect and contradictory – it does seem clear that
the Vietnamese readily sought it out as a curative drug, particularly to
treat episodes of fever. The Vietnamese were said to appreciate its fever-
reducing and tonic properties; some even used it recreationally as a
complement to opium and purchased it "on the side," sometimes through
illegal channels.[66] Yet AMI doctors repeatedly complained that the drug
was refused outright for preventive purposes, or was taken in smaller
doses or for shorter periods than recommended.[67] Their main explanation referred to apprehensions about the toxicity of quinine, especially if
taken for long periods of time. Colonial doctors did, indeed, report some-
times-serious adverse effects that patients may have experienced or witnessed. They may also have heard rumors that the drug could cause fatal
suffocation and female infertility – which colonial reports asserted were
spread by traditional therapists in order to counter biomedical competition. Regardless, such stories may have kindled vivid fears among some
segments of the population, reinforcing already negative assumptions
about QE.[68]

Here, as in the provided examples of resistance, I am not claiming that
the Vietnamese were ignorant of modes of disease transmission, refused
biomedical explanations, or were indifferent to protective measures. I
am suggesting that they saw modern medicines as adequate tools for
some purposes and not for others, notably for the prevention of infectious illness. This is supported by the persistent and widely reported
Vietnamese ambivalence toward vaccination. Furthermore, BAYB
readers hardly ever mentioned preventive uses of medicines; however,
these were generally evoked in terms of their immediate restorative
effects on equilibrium, strength, and vitality. Concerns about toxicity
and the possibility of adverse effects were likely also a motivation for
abbreviating the duration of drug therapy, whether preventive or curative, which suggests an alternative explanation to that of an Vietnamese
"impatien[ce] to get better" that colonial doctors denigrated and the
frequent abandonment of long treatment courses for syphilis or recurrent amoebic infection.[69]

[66] "Rapports mensuels du fonctionnement des services sanitaires et médicaux en Annam, 1912," VNA, centre no. 1, IGHSP 12.
[67] Dr. Hénaff, "Rapport annuel sur le fonctionnement du service médical de la ville de Saigon pendant l'année 1910," AHMC 15 (1912): 223; J. Mesnard and L. Bordes, "L'importance du réservoir de virus autochtone dans la lutte contre le paludisme en Indochine," BSPE 23 (1930): 811–20.
[68] ANOM, Gougal 65324.
[69] A. de Raymond, "Le traitement des lépreux au Tonkin par injections intraveineuses d'un savon total de chaulmoogra," BSMI 9, 7 (1931): 592; Dr. Normet, "Les traitements pratiques. La dysenterie amibienne," AMPC 21 (1923): 338–45.

These points of intersection and divergence between Vietnamese/lay and colonial/biomedical views concerning which diseases were worth treating and which medicines were worth taking were far from fixed. Over time, new sites of potential inter-comprehension emerged. The array of pharmaceuticals available in Vietnam expanded, with a general trend toward safer and more effective products. In addition, knowledge – about both specific drugs and biomedical models of disease and therapy – continued to spread, perhaps faster and more widely, through multiple routes ranging from personal experience to virtual consultations. Medicines were crucial mediators in this communication. Yet while the AMI did make some concessions in order to broaden access to therapy, including both essential medicines and traditional therapies, as we will see in Chapter 8, the continued reluctance of colonial doctors and health authorities to mobilize medicines as tools of medicalization limited their ability to hinge the strong Vietnamese demand for some drug therapies to the official goals of conversion and sanitation.

7.5   (In)compatible Representations (Part II): Medical Consultation as Gateway to Treatment?

Many AMI doctors reprovingly noted that, although the Vietnamese "liked" medicines, they avoided attending medical consultations except as a "last resort" and often did not follow treatment instructions. In other words, they were convinced of the value of colonial medicines, but not necessarily of the value of biomedical advice and supervision. Let us reexamine this statement, first by considering what consultations in the public health care system entailed, then by examining the possible forms of therapeutic relationship that may have arisen at these sites of interaction. The therapeutic relationship had, by the late nineteenth century, been enshrined in institutions and law as a crucial step for obtaining medicines, and has since been regarded by anthropologists and sociologists as key to compliance with treatment. How might this relationship have played out in a colonial context? Might Vietnamese quests for relief and cure led to an increasing use of biomedical facilities, and thus to growing contact with and perhaps embracing of the principles of etiology, diagnosis, and therapy advocated within them? The rising popularity of private clinical consultation services in urban Vietnam from the 1920s might offer some clues.

The scarcity of biomedical doctors in Vietnam was perhaps the biggest, but certainly not the only, obstacle to seeking medical advice and obtaining prescriptions. Even as AMI doctors chastised patients for failing to recognize the importance of prompt clinical consultation, they hinted at many possible causes of misunderstanding in the doctor-patient encounter. The majority of French doctors, as well as auxiliary doctors posted outside Vietnamese-speaking communities, were not fluent in their patients' language, and the mediation of interpreters posed challenges to communication and confidentiality.[70] But when, in 1926, Dr. Motais described the language of his patients as being "very difficult for us to understand," he referred not only to literal linguistic barriers, but also to how their modes of self-expression failed to meet biomedical expectations of the information required for diagnosis. In other words, patients were, unsurprisingly, unfamiliar with the conventions of Western doctor-patient communication. Motais also complained: "The native patient is completely unaware of the possible connection between present and past symptoms. He more easily resigns himself to tolerate infirmities [. . .] and rarely consults a European doctor for insidious and chronic conditions, like tabes [dorsalis]."[71] Two years later, Drs. Montel and Veille criticized patients' failure to grasp the purpose of interrogation: they refused to answer questions, described only present and bothersome symptoms, and failed to disclose or even remember prior signs and symptoms of disease, "believ[ing] that the skill of the doctor is [the ability] to guess."[72]

As this last comment suggests, most Vietnamese patients had prior expectations of how therapeutic relationships were meant to play out. In pre-colonial Vietnam, as well as outside the AMI, patients generally chose their therapists and met them in an intimate and familiar space. Therapists sought to gain their patient's trust, and were often compensated on the basis of the latter's perception of therapeutic outcomes. This may explain the observation found in some AMI reports that patients were skeptical of free care, given that the cost of treatment should be proportional to its efficacy. While biomedicine and its regulation made increasingly rigid distinctions between the roles of

---

[70] Although colonial authorities tried to impose on doctors courses in at least one "Indochinese language" in 1910, the proposal was quickly abandoned due to the high mobility of doctors: the majority of military personnel was posted only temporarily, for a few years, in Indochina, while civil French and Vietnamese AMI health care professionals were frequently moved from one post to another around the Union, and thus worked with groups, including ethnic majority and minority groups, who spoke very different languages (Văn Thế Hội, "La valse des médecins indigènes," *La tribune indigène*, no. 344, September 16, 1920).
[71] Dr. F. Motais, "Le tabès en Cochinchine," BSPE 19 (1926): 81.
[72] M. L. R. Montel and A. Veille, "Un cas d'amibiase cérébrale," BSPE, 21 (1928): 231–39.

doctors and of pharmacists, many Vietnamese therapists combined them: they diagnosed as well as prescribed, prepared, and dispensed remedies.[73] And while the emergence of biomedicine shifted the distribution of power in the therapeutic encounter, emphasizing doctors' mastery of scientific language, knowledge, and technologies over patients' narratives and experience, Vietnamese therapists continued to attend closely to individual histories and characteristics such as age and gender.[74]

Patients also complained about their experiences with biomedical doctors. Even the well-educated correspondents of the BAYB told Nguyễn Văn Luyện that they had not fully understood their doctors, or that their doctors had failed to understand them and their problems. For example, in 1936, a man from Hanoi asked the editor for an explanation of the cryptic note he had received after an examination and blood analyses at the hospital: "E. Elles pustulo squamous [. . .] R.V.F. 99," to which he added: "What am I to make of this?"[75] Others were annoyed that it had been impossible to consult the same doctor over several visits to an AMI hospital or clinic. Medical examinations, which often required undressing and palpation, were likely seen as offensive.[76] Contemporary photographs also show that consultations were often held in open spaces, without any privacy, under the gaze of strangers, thus making a confidential interaction unlikely (Figure 7.2). BAYB readers also resented doctors' scorn for Vietnamese medicine, complaining that they were mocked for their beliefs, or chided for admitting that they had used a traditional remedy.

Doctors' esoteric language and lack of respect for patients' knowledge, practices, and privacy was puzzling even to Western patients, while doctors' authority as experts was often reinforced by their dominant social

---

[73] This does not mean that all Sino-Vietnamese therapists were merchants of medicines or vice versa. A number of Sino-Vietnamese drugstores also offered the services of a resident therapist.

[74] With the rise of biomedicine, the therapeutic relationship was no longer centered on the patient as it had been in the late eighteenth century. It was, on the contrary, increasingly centered around the doctor's knowledge and capacity to intervene. The development of effective yet toxic synthetic drugs confirmed and justified this authority: Irving Kenneth Zola, "Structural Constraints in the Doctor-Patient Relationship: The Case of Noncompliance," in *The Relevance of Social Science for Medicine*, ed. Leon Eisenberg and Arthur Kleinman (Rordrecht: Reidel, 1981), 241–52.

[75] Readers' correspondence, BAYB, no. 22, March 1936, 23–25.

[76] In the Confucian tradition, patients, especially women, did not undress, and were barely touched, only for taking the pulse. The forced complete undressing of individuals afflicted by scabies, whose whole bodies were then vigorously rubbed with Helmerich's ointment, was apparently not terribly popular with patients: Dr. Paucot, *Notions d'hygiène à l'égard des indigènes* (Paris: Challamel, 1908), 32–33.

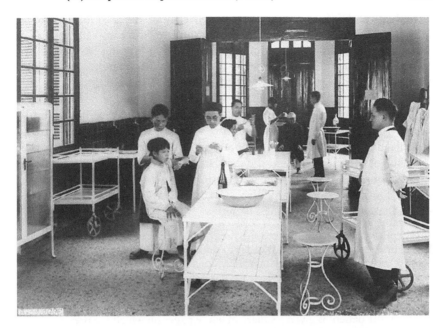

Figure 7.2 Hanoi Native Hospital Bandage Room, 1920s to 1930s (Archives nationales d'outre-mer [ANOM], Agence économique de la France d'outre-mer/Gouvernement général de l'Indochine 30Fi117/25. Reproduced with the authorization of the ANOM)

positions based on class and gender.[77] Yet the conditions of colonial domination created a particularly stark inequality between the expert, who was backed by foreign rule and knowledge, and the patient, whose political subjection was amplified by physical suffering and social vulnerability. In his famous essay on "Medicine and Colonialism," the Martinican psychiatrist Frantz Fanon described the medical consultation as a battleground in which patients – who often consulted late and were thus seriously, even fatally, ill by the time they did – were mistrustful and defiant. Doctors' often-explicit complicity with acts of dispossession and exploitation, as well as their claims to superiority, made the promise of biomedicine indissociable from colonial oppression.[78] In Vietnam, some AMI doctors made particular efforts to dissolve this assumption of

[77] Sally Wilde, "The Elephants in the Doctor-Patient Relationship: Patients' Clinical Interactions and the Changing Surgical Landscape of the 1890s," *Health & History* 9, 1 (2007): 2–27.

[78] Frantz Fanon, "Médecine et colonialisme," in *L'an V de la révolution algérienne* (Paris: François Maspéro, 1959), 111–40.

complicity and to regain their patients' trust, for instance by learning local languages and cosmologies. Yet such examples were so rare that they attracted special attention from the media: Dr. Lemoine learned about Vietnamese medicine in order to better treat his patients, while Dr. Sambuc was known for his commitment to his Vinh Long patients and his fluency in both Vietnamese and Cantonese.[79]

The potential for misunderstanding and mistrust was probably amplified by the particularly rigid structure of medical consultations in the colonial health care system. The combination of heavy-handed regulation and lack of oversight created the conditions for impersonal, even hostile, interactions.[80] The following description of the consultation system in one of Tonkin's largest hospitals in 1915 is illustrative of the strict protocols adhered to by most public facilities:

Prescription card system: consultants, registered in order of arrival [. . .] by the head nurse, are presented in this order to the doctor who questions and examines them. Once this is done, the patient receives a red card if he is diagnosed with a surgical condition, and a blue card for a medical condition. On the back of the card is recorded the civil status he declared, as well as the diagnosis of the condition; on the front, the prescription that has been ordered. In addition to the card, the patient is given a square of white paper on which the prescription is also written. This [. . .] paper must be given by the patient to the nurse in charge of the Pharmacy who will, in exchange, give the prescribed medicines.[81]

In large hospitals, patients were sometimes triaged following a brief initial consultation. Consultation times were fixed. The consumption of medicines was also closely controlled. Sometimes patients were made take their treatment under direct observation by a nurse; often, they were dispensed only enough medicines, especially if these were toxic drugs and medical specialties, to cover twenty-four hours of treatment (due to both mistrust of patients and budgetary concerns), thus forcing them to return and go through the consultation system again.[82] The administration of castor oil, eye drops, and quinine was sometimes obligatory. This was resisted in various ways, including by taking traditional medicines in order to counter the drugs' effects, even if only symbolically.[83] Hospitalized patients were also closely watched and were sometimes subjected to therapeutic experimentation without any

---

[79] *L'Écho,* no. 1224, June 19, 1929.
[80] "On se plaint du médecin indigène de l'Institut de puériculture de Saigon," *La tribune indochinoise,* no. 647, December 17, 1930.
[81] ANOM, RST NF 4014.
[82] "Rapport sur le fonctionnement de l'Assistance médicale dans la province de Hai Duong, 1915," ANOM, RST NF 4003.
[83] "Service médical de la colonisation, Rapport sur le service médical, 1er trimestre 1939," ANOM, RST NF 382; Léon Robin and Tru'ờng Văn Huân, "Essais comparés de

explanation, or to long and painful courses of treatment that sometimes turned out to be ineffective or harmful. The experience of hospitalization itself was often pervaded by the fear of surgery – a fear that, according to AMI reports, was occasionally "exploited" by Sino-Vietnamese therapists.[84] Indeed, on several occasions, BAYB readers asked the editor to recommend drug-based therapeutic options as an alternative to surgery. Strict visiting hours, and other rules, isolated patients from family networks through which therapy was usually managed collectively.[85] The popular press also, as we have seen, frequently depicted public hospitals as dirty, rundown, and overcrowded, staffed by unwelcoming and negligent personnel, and lacking in equipment and supplies, especially medicines. The Vietnamese were thus given many good reasons for avoiding hospitals as well as other public consultation services.

And yet, despite all these good reasons for avoiding AMI facilities, there are hints of a growing demand for, and thus perhaps of familiarization with and acceptance of, biomedical consultation services, especially those that offered convenient hours, employed Vietnamese doctors, and distributed free treatment for all. Already in 1903, Dr. Déjean de la Bâtie reported that a free consultation service in Hanoi, which employed only Vietnamese personnel and was open every morning, even on weekends, had welcomed 2,353 patients in its first year, with an average of 8 visits per patient – that is, 4 times more than in the average AMI facility. By 1907, the number of patients had more than doubled.[86] A free clinic established in 1905 by missionaries in Vinh Long's Hôpital indigène, which also opened every morning, soon attracted more than 300 patients each month; it was then taken over by the AMI.[87] In 1910, Dr. Hénaff described how the "native public," having grown familiar with and appreciative of the Saigon medical service's charitable consultations, "flock[ed] to it in ever greater numbers," reporting 6,684 patients, an average of 100 each day, for that year.[88] The press also remarked on the popularity of specific outpatient consultation services. In 1929, the Tan Dinh free clinic, recently established within Saigon's municipal polyclinic and supervised by Dr. Lê Văn An, was said to be already attracting more

prophylaxie médicamenteuse antipalustre en région hyperendémique par la praequine, associée à la quinine ou à la quinacrine," BSPE 28 (1935): 651.

[84] Reportedly, some even spread the idea that all hospitalizations were inevitably associated with surgical operations (ANOM, Gougal 65324; RST NF 4014).

[85] Several AMI reports also deplored the difficulty of making patients and their families understand the need for regulated visiting hours; others explained escapes from the hospital in terms of the need to reunite with kin.

[86] VNA, centre no. 2, Goucoch IA.8/077(4).

[87] "Les œuvres de bienfaisance en Cochinchine," *La quinzaine coloniale*, 17 (1905): 625–26.

[88] Hénaff, "Rapport annuel."

than 200 patients each day, more than half of which consulted more than once. In a single month, the clinic had dispensed medicines to 8,125 of its 10,327 patients.[89] While urban clinics provide the most striking numbers, there is evidence that some rural consultation services were also popular. The auxiliary doctor Phạm Gia De calculated that, within a month of opening in 1923, the health post of Nha Nam (Bac Giang) received an average of 75 patients per day.[90] Some village communities even established their own consultation services instead of waiting for the AMI to do so.

Although hospitalization was never made compulsory in Vietnam, it was clearly not seen as a personal choice. By contrast, outpatient consultations appear to have been perceived as less constraining, and as more adaptable to patient needs and demands. Indeed, clinics were, it was said, more attractive to patients when they were physically separate from hospitals. For example, when a Hanoi tuberculosis consultation service moved from the hospital to Richaud Street, its consultation rates increased fourfold within weeks.[91] The small size and staff of many consultation services might allow for greater continuity of care and, in some cases, for more flexibility in access to medicines.[92] Dr. Koun, who supervised the free consultation service in Hué in 1913, allowed patients, including patients with syphilis, to take away a full course of prescribed medicines, noting that this increased adherence to treatment.[93] From the 1920s, patients increasingly came to consultations with specific requests for medicines (of which many AMI doctors were still suspicious, while, as seen in Chapter 5, such requests could also put pressure on nurses to provide the medicines illegally).[94] Free public and charitable outpatient clinics thus appear to have become increasingly important sites for negotiating access to colonial medicines. Alongside the colonial state's framing of health as a collective obligation emerged understandings and practices of health care as a right and as a choice.

---

[89] Lê Trung Nghĩa, "A la clinique de Tan Dinh," *La tribune indochinoise*, no. 469, September 27, 1929.
[90] "Rapport annuel du poste médical de Nha Nam, 1923," ANOM, RST NF 4021.
[91] "Pour les tuberculeux."
[92] Although small facilities could also be overcrowded, which might affect quality of care, as was probably the case for the Hung Yen clinic described by its director in 1915 as follows: "everything has already been said about the one and only room that is serves as a waiting room, a consultation room, a pharmacy, for the arsenal, for operations, for bandages and in which each morning jostle school pupils, [. . .] prisoners and outpatients with no bench to sit on." (ANOM, RST NF 4003).
[93] Koun, "Fonctionnement du deuxième service," 423.
[94] Grenierboley and Nguyễn Hữu Phiếm, "Utilisation des sulfamidés," 604.

7.6   Private Doctors and Problems of Quality and Access

This was, of course, particularly true for those who were willing and able to pay to consult a private practitioner. Until the 1920s, few doctors practiced privately in Vietnam – fewer than private pharmacists. Their patient pool was largely confined to the small European community and to a few wealthy Chinese. During the interwar period, however, the number of private practitioners grew rapidly, again especially in the major urban centers: business tax records for 1937–38 list 22 private doctors in Hanoi and 65 in Saigon-Cholon. By this time, according to Cochinchina's Local Directorate of Health, of all doctors in the colony (a total of 212), about 40 percent (82) were private practitioners. As with pharmacists, the majority was of Vietnamese origin, accounting for 70 to 75 percent of all private physicians in the 1930s, and up to 80 percent in Saigon.[95] Despite the restrictions placed on Vietnamese doctors trained in Hanoi who, until the 1930s, were required to obtain a (revocable) administration authorization to practice outside the AMI, and only after ten years of public service, a significant number chose to enter private practice.[96]

Many of these doctors were well-known public figures: several held political offices or positions in professional organizations, or, as we have seen, founded, edited, and wrote for popular magazines. These figures were also written about in the press: they were congratulated for illustrious careers or for charitable service, were praised in open letters, and were, on occasion, reported on as victims of theft or kidnapping. Such media attention suggests that private practice was a thriving, well-respected, albeit highly competitive, business by the late 1930s. Discontent with working conditions in the public system (low pay, frequent transfers, slow promotion, restricted practice rights, and racial discrimination) was surely a factor in the decision to leave the AMI.[97] These practitioners must also have been motivated by the prospect of an expandable market for medical services outside the public system. Thus, the rise of Vietnamese private practice is a significant indicator of new demands for biomedical advice and solutions – including for medicines –

[95] ANOM, RST NF 2833.
[96] It is nevertheless difficult to evaluate the proportion of Vietnamese doctors who worked in private practice. I counted 508 biomedically trained Vietnamese doctors between 1905 and 1940. Of these, from 150 to 200 appear to have worked in private practice at some point in their career: Laurence Monnais, "Le Dr Nguyen Van Luyen et ses confrères. La médecine privée dans le Viêt nam colonial," *Moussons. Recherches en sciences humaines sur l'Asie du Sud-est – Social Science Research on Southeast Asia*, 15 (2010): 75–95.
[97] Yet many of them capitalized on their prior public sector experience, putting this forward as a guarantee of their expertise when advertising their practice, or using it to build up a client base in smaller urban centers where they practiced as AMI doctors.

from the emerging Vietnamese urban middle class. In 1935, Nguyễn Văn Luyện brought up the idea of subsidies as an incentive for private practitioners to set up in the countryside (and to also act as "propharmacists"), as well as to offer consultation rates that would include prescription fees in order to broaden access to biomedical care.[98] The proposal was taken into consideration by the authorities in Hanoi. This suggests, albeit indirectly, that private practitioners played an important role in health care at the time.

Many of these private practitioners offered one or even several specialized services, often in combination with general practice, as was also common among metropolitan doctors.[99] This suggests that their (potential) clientele was familiar with biomedical divisions of bodily systems and their pathologies. While some forms of specialization existed in precolonial Vietnamese medicine, these divisions in the private biomedical sphere were clearly modeled on metropolitan practices and institutions, and largely based on Western scientific, technological, and nosographic criteria. Of forty to fifty private specialists in my database, the largest group, of nine, offered venereal and dermatological services. Other popular specialties were obstetrics-gynecology, pediatrics, ophthalmology, and otorhinolaryngology (ENT).[100] This offer likely more or less reflects clients' health priorities. Some advertised therapies, such as Lê Văn Huế's "new therapeutic procedure for gonorrhea – no pain, complete cure," while others invested in expensive technologies such as x-rays, demonstrating not only their ability to mobilize significant resources, but also their confidence in potential clients' eagerness to adopt new conceptions and technologies of diagnosis and treatment.[101] This eagerness extended to adopting certain therapeutic vogues. For example, no fewer than seven private practitioners, of which six were Vietnamese, offered electrotherapy; popular also in France at the time, this technique was used to treat a

---

[98] Editorial, BAYB, no. 8, February 1935, 1.

[99] In the 1930s, half of Parisian clinics were said to offer specialized consultation services, even though there were not yet clear rules about specialized training, certification, and diplomas, which would only come in 1947: George Weisz, "Regulating Specialties in France during the first Half of the Twentieth Century," *Social History of Medicine* 15, 3 (2002): 457.

[100] I also found mentions of two pneumologists, two radiologists, two stomatologists, a hematologist, a cardiologist, and even a diabetologist.

[101] Advertisement, *La dépêche d'Indochine*, March 31, 1938. BAYB readers' correspondence suggests that the uses of electrotherapy in Vietnam were similar, often offered in conjunction with physiotherapy but also acupuncture, not as a return to Chinese traditional techniques but as an echo of its contemporary popularity in Western settings: Linda L. Barnes, *Needles, Herbs, Gods and Ghosts. China Healing and the West to 1848* (Cambridge: Harvard University Press, 2005), 311–29.

range of conditions, including hemorrhoids, gonorrhea, eczema, neuro-muscular pain, and neurasthenia.

In fact, the most prosperous doctors seem to have been specialists. Some owned a clinic, or even a maternity service –as was the case of Nguyễn Văn Luyện – or a medical laboratory, in addition to their general practice. They earned 600 to 1,500 piasters per month in 1922, according to *La tribune indigène*. By comparison, a Vietnamese doctor in the AMI system, depending on whether he was an auxiliary or a full doctor, had a starting salary of 100 to 300 piasters per month. Knowing that the average cost of a consultation was 2 to 5 piasters, we can estimate that most private practitioners saw about 12 to 16 patients per workday, 5 to 6 days a week.[102] Efforts to increase the availability of private consultations is also revealing: From 1940, the Syndicat des médecins civils de Cochinchine (Syndicate of Civilian Doctors of Cochinchina) organized a night-duty system so that a doctor-prescriber would be available in Saigon at all times, even during holidays. The coordinates of the doctor on call were published every day in *L'Écho*. This "out-of-hours" medical service was occasionally coupled with an analogous pharmacy service.

Letters of gratitude to private doctors were published in the press; most were written by urban, well-educated men such as public servants, tra-ders, students, and intellectuals. Some doctors made efforts to attract women and children, whether by offering specialized consultation ser-vices or lower fees.[103] For example, Dr. Bigo charged these patients, as well as public servants, two rather than three piasters. This was still quite expensive.[104] For those who could afford them, however, private con-sultations offered a privileged and flexible space in which to negotiate access to medicines. In parallel, some public outpatient services, as we have seen, also came to be seen as acceptable, or at least tolerable, routes for obtaining free and/or effective treatment. By 1940, a growing number of Vietnamese were willing to engage in a biomedical doctor-patient relation as part of their quest for therapy.

All this suggests that medicines played a pivotal role in Vietnamese appropriations of biomedicine, which involved a broad process of medical

---

[102] Consultations costing five piasters were for exceptional cases, such as night-time con-sultations or house calls far from the doctor's office. Rates for specialized interventions such as deliveries or minor surgery varied between five and fifty piasters.

[103] "Hommage à la science d'un docteur," *L'Écho*, no. 440, February 10, 1923.

[104] In 1929, at the private Drouhet Hospital, the rate was initially set at 5 piasters, but it was soon realized that this was unaffordable, or nearly so, even for the wealthiest patients (Dr. Déjean de la Bâtie, "A l'Hôpital Drouhet. Les Annamites y sont admis," *L'Écho*, no. 1312, October 3, 1929). A 1933 advertisement for the private Clinique Angier mentions a hospitalization rate of 3.50 piasters per day for Vietnamese patients and of 7 piasters for others (PNTV, no. 196, April 20, 1933).

education that entailed "cultural translation."[105] By learning about (many different) medicines and seeking out some of these, the Vietnamese probably came to learn about and, to some extent, to accept and even adhere to (colonial) biomedical principles, institutions, and practitioners; their models of disease and therapeutics; as well as their conventions and rules of care. Yet, as should by now be clear, access to doctors, public or private, remained limited during this period. This means that any question about the nature and magnitude of medicalization under colonial rule in Vietnam must take into account highly differentiated modes of access to biomedical advice and therapy, marked both by stark contrasts between urban and rural health care provision, and by the enduring, yet changing and flexible, presence of both traditional and private-biomedical products and services. Looking beyond these persistent disparities, which may even have been growing during the economic turmoil of the 1930s, a close look at the consumption, as well as the nonconsumption, of medicines is revealing of pathways of colonial medicalization that have attracted very little attention until now – be it from contemporary medical authorities or from historians. These pathways were highly varied, ranging from the "updating" of a Confucian duty of health self-education within a vibrant press, to the growing popularity of specialized (bio)medical practitioners able to respond to prevalent expectations and anxieties, as well as a growing demand for specific, effective, and fast-acting remedies. Viewed from outside a normative biomedical frame, without the prejudices of Western, colonial medical attitudes, this complex and uneven medicalization clearly appears to have flourished in interaction with other medical systems, in environments and practices characterized, at both individual and collective levels, by therapeutic pluralism.

---

[105] On medical education as cultural translation in Southeast Asia, see Hans Pols, C. Michele Thompson, and John Harley Warner, ed., *Translating the Body. Medical Education in Southeast Asia* (Singapore: NUS Press, 2017).

8   Therapeutic Pluralism under Colonial Rule

The intersection between local demands for therapy and what was on offer in colonial Vietnam gave rise to diverse forms of accommodation, combination, and hybridization. These forms of therapeutic pluralism are at the heart of this final chapter. There is no stable or precise definition of medical (or therapeutic) pluralism. Elements – therapeutic objects, models and representations, symbols, practices – from more than one medical tradition or therapeutic system can be combined, on the basis of ideological, empirical, and/or pragmatic considerations, at the level of individual practices of care, whether synchronously, sequentially, or from one episode of illness to another. Medical pluralism can also characterize specific spatial environments; it can arise from coexistence and interaction at the level of a city or region (that do not necessarily extend elsewhere), or might be defined at the level of a health care policy or system, usually on a territorial scale, for example, of a colony or a nation, either in terms of the orientations and convictions that govern these, or of the forms of care that they provide.[1] Whether it arises from individual practice, spatial interaction, or integrative policy, pluralism always entails a mutual transformation of the medical systems it draws upon, blurring the boundaries between them in ways that go beyond their legal or governmental regulation. By examining these different layers of pluralism, I revisit many of the themes developed throughout this book: the accessibility of biomedical care or lack thereof, a dense and vibrant private health sector, and emerging demands for certain kinds of medicines and therapeutic effects. I examine the extent to which these factors converged by 1940, and how they interacted with a growing politicization of both access to drugs and to health care, as well as the *reinvention* of Vietnamese medicine as a national medicine, to shape a precocious, and profoundly dynamic, integrative health care system.

[1] On the importance of this kind of nuance when it comes to look at medical pluralism and its local variants, see Robert Frank and Stollberg Gunnar, "Conceptualizing Hybridization: On the Diffusion of Asian Medical Knowledge in Germany," *International Journal of Sociology* 19, 1 (2004): 79–88.

8.1   Mapping Medical Proximities and Cosmopolitanism

In 1931, the inspector of pharmacies for Annam, Antonini, estimated that only fifteen thousand to twenty thousand of Tonkin's nine million inhabitants (0.2 percent) were able to purchase what he called "French medicines."[2] A few years later, in 1936, the local director of health for Tonkin declared: "to ask an Indochinese whose [revenue] is under five piasters a month to find money to pay for a medical consultation worth two piasters [. . .] and for a prescription that never costs less than four is a cruel joke."[3] Even earlier, from the 1920s, the press had denounced the financial inaccessibility of colonial medicines. Over the next decade, some journalists and traditional therapists' associations suggested that this situation was forcing people to use Vietnamese medicine. An article in *L'Annam nouveau,* for instance, estimated in 1934 that 99 percent of the Vietnamese population still used Vietnamese medicine primarily because it was less expensive than biomedicine.[4] One editorial calculated in 1939 that a simple case of bronchitis cost 7 piasters to treat with biomedicine (including the cost of consultation) and only 0.50 piasters if one opted to purchase a remedy (containing guaiacol, just like the French specialty one was likely to be prescribed) directly from the local Chinese druggist.[5]

Such comparisons should, however, be qualified. Chinese medicine could also be very expensive, and only the elite could afford the most renowned specialists. On occasion, AMI doctors were shocked by the fact that some individuals were ready to pay "a lot" for Chinese remedies, while the popular press denounced various "charlatans" who charged their patients tens of piasters for treatment.[6] Furthermore, the price of pharmaceuticals outside the public health system appears, on the basis of fragmentary information such as occasional displays in publicity, to have varied widely. On the eve of World War II, Dagénan pills were sold for up to 20 to 30 piasters on the black market (see Chapter 5), but some commercial specialties were relatively affordable; in addition, they were obtainable without paying for consultation fees. For example, Oxymenthol cough tablets sold for 0.35 piasters for the equivalent of eight days of treatment in 1930, Gastrol sold for 0.40 piasters for a tube in 1932, and Potion Peschier sold for 0.60 piasters for a bottle in 1926. Some local specialties were also relatively cheap: Collyre Jaune and other

---

[2] ANOM, RST NF 4683.
[3] ANOM, RST NF 3686.
[4] "Réglementation de la vente des médicaments de la pharmacopée sino-annamite," *L'Annam nouveau,* no. 311, January 28, 1934.
[5] Cited in Nguyễn Văn Ký, *La société vietnamienne face à la modernité. Le Tonkin de la fin du XIXe siècle à la seconde guerre mondiale* (Paris: L'Harmattan, 1995), 92.
[6] ANOM, RST NF 4003.

brand eye drops cost 0.20 to 0.30 piasters a flask between 1920 and 1930, Sudol cost 0.50 piasters a tube in 1927, and Robur pills cost 0.40 piasters for a box of twenty pills. In 1940, the Lôc Hà drugstore charged only 20 cents per packet for an antimalarial drug; a full treatment, it was said, required two packets. Other specialties, however, sold for more, including hybrid specialties, which were not necessarily cheaper than imported pharmaceuticals. For example, in the late 1920s, Ablennol cost 1.30 piasters a box and Sensal depurative sold for 1.70 per flask, Maubar or Vin 33 500 cost more than 2 piasters a liter, and a tonic sold by the Pharmacie chinoise de Shanghai in Cholon sold for 1.80 piasters for a box of tablets.

While the controlled price of QE and essential medicines sold in rural outlets was much lower (0.10 to 0.20 piasters for a single dose of Antipyrin, and 0.18 piasters for a tube of quinine), even these were reported to be unaffordable for many. Available figures on salaries indicate that a mid-ranking Vietnamese employee of the colonial civil service could afford an occasional commercial specialty, but certainly not a medical specialty, and probably not the added price of a medical consultation, except, perhaps, in cases of serious illness. In 1920, a commission investigating pay in the civil service estimated that a bachelor might spend 2 piasters a month on "pharmacy," and a couple would pay 4 piasters, while the salary of a government clerk such as an accountant ranged from 40 to 60 piasters. Average spending on lodging and food was estimated, respectively, at 12 and 15 piasters.[7] Even the relatively well-off readership of the VSB and BAYB might thus welcome the advice regularly provided by editors on how to treat minor problems cheaply, without a doctor, often including do-it-yourself recipes for remedies, which might, for example, call for plants sold in local markets.[8] An unskilled worker was paid on average 15 piasters per month, which would have made it hard to buy even the cheapest specialties. Comparisons with potential spending on other consumer products and "entertainment" services are suggestive: the services of a prostitute were priced between 0.10 and 0.50 piasters in the 1930s, while a good quality suit cost from 6.50 to 15 piasters.[9]

Besides the question of cost, there was also that of proximity. As noted previously, it is quite clear that the majority of the Vietnamese population did not have geographical access to biomedical treatment into the 1930s,

[7] "Relèvement des soldes du personnel indigène," *La tribune indigène*, no. 252, January 22, 1920.
[8] Nguyễn Văn Luyện was surely aware of this demand for more affordable alternatives, yet he also insisted, in his editorial of October 1934 (BAYB, no. 4), that while the cost of prescriptions and of Western drugs was indeed high, this should be seen as a worthy investment, which would save money in the long run.
[9] Brocheux and Hémery, *Indochine*, 203, 209; Roger Charbonnier, *Contribution à l'étude de la prophylaxie antivénérienne à Hanoi* (Paris: Jouve & Cie, 1936), 17.

suggesting that the selective and partial Vietnamese consumption of colonial medicines was shaped by the "tyranny of distance."[10] Private doctors and pharmacists were few, and mostly based in the major cities, thus accentuating the gaps in services offered by AMI facilities, particularly in rural areas. By contrast, Sino-Vietnamese therapists and traders were, as we have also seen, much more numerous and widely spread out across the territory than distributors of biomedical drugs. The ratios found by pharmacy inspections and surveys are striking. In 1931, Tonkin was estimated to have a ratio of sites of sale of Sino-Vietnamese medicines against authorized distributors of colonial medicines of 1,799:65, whereas Thai Binh Province's ratio was 188:5 (the latter exclusively composed of essential medicines outlets) and Sontay City's ratio was 20:1 (a Vietnamese pharmacist). My Tho Province in Cochinchina was estimated to have four thousand sellers of traditional medicines in 1942, but only three private pharmacies (all in the provincial capital) and two private medical practitioners.[11] In fact, as Vietnam's biomedical network expanded, regional disparities in access to biomedicine probably grew. Readers of the BAYB confirmed that in the mid-1930s, being far from the city meant having little access to effective medicines.[12]

In cities, especially in Saigon-Cholon and Hanoi, traditional and non-professional traders of medicines took part in an increasingly dense and "cosmopolitan"[13] market for health care. By 1931, in Hanoi, there was approximately one point of access to medicines for every four hundred inhabitants: 180 of these were Sino-Vietnamese drug traders, while private pharmacists and doctors, AMI facilities, and some illicit distributors added up to no more than a few dozen. According to municipal figures for 1938, of 497 individuals with registered businesses in the city, fifty-four, or nearly 11 percent, dealt in medical goods and services – this figure included Sino-Vietnamese druggists but not, of course, itinerant and illicit traders in medicines.[14] The proximities between private and public urban health actors can also be mapped; their distribution crisscrossed the heart of

---

[10] Geoffrey Blainey, *The Tyranny of Distance: How Distance Shaped Australia's History* (Melbourne: Sun Books, 1966).

[11] "Lettre de l'Inspection des services de santé au Gouverneur général de l'Indochine, Saigon, 18 septembre 1942," VNA, centre no. 2, S52-8, Tòa đại biểu chính phủ Nam Việt, Dông y si, dông y, 1942–43.

[12] Readers' correspondence, BAYB, no. 18, December 1935, 30.

[13] Frederick L. Dunn, "Traditional Asian Medicine and Cosmopolitan Medicine as Adaptive Systems," in *Asian Medical Systems: A Comparative Study*, ed. by Charles Leslie (Berkeley: University of California Press, 1976), 133–58. See also Zhang Yuehong E., "Switching between Traditional Chinese Medicine and Viagra: Cosmopolitanism and Medical Pluralism Today," *Medical Anthropology* 26 (2007): 53–96.

[14] ANOM, RST NF 2833.

these cities' colonial and Asian business districts, dotting the main streets in spaces of intense traffic and commerce. In Saigon, seven doctors set up private clinics on Mac Mahon Street, and seven more on Chasseloup-Laubat Street, where the offices of the IGHSP were located. Another six worked near four retail pharmacies, as well as several dentists and midwives, on Bonnard Boulevard, known to attract a dynamic indigenous clientele (see Figure 4.1).[15]

In this vibrant urban space, recognized professionals brushed shoulders with traditional and neo-traditional therapists and traders. In Hanoi's old commercial district, seven Vietnamese-owned private pharmacies did business side by side with dozens of shops and stalls selling Chinese and Vietnamese, as well as Japanese and Korean medicines. In Saigon, in 1935, more than twenty health care businesses had their address on the famous Catinat Street: two Vietnamese doctors, the city's four biggest pharmacies (Pharmacie de France, Pharmacie Normale, Pharmacie Centrale, and Pharmacie Principale) and a few Vietnamese-owned pharmacies, several Chinese druggists, and Rhône-Poulenc's Indochinese branch. When the pharmacist Lê Văn Minh moved from Catinat Street to Sailors Street in Cholon, he found half a dozen other Vietnamese pharmacists and dozens of traders of remedies of all sorts. While traditional actors sought to enter iconic spaces of colonial consumption, biomedical ones also moved toward old commercial neighborhoods, shaping and responding to a changing demand for care. Within this cartography of proximities and interpenetration, practices of medical pluralism could take a variety of forms, which were shaped by mutual competition as well as cross-fertilization between medical systems and especially practitioners. All this happened largely beyond the control of colonial health authorities.

8.2   A Right to Health: Vietnamese Medicine to the Rescue

While official discourse minimized the value of medicines for colonial medicalization, several actors and observers – including colonial doctors, journalists, and traditional therapists – saw problems of pharmaceutical supply, distribution, and cost as threats not only to the spread of biomedicine but also to the accessibility of health care of any kind. Increasingly, positive claims were made for the value of traditional medicine as a readily available and appropriate means of providing effective care, but also as a modernizing force. In other words, these individuals promoted an early version of an integrative health care system.

---

[15] VNA, centre no. 2, S52-7, Hội ái hữu nha sĩ Việt hoa ở nam kỳ, 1935–40.

A few AMI and private biomedical doctors occasionally offered traditional therapies as an alternative to costly or scarce colonial medicines, or because they had seen that these worked and helped to attract and retain patients. Their physical proximity to traditional practitioners probably played a role in this, by stimulating interaction and a level of familiarity with them. Dr. Henriette Bùi Quang Chiêu recalled rediscovering Chinese medicine after she opened a clinic in Cholon in 1938, and hinted that other doctors were, like her, both curious about local medical traditions and persuaded that these constituted a potential resource for bridging gaps in AMI care. Posted in Quang Ngai, a fairly remote region known for its lack of AMI services in 1935, Dr. Hoang Mong Long openly identified himself as an expert in "Chinese acupuncture and Sino-Annamese pharmacopeia."[16] Some qualified dentists and midwives reportedly offered their urban clientele a combination of traditional and biomedical services. This was the case of Lâm Quang Sì, who established a "mixed" dental practice in Saigon in 1918, first on Vannier Street, then moving to 34 Bonnard Boulevard in 1935. Records indicate that he first came to Saigon from Gia Dinh in 1910 as the assistant of a Japanese dentist, went on to study dentistry for three years (it is not said where), and was hired as an assistant by a dental surgeon by the name of Déjean before opening his own clinic.[17]

In 1935, Dr. Lê Văn Phấn, a recent graduate of the Hanoi Medical School, advertised his private clinic as having gained the approval of the country's high authorities and intellectual elite, and as offering lower consultation rates to those who opted for a combination of traditional and biomedical treatments.[18] The same year, he also requested support from the superior resident of Tonkin to open a "house of medicine" in Hanoi "to counter [. . .] the harmful influence of quacks and charlatans [and] secure the triumph of Western medicine by complementing it through the rational study of Sino-Annamese medicine," which was denied when it was discovered that Lê Văn Phấn was collaborating with a Sino-Vietnamese pharmaceutical firm.[19] Although there is little further information about Lê Văn Phấn and other doctors who offered integrative care, we can postulate that combining and moving between medical

[16] "Rapport sur les résultats obtenus et les possibilités d'organisation dans les différentes provinces de l'Annam, signé Terrisse, Hué, 15 janvier 1936," VNA, centre no. 2, RSA 3362.
[17] VNA, centre no. 2, S52-7.
[18] Advertisements, BDP, no. 3081, November 2–3, 1935, and no. 3082, November 4–5, 1935.
[19] "Demande de création d'un office de propagande pour la médecine française à Hanoi formulée par Le Van Phan, médecin indochinois à Hué, 1935," VNA, centre no. 1, RST 47950.

systems was a way of carving out a niche in a highly competitive health care market.

The progressive press also insisted, from the late 1910s, on the crucial importance of broadening access to medicines in order to meet the goals of colonial medicalization. Given the scarcity of facilities and personnel, especially of mobile teams, journalists suggested that medicines were the best tool for expanding the provision of care and even improving public health.[20] Some warned, accusingly, that the colonial administration would lose ground if it refused to make medicines more readily available, notably by leaving the door open for Sino-Vietnamese therapists and traders to take advantage of the growing demand for pills and injections. Much of the press, however, adopted a more moderate position on the role that traditional medicine should be given in colonial health policy. Nguyễn Văn Luyện, as BAYB editor, accepted the inevitability of continued recourse to Vietnamese medicine, and thus advocated its "intelligent" promotion. Frequent denunciations of "bad" – that is, incompetent, venal, and harmful – traders and therapists in the interwar media can be seen as part of a broader effort to protect the reputation of an authentic Vietnamese medicine, practiced by honest and competent individuals. Some journalists went even further in promoting traditional medicine, advocating for official recognition by colonial health policy.

This promotion depended on identifying, selecting, and improving its "good" elements – substances and remedies, principles and practitioners – through scientific research and validation, as well as professionalization. The editors of L'Écho argued, in a commentary on a paper on a local snakebite remedy delivered before the French Academy of Sciences in 1922, that "not all of Annamese medicine must be rejected."[21] Local pharmacopeias were a source of potential discovery to be unleashed by methodical research. This was followed by a full-page article entitled "Sino-Annamese Medicine," in which the newspaper's editor-in-chief, Nguyễn Phan Long, proposed to update (by means of the scientific method) a "lagging" but promising "ancestral" medicine, with its incredibly rich pharmacopeia and its suitability to local climate, constitutions, and cosmologies, as well as by means of rigorous training, to ensure that its practitioners were trustworthy and competent.[22]

Such arguments for the modernization of Vietnamese medicine, via scientific validation and professionalization, also began to appear in

[20] N.H.Y., "La crise des médicaments"; Trần Đình Nam, "Le problème de la souffrance physique et le peuple d'Annam," L'Écho, no. 457, March 29, 1923.
[21] L'Écho, no. 418, December 16, 1922.
[22] Nguyễn Phan Long, "La médecine sino-annamite," L'Écho, no. 421, December 23, 1922.

nationalist discourses and the claims of some traditional therapists' associations in the 1920s and 1930s.[23] Nationalists hinged this argument to the imperative of preserving the legal and competent practice of Vietnamese medicine in order to protect a universal right to high-quality health care, or even just to the possibility of relief and cure provided by a well-trained practitioner of any medical tradition. This was especially needed to compensate for the AMI's rural gaps, Nguyễn Văn Luyện pointed out in 1936.[24] Representatives of traditional therapists also used this argument to support their claims for official recognition. In January of 1940, an association of Sino-Vietnamese therapists from Tonkin requested, in a press release addressed to Governor General Georges Cartroux, the resumption of work on laws pertaining to Sino-Vietnamese pharmacy, which had been suspended.[25] As seen in Chapter 6, therapist associations managed to gain enough political clout to make the administration back down from attempts to impose drastic legal restrictions. At the same time, they proposed to boost the legitimacy of Vietnamese therapy by modernizing it and regulating it.

Another association, the Viêt nam y dược hội, recommended particularly concrete and immediate measures: to conduct scientific work on selected medicinal plants, to promote high quality publications on Vietnamese medicine, and to ensure the widest possible distribution of scientifically validated, locally produced, and cheap medicines.[26] In a less polemical tone, the PNTV and health magazines also made Vietnamese medicine part of claims to a universal right to health, or at least to basic health care, by offering recipes and advice that presented traditional medicine as a pragmatic and valid source of therapy. In 1929, its first year of publication, the PNTV published nine articles written by the "Annamese doctor" Nguyễn Tư Thức that provided information on women's health, hygiene, and even microbes, as well as recipes for simple

---

[23] There are also examples in other colonies of similar appropriations of Western science for political purposes: Projit Mukharji, *Doctoring Traditions: Ayurveda, Small Technologies, and Braided Sciences* (Chicago: University of Chicago Press, 2016). What might set the case of Vietnam apart is that the defense of "honest" practitioners of Vietnamese medicine was oriented toward the goal of gaining definitive autonomy from the Chinese model and delineating the contours of a distinctively national medicine: Monnais, Thompson, and Wahlberg, *Southern Medicine*.

[24] Editorial, BAYB, no. 26, August 1936, 1–2. See also "La médecine sino-annamite dans nos campagnes," *L'Écho*, no. 269, December 1, 1921.

[25] ANOM, Aff Po 3242.

[26] Among the active members of this association were Nguyễn Di Lûan and Đặng Thúc Liêng, who, together, would also encourage the publication of several manuals of traditional medicine, some of which insisted on the importance of modernizing the traditional pharmacopeia while still preserving its local patrimonial characteristics: Guénel, "Nationalism and Vietnamese Medicine."

remedies, including those of the famous traditional therapist Nguyễn An Cư, who was also praised by the editors. The description of a visit to a Chinese hospital in Cholon published in the VSB in 1926 described its diagnostic and therapeutic practices as "outdated," but then called for the scientific validation and professionalization of Chinese medicine in order to harness its cultural and practical value.

VSB editors then began to promote the modernization of Vietnamese medicine even more explicitly. The goal was not only to improve its efficacy and to broaden access to quality care, but also to bring it closer to Western medicine. Thus, in 1929, a change in the magazine's format was announced as aiming to provide more "content that explains Western medicine to then better develop Vietnamese science," while Nguyễn Văn Luyện wrote about "Western medicine and our own," proposing to make these mutually legible by applying the "scientific method." The benefits would include both improvement in Vietnamese remedies and the promotion of trust in, and a better understanding of, Western ones:

Western medicine uses many of the same remedies as ours. What we gain is in the active ingredient [in French in the original Vietnamese text]. Our scientists must focus on the analysis of the efficacy of our remedies according to the Western experimental method [. . .] Experience will be the basis and tests the proof [needed] to practice medicine. The use of Western remedies increases every day but we cannot abandon the remedies that we have inherited.[27]

Another argument Nguyễn Văn Luyện made to justify preserving this legacy was the suitability of these remedies for "Vietnamese constitutions." To my knowledge, this is the first explicit proposal made by a Vietnamese doctor to regenerate and modernize Vietnamese medicine. That it was published in a pro-biomedical publication that also served as a marketing tool for one of Hanoi's largest French pharmacies is remarkable. While, in the 1920s, this type of rhetoric was still fairly marginal, it conveyed, via sometimes surprising tribunes and interlocutors, a budding movement that would take off in the late 1930s. This was a movement for the reinvention of Vietnamese medicine as distinctively and authentically Vietnamese and, especially, as worthy of recognition due to its openness to the scientific improvement and validation of its therapies, particularly of its medicines. This *neo-traditional* medicine would then be poised to become an integral part of a health care system adapted to the needs and means of the local population.[28]

---

[27] "Thuốc tây và thuốc ta," VSB, no. 40, May 1929, 3–7.

[28] In his *Histoire de la médecine*, Dương Bá Bành went as far as defining the interaction between the systems as "medical syncretism," at the level of both theory and practice, especially concerning therapeutics. At the same time, he insisted on limiting the integration of Western concepts so as not to infringe on Vietnamese cosmogonic theories.

8.3   From Compensating for Scarcity to Potential Therapeutic Treasure

In the 1930s, Vietnamese medicine was increasingly, and explicitly, seen as a potential resource for bridging gaps in the AMI's provision of medicines and services (i.e., as a *complementary* solution to insufficient "best" biomedical care), but also, especially under conditions of wartime shortage, identified by some as a source of real value by some colonial experts and AMI officials.

The creation of the AMI in 1905 had relegated Vietnamese medicine to the status of barely tolerated traditional practice on the margins of an institutionalized biomedicine. Yet the care provided within its facilities was, in practice, at least in some facilities and regions, discretely plural from the outset. The Hôpital indigène of Bac Giang, which was built in 1904 with financial support from local merchants and entrusted to an "unqualified Annamese doctor" in 1907, maintained as part of its objectives: to offer "consultation[s] for natives wanting to follow Sino-Annamese therapy," even after it was placed under the supervision of a French doctor.[29] In other cases, the desperate need for staff made it hard to refuse the help of local therapists. In the 1910s, several Vietnamese physicians (*thầy thuốc*) trained in Chinese medicine at the court of Hué were employed in AMI hospitals in Annam.[30]

The loosening of restrictions on authorizing Sino-Vietnamese drug traders as managers of essential medicines and specialty outlets is also indicative of the pragmatic emergence of plural practices. Proposals to regulate the practice of Vietnamese medicine aimed for restriction, yet they also implied an acknowledgment of the mismatch between Vietnamese demands for therapy and what the colonial system provided. The 1920 bill had set the maximum number of Sino-Vietnamese therapists authorized to practice in Cochinchina at 500 (see Chapter 4); while this figure clearly underestimated the real demand, it largely exceeded the number of AMI doctors and pharmacists. When the abandoned proposal was revived in 1942, the number had doubled and further conditions were specified, including the imposition of minimal, homogeneous training standards. We might see this as an explicit response to the growing gap

---

[29] ANOM, Gougal 65324.

[30] However, they were enlisted as "volunteer nurses" ("Rapports sanitaires annuels sur le fonctionnement des services de l'Assistance médicale en Annam, 1913–1914," VNA, centre no. 2, RSA 778). There were also several (failed) initiatives to "reeducate" these traditional therapists (creation of an exam to weed out "charlatans" in Tonkin in 1898; creation of an applied school for "traditional Annamite doctors" in Hué in 1908), before efforts were turned toward a program of reeducation focused on subaltern personnel, in particular on local midwives, the bà mụ.

between the population's rising expectations of care and the inaccessibility of AMI services and of expensive medicines.[31] By the 1930s, the combined pressures of local budgetary constraints, global economic crisis, and powerful nationalist movements pushed colonial health authorities to find an official place for Vietnamese medicine within the system. In 1935, Dr. Terrisse, as part of his innovative Rural Assistance program in Annam, openly suggested that traditional health actors be implicated in the medicalization project. He sought out the collaboration of the auxiliary doctor Hoàng Mộng Long as well as Phó Đức Thành, owner of the Grande pharmacie sino-vietnamienne in Vinh (whose knowledge and openness of mind he said he admired).[32]

Despite such proposals, and the widely acknowledged limits of the AMI, the officially recognized role of Vietnamese medicine remained, by and large, confined to minor interventions and rural areas. In a 1937 plan to reorganize the health services of Indochina, Pierre Hermant, whose knowledge of Southeast Asian health and especially of rural health was extensive, stated that the AMI, in its current state, was inadequate. In order to finally extend its reach into the countryside, he wrote, "the tolerance of traditional medicine is not only a moral and political obligation [. . .] it is also a material imperative."[33] In 1938, the Grand Council of Economic and Financial Interests proposed to regulate the status of Vietnamese medicine, but *only* in the cities, so that rural populations could be given the choice and flexibility they needed.[34] The following year, the Council stated:

Traditional medicine no doubt has an effect on some common ills; it can make a contribution alongside the action of medical assistance. The field of operation of the Assistance is the battle against contagious disease, and the treatment of patients whose conditions exceed the resources of the local pharmacopeia and, especially, we could almost say [. . .] the improvement of the health status of populations wherever it seems poor because of the main endemic diseases.[35]

The 1942 law on the "regulation of the Sino-Indochinese pharmacopeia" would finally, after a long series of discriminatory and aborted legislative projects, legally recognize traditional medicine, but only as

---

[31] "Note postale de l'administrateur de Chaudoc au Gouverneur de la Cochinchine, 28 décembre 1942," VNA, centre no. 2, S 52–8, Tòa đại biểu chính phủ Nam Việt.

[32] "Dr. Terrisse, Programme de développement de l'Assistance rurale en Annam, 1935, dactylo, 43 p," VNA, centre no. 2, RSA 3362.

[33] "Programme d'organisation des services d'Assistance médicale en Indochine, 1938," ANOM, CG Folder Bc.

[34] "Grand conseil des intérêts économiques et financiers de l'Indochine, 12e séance plénière, mercredi 9 novembre 1938," ANOM, Indo NF 2300.

[35] ANOM, NF Indo, Box 410, Folder 3569.

a complementary, second-class medicine.[36] A few years earlier, a course on the Sino-Vietnamese pharmacopeia was made compulsory for Hanoi's medical and pharmacy students. Its objective was to provide them with the knowledge and objectivity to "take advantage, and avoid the dangers, of this pharmacopeia."[37] While colonial administrators seem to have taken a growing interest in a "rediscovery" of Sino-Vietnamese remedies during this period, their curiosity was directed toward very specific goals. The most obvious was to identify alternatives to the importation of often-expensive medicines and to offer basic solutions for minor health problems for the majority of the population. While colonial health care professionals had occasionally sought out local remedies to treat conditions for which Western medicines were unavailable or ineffective, as in the case of leprosy treatment (see Chapter 3), this new interest heralded a more systematic approach to the local pharmacopeia. State-employed pharmacists and doctors engaged in pharmacological research and development in Indochina. The first group played an important role in the extraction of alkaloids from local substances, some of which were eventually used in the composition of new drugs. They also developed new therapeutic forms and analyzed the pharmacological properties of both biomedical and Vietnamese ingredients and medicines, thus contributing to an embryonic bioprospection effort.[38]

Indeed, Vietnam's biodiversity was seen as a rich trove of pharmacological treasure that the colonial government was eager to explore. One of the clearest expressions of this "recuperative" impulse was the creation, in 1942, of the Comité d'étude et d'utilisation des drogues indochinoises (Committee on the study and use of Indochinese drugs), based at the University of Hanoi. It had four main objectives: to prospect and sample the local flora; to study plants in the laboratory in order to identify their physiological effects and therapeutic properties; to study their effects on disease in clinical settings; and, finally, to develop the cultivation of the most useful plants on an industrial scale.[39] Wartime conditions increased the priority level of these projects, while also exposing the ambiguities and utilitarianism of late-colonial efforts to draw parallels between the two medical systems. These actions also presaged some of the conditions and directions that would continue to shape the postcolonial pharmaceuticalization of Vietnam, and its path toward a model integrative health care system from 1954.

---

[36] ANOM, Gougal SE 213.
[37] Gougal SE C49 c2(2).
[38] Monnais and Tousignant, "The Values of Versatility."
[39] "Plantes médicinales. 1. Comité d'études; 2. Production et commerce; 3. Renseignements techniques sur les diverses plantes médicinales, 1942," ANOM, Gougal SE 2293.

8.4   Therapeutic Itineraries through Hybridity

It should be clear by now that, for the majority of the population, Vietnamese medicine was the only treatment option. Indeed, this reality was put forward to argue for its transformation, selective recognition, and subordinated integration into a two-tiered health care system. That being said, a small but significant segment of the population did have access to the multiple, contiguous, often intersecting therapeutic options offered by the cosmopolitan medical markets described herein, or around the nodes formed by AMI facilities and a few outlets and private practitioners in provincial centers. Itineraries through these therapeutic options gave rise to individual practices of pluralization that were rich and diverse, and in which colonial medicines played an increasingly central role. In the last sections of this chapter, I turn to this *pluralism in practice* as it is revealed "from below"[40] – that is, from therapeutic itineraries – in order to explore the complex lay rationalities that underpinned them.

As mentioned on several occasions, AMI reports, especially in the early years, were full of disparaging remarks about Vietnamese patients' sequential or simultaneous recourse to biomedical and traditional therapies. Doctors deplored the fact that patients came to the AMI as "a last resort" after having exhausted the possibilities of "traditional empiricism."[41] They discovered Chinese, or Vietnamese, pills hidden under hospital mattresses, proclaiming that the "Annamese, impatient to get better," did not hesitate to combine "every possibility at once, European and indigenous medicine, exorcism, etc."[42] The press also reported plural therapeutic practices: *La tribune indochinoise* noted, in 1930, that some sought out vaccination yet continued to wear amulets.[43] These observations suggest that such modes of hybridization were quite common in therapeutic practices throughout the period of colonial rule. Yet they tell us little about the individual itineraries and the logics that guided them. For this information, we need, once again, to turn to readers' correspondence in the BAYB, examining it even more closely to "close the loop."

The narration of individual therapeutic experiences reveals different types of plural itineraries. BAYB correspondents frequently described practices of simultaneous recourse to different therapeutic systems. One

---

[40] Roy Porter, "The Patient's View. Doing Medical History from Below," *Theory & Society* 14, 2 (1985): 175–98.

[41] Dr. Beaujean, "Un cas d'intoxication par absorption de drogues indigènes à base de mercure," BSMI 5, 4 (1914): 129–31.

[42] Massias, "La fièvre typhoïde"; ANOM, RST NF 3683. It should be mentioned that there were also reports of European hospitalized patients who used Sino-Vietnamese remedies.

[43] *La tribune indochinoise*, no. 548, April 19, 1930, and no. 562, May 24, 1930.

illustrative case was brought by a public works employee, who wrote to the editor in chief in 1935 on behalf of his twenty-year-old son. The son had taken "many" Vietnamese and Western medicines to relieve chronic stomach pain, but although his pain had abated, he still looked pale and unhealthy: the father asked for the name of a good tonic.[44] There was also a letter from a Mr. Lưu, who, suspecting that his twelve-year-old son had either "worms or bacteria," had given him both castor oil and a Chinese product, which got rid of the worms, but not of the stomach pain.[45] Thành Xuân had given his young son, ill with whooping cough, "Annamese and Western remedies for almost a month." Finally, the cough went away but the boy developed asthma, for which his parents "treated him with many medicines over the next year."[46] Another common type of plural itinerary described in the BAYB was made up of successive recourse to different therapeutic systems. A typical example is of Mr. Ninh's nephew who, he wrote in 1935, "has asthma and has coughed for years; he has taken traditional remedies but does not get better," and for whom he now sought the editor's recommendation for Western medicines.[47]

While successive itineraries were often, as in these cases, quests for new options after the failure of prior treatment, others continued to move back and forth between "traditional" and "Western" therapeutic options. Recall the young intellectual who thought he was suffering from neurasthenia (see Chapter 7). Having suffered for years, he first tried a range of pharmaceutical specialties, including several barbiturates. He then consulted a traditional therapist who diagnosed overheated internal organs, which required cooling in order to restore balance. Dissatisfied with both types of drugs for their lack of efficacy, and distrusting the therapists' diagnosis, he turned to Nguyễn Văn Luyện in 1936 for guidance toward more appropriate Western products.[48] Ông B. H., from Haiphong, recounted an even longer and more tortuous quest for therapy. It began with skin eruptions and itching for which he took various medicines to "cleanse" his organism. His traditional therapist then told him he had "too much heat inside" and needed to take tiger bone gelatin. Unconvinced, he went on to consult a French doctor named Dr. Fesquet, who prescribed medicines in a water solution for injection. After this treatment, Mr. B. H. developed a high fever, so he went back to traditional medicine. A friend then suggested he might have syphilis and

---

[44] Readers' correspondence, BAYB, no. 30, December 1935, 29.
[45] Readers' correspondence, BAYB, no. 37, August 1937, 28.
[46] Readers' correspondence, BAYB, no. 9, February 1935, 27.
[47] Readers' correspondence, BAYB, no. 11, April 1935, 28.
[48] Readers' correspondence, BAYB, no. 19, January 1936, 32–33.

recommended a calomel ointment. The effect of the ointment, to which B. H. added tonics, did not last, so he took some Chinese medicines followed by a Vietnamese drug, Tự Ngọc Liên, a product of the eponymous local drugstore. His symptoms had then changed from pain upon urinating to pain in the anus. Finally, he went back to Fesquet, who prescribed sandalwood and an injection of Gonacrine, a powerful antiseptic. He felt much better, but, as a precaution, had also consulted a doctor by the name of Dr. Dê and occasionally gave himself an enema of silver nitrate.[49]

Plural recourse to therapy was only one among, and often combined with, several types of practice defined as irrational from a biomedical vantage, including, as can be seen in the above cases, self-medication, overconsumption, "off-label" use, and non-adherence. At the same time, these various practices can be seen as manifestations of self-directed quests for healing that critically evaluated and navigated a proliferating number of therapeutic options and sources of advice. With rapid growth, over the span of only a couple of decades, in the quantity and diversity of medicines on the Vietnamese market, some consumers crafted therapeutic combinations that were increasingly varied, complex, and often risky. Some of Nguyễn Văn Luyện's virtual patients confessed to having consumed ten to twenty different medical specialties, which were theoretically prescription-only, sometimes over the space of only a few months or even weeks.

A reader thought he had gonorrhea; after trying a huge variety of medicines (which included copaiba, horse chestnut extract, belladonna ointment, injectable sandalwood-based medicines, as well as brand-name products, including Kitine, Gonacrine, Peyrard injections, Argyrol, and Gonagone), he asked Nguyễn Văn Luyện to help him find a definitive cure.[50] In 1936, "N. V. T." described himself as overworked. For his digestive problems, pain, and fatigue, he had taken Gastrol "and a few medicines from here," but to no avail. He then tried "all the medicines of the Vo Van Van pharmacy," but the results were no better.[51] A few months earlier, "V. V. Ch.," a nineteen-year-old student living in Nam Dinh, recounted: "last January, I noticed that each time I eat a bowl of rice, I have violent stomach pains. I took Gastrosodine, Gastrol, Tricarbine as well as all the Vietnamese remedies."[52] Another correspondent, Ông T. B. K., described his itinerary as follows:

[49] Readers' correspondence, BAYB, no. 25, July 1936, 30.
[50] Readers' correspondence, BAYB, no. 21, March 1936, 29.
[51] Readers' correspondence, BAYB, no. 28, October 1936, 26.
[52] Readers' correspondence, BAYB, no. 13, July 1935, 27.

From the ages of 15 to 19, I was healthy, had good skin and liked to exercise. When I turned 20, my health started getting worse and my skin got darker. At that time, I had a tertian fever [type of malaria] on top of spermatorrhea. At 19, I had nasal surgery; at 20, I took Hémoglobine Deschiens, Histogénol, Quina Laroche, etc., each time to no avail, during three, four months. At 21, I had injections of quinine with Histogénol, Plasmochine, Quina Laroche; at 22: injections of 914 [. . .] I also took Opocalcium and sparteine. At 23: injections of sodium cacodylate, Acétylarsan, strychine sulfate.[53]

These readers sought advice from the BAYB editor only after unsuccessfully trying out a wide range of medicines, usually including several specialties. They did so at a time of change in Vietnamese society, when colonialism and modernization brought new pressures. Yet these coexisted with persistent co-occurring pathologies that were difficult to treat, and against which most medicines were ineffective. Still, some products were considered, and consumed, as panaceas that were good for multiple conditions. Pluralistic practices emerged in the encounter between patients' anxieties, their experiences of serious or debilitating illnesses, and their therapeutic hopes.

8.5   Irrational Therapeutic Practices: Myths and Realities

The plural therapeutic itineraries that arose from these underlying logics and practices deviated from biomedical norms and prescriptions for taking medicines. As seen over the previous chapters, there were many reasons for individuals to avoid or to discount medical advice, including miscommunication, fear of adverse effects – which was sometimes well-founded – the mismatch between prescribed treatments and patients' financial means, or a lack of time for hospitalization, recovery, or frequent doses. Indeed, some of the instructions given in the Vidal repertory for taking medicines properly were clearly unsuited to Vietnamese lifestyles. Some medicines were to be taken six to eight times a day, in water; for others, it was recommended to rest or to avoid exposure to heat and sun.

New demands for more rapid relief and cure, or for antidotes to the effects of the pressures of modern life, also gave rise to practices of prolific consumption and of therapeutic "sampling." Experimental, trial-and-error itineraries through multiple therapeutic options were also sometimes prompted by a wrong diagnosis or prescription, and the ensuing failure of therapy, as in the case of the biomedically trained nurse Nguyễn Van S. The latter told the editor of the BAYB in April 1938 that, having been diagnosed, despite lack of any positive test results, with renal

---

[53] Readers' correspondence, BAYB, no. 4, October 1934, 28.

tuberculosis by his doctor, he had taken five flasks of Sirop Famel, another five of Sirop Lebrun, and ten of Pulmosérum. He had also been injected, at the hospital, with eight doses of Cinnozyl, two of Antigène, forty of guaiacol and iodoform oil, twelve of Sandoz calcium (mixed with Cadior and administered intravenously), twenty of Francalcium, ten of Laroscorbine, five of Panxylon, and two of Vitadone. Finally, his doctor advised him to take Histogénol, a tonic recommended for cases of tuberculosis; he had consumed fifteen boxes.[54] Some readers, as we have seen, did seek expert advice but were unable to obtain, whether from Chinese medicine, Vietnamese medicine, or biomedicine, a persuasive or therapeutically useful explanation for their illness. It was not only "ignorant" or "resistant" patients who consumed medicines in ways that might be judged as irrational.

In addition to such excessive drug consumption and to practices of diluting the strength or shortening the duration of recommended therapies, there were also cases in which therapeutic indications were ignored or, most often, broadened. The itineraries described by BAYB correspondents confirm that some medicines were used for a very wide range of purposes. Some, indeed among the most popular, were adopted as veritable panaceas. Although Compound 914 had multiple "official" indications for treating infectious disease, it was used, in interwar Vietnam, not only to treat syphilis, gonorrhea, malaria, and tuberculosis, but also hemorrhoids, headache, toothache, renal problems, eczema, fatigue and overwork, nervousness, spermatorrhea, muscular paralysis, menstrual problems, constipation, and all kinds of itching. Another arsenical compound, Acétylarsan, was also used – in addition to its recommended uses – for the treatment of head colds, headaches, skin cruptions, anal fistulae, insomnia and epilepsy, and in its pediatric formulation, for rickets, vomiting, malaria, perspiration, teething pain, parasites, and nasal congestion. Again, the BAYB editor cautioned readers against these therapeutic "diversions," emphasizing the risk of therapeutic failure or toxicity.

The editor was particularly worried about the prevalent misuse of injectable products. As mentioned in Chapter 6, the widespread association between injections and tonic effects was a significant reason (among others) for the overuse or off-label use of some medicines. A few arsenical compounds and arsenic- or mercury-based products such as Épicral were prescribed both as syphilis cures and general tonics; the majority were not officially indicated as such, but were nevertheless consumed for this effect.[55] Conversely, products with tonic effects were used to treat serious

[54] Readers' correspondence, BAYB, no. 40, April 1938, 27.
[55] Readers' correspondence, BAYB, no. 5, November 1934, and no. 21, March 1936, 25.

infectious diseases. In 1935, the BAYB editor told a recently discharged tuberculosis patient that the medicines he was given at the hospital (injections of Angiolymphe, Lipocire, and Biocholine) were merely tonics and not, "as people often think," specific medicines, which were needed to treat this "very serious" disease.[56] The editor repeatedly warned that tonics, especially the apparently very popular Biocholine, which was often used by tuberculosis sufferers, could not do everything: their main function, when used appropriately, was to preserve an already disease-free state of health.[57] The questions asked by Ông P. T. C., from Phan Rang, in the BAYB in 1937 are particularly revealing: "Do all medicines made with arsenic (Stovarsol, Acétylarsan, 914) tonify the blood and how? Do they not work like tonic potions and other injections? Or do they purge the blood of microbes and tonify it? Is it true that arsenic-based medicines are excellent to reinforce the heart and thus help the patient recover?"[58] This conflation of injection, tonic, and anti-infectious drug marked a parallel association between symptomatic or adjuvant treatment (to relieve symptoms quickly and boost the organism) and specific curative treatment (targeting the pathogenic cause of disease).

These different ways of stretching official therapeutic indications show, once again, the capacity of Vietnamese patients to develop their own expectations of what medicines should do, independently, to some extent at least, of what colonial health care policies and professionals prescribed and made available. Advertising stimulated this creative capacity, but it also made the Vietnamese into active agents who shaped the health market in which they participated. In just two sentences about Dagénan written in 1949, Dr. Dương Bá Bành captured this autonomy and agency, which facilitated a very rapid assimilation of new medicines into plural and self-determined health practices: as soon as they were introduced to Vietnam, he wrote, modern drugs had been the object of "a formidable vogue among families, who always have a few tablets at their disposal, convinced that this true panacea cures all. And thus is it used in Sino-Vietnamese medicine, more or less combined with other drugs."[59]

This did not exclude a desire to learn about and to apply therapeutic rules as defined by biomedical experts. In July 1936, Ông T. S., from Haiphong, told the BAYB that he had been cured of gonorrhea by a four-month course of Gonacrine injections and "a vaccine." "Now," he wrote, "I want to do things properly; I want to receive a yearly injection.

[56] Readers' correspondence, BAYB, no. 15, September 1935, 34.
[57] Often mentioned in the readers' correspondence, Biocholine is in fact a tonic that is supposed to help prevent several diseases, including tuberculosis and pneumonia.
[58] Readers' correspondence, BAYB, no. 37, August 1937, 24.
[59] Dương Bá Bành, Histoire de la médecine, 80.

So I would like to know, in particular: should I really start the injections again? If so, how many? Some say that now injections of mercury cyanide and bismuth are recommended, is this so?"[60] Besides revealing a desire to prevent disease and to toe the biomedical line, these questions suggest that new interpretive grids were being constructed in order to grasp and categorize the indications and effects, and especially the efficacy, of medicines. These grids were modulated according to the origins – "Western" or "traditional" – of medicines. They were shaped, on the one hand, by the introduction of, and a familiarization with, a growing range of therapeutic options, including some highly effective colonial medicines. On the other hand, they took form in interaction with the emergence of deeply politicized discourses on Vietnamese medicine that emphasized its indispensability, but also its amenability to scientific improvement, even as it remained true to its deeply-rooted local, time-proven, and traditional character, which made it suited to Vietnamese bodies and cosmologies. From this colonial encounter, there arose a popular representation of Vietnamese medicines as "mild" and slow acting. This representation, key to the reinvention of a distinctive Vietnamese medicine, was constructed in opposition to Western, but also to some Chinese (and Japanese) medicines, which were seen as "strong": effective but also toxic.[61]

As a result of this emerging binary, Western medicines were increasingly prioritized, or exclusively used, for the treatment of serious or acute disease. Vietnamese medicines were preferred for problems identified as benign, chronic, or "specifically Vietnamese" (or of supernatural origin), or for individuals who were seen as needing gentler treatment, such as children and women, especially if they were pregnant, breastfeeding, or infertile.[62] This is a form of therapeutic pluralism, "segmentary pluralism"[63] – that is, different from those described previously in which medical systems were brought into interaction (whether as simultaneous, successive, or back and forth recourse) – in response to a single episode of illness. Here, the choice of medical system is made in response

---

[60] Readers' correspondence, BAYB, no. 24, July 1936, 25.

[61] As early as 1902, Dr. Vialet drew attention to similarities in local representations of Chinese, Japanese, and Western medicines: "Médecine et chirurgie indigène au Tonkin," AMN 77: 34–36. But these connections became more widespread in the 1930s.

[62] Indeed, "feminine" troubles, such as menstrual cycle irregularities or infertility, were rarely among the indications of advertised Western specialties, except for certain tonics. By contrast, a significant number of hybrid specialties and Vietnamese remedies did address such problems.

[63] Robert Debusman, "Médicalisation et pluralisme au Cameroun allemand: autorité médicale et stratégies profanes," Outre-mers. Revue d'histoire 90, 1 (2003): 241–42.

to an episode of a particular type of illness or a specific "constitution," gender, or age. When, however, "gentle" Vietnamese medicines proved ineffective, some readers sought recommendations from the BAYB editor for other (Western) therapeutic options. One reader wrote on behalf of his sister, who remained childless after eight years of marriage and had spent a lot of money on Vietnamese medicines: "What should she do now?," he asked.[64] A father asked what Western medicine "thinks" of the unexplained bleeding of his twelve-year-old daughter, for whom traditional remedies did nothing.[65] Lê V. H., from Hanoi, asked: "My wife has already had two children but delivered early. She is pregnant again [. . .] but she feels weak, lacks energy and coughs [. . .] She would like to take a Western tonic wine. We would like to know which one to take. Before she took our traditional remedies [. . .] but all were ineffective. She would now like Western remedies and awaits your response."[66]

The labeling of Western medicines as "hot" motivated, in some cases, the use of Vietnamese medicines as adjuvant, rather than as alternative, therapy in order to counter the potential toxic effects of modern pharmaceutical specialties: an instance of what anthropologist Nina Etkin has called "calculated syncretism."[67] The simultaneous popularity of French, traditional, and hybrid or neo-traditional specialties to treat spermatorrhea provides a striking illustration of how the goal of maximizing efficacy, while minimizing adverse effects was managed through plural health practices. Some situations nevertheless continued to create dilemmas: for example, the treatment of syphilis in women, or the prevention of malaria in children. These last examples also show that recourse to Western medicine as an "alternative medicine," to echo the medical historian Donald Bates, was not, or no longer, excluded. Yet if biomedical therapies were increasingly solicited as the first or preferred option, especially for treating infectious diseases (above all STIs), they were also seen as having their limits and disadvantages.[68]

Such varied therapeutic itineraries provide elements for better understanding the selectivity of Vietnamese therapeutic demands, hinting at the complexity and dynamism of the logics underlying the consumption of medicines under colonial rule. These logics were informed by deeply anchored representations – which continued to be denigrated by many

---

[64] Readers' correspondence, BAYB, no. 28, October 1936, 28.
[65] Readers' correspondence, BAYB, no. 9, March 1935, 28.
[66] Readers' correspondence, BAYB, no. 30, December 1936, 35.
[67] Etkin, "Side Effects," 104.
[68] Donald G. Bates, "Why Not Call Modern Medicine 'Alternative'?," *Perspectives in Biology & Medicine* 43, 4 (2000): 514–25.

biomedical actors – as well as by new experiences, knowledge, and tools as they were integrated into individual health management strategies.

Medical discourses on Vietnamese recourse to biomedicine and consumption of medicines also changed. Prior to World War I, official reports usually blamed Vietnamese populations' mistrust, ignorance, and inertia as the reasons why they avoided biomedicine and why they persisted, "by default," in using their "ancestral" medicine.[69] From the 1920s, however, colonial authorities and doctors increasingly acknowledged the rationality of recourse to "traditional medicine," whether as a necessity in the face of the inaccessibility of colonial medicines, or as a choice motived either by political rejection of Western, colonial medicine or by the positive value given to a medical tradition that was both deeply rooted and capable of progress.[70] The recognition of these factors highlights, even if unintentionally, the agency of Vietnamese patients, their capacity to accept or to refuse, to negotiate, and to choose among available therapeutic options. AMI doctors were unable or unwilling to see Vietnamese practices of therapeutic pluralism as a sign of their acceptance of biomedicine. But I suggest that we might consider these mosaic therapeutics as such proof, given the practices and rationalities described in the previous three chapters. Practices of non-compliance, and even the refusal of (some) Western drugs, were not manifestations of a static culture. They were embedded in, and illustrative of, a fast-changing socioeconomic context, and part of a dynamic, changing set of health practices and representations in interwar Vietnam.

[69] ANOM, RST NF 896 and 4014; Gougal 17171.
[70] ANOM, NF Indo 2298.

Conclusion: From Colonial Medicines to Postcolonial Health

Exploring the logics and practices of pharmaceutical production, distribution, and consumption in colonial Vietnam, this book shows that therapeutic consumption practices of therapeutic pluralism and self-medication, which are now prevalent in this location, emerged in the early twentieth century, and became well established before the end of French rule. This does not mean that the (colonial) past can fully elucidate or explain the present, much less generate solutions. Nor can the Vietnamese history of colonial medicines serve as a template for understanding a global process of pharmaceuticalization that took off in the 1950s and 1960s with the diffusion of antibiotics. Pharmaceuticals entered Vietnam in a very particular context. This was a terrain marked by the intensity of colonial domination and medicalization – even in comparison with other French colonial territories – which coincided with a time of transition in the modes of production and consumption of medicines. It was also a space in which traditional therapeutics had deep roots; its pharmacopeia was fueled both by a remarkably rich local pharmacopeia and by long-standing networks of therapeutic exchange. Last but not least, Vietnam continued to be shaped, more broadly, by its spatial, historical, and cultural proximity to China. This sparked a highly localized and particularly early, complex, and dynamic process of selective appropriation that was hybridized through and through.

Despite these specificities, the little-explored history of medicines in Vietnam nevertheless offers keys to a broader understanding of the initial phases of the pharmaceutical industry's global expansion. By this time, processes of globalization (that is, of global commercial and economic circulation) were clearly already underway. As the Western, and especially the French pharmaceutical industry, epitomized by Rhône-Poulenc and its affiliates, grew, it engaged in a highly mobile race to markets as well as to sites and populations of therapeutic experimentation. This mobilization heralded what would later, in the 1970s, be demonized under the label of pharmaceutical invasion. Yet this spatial mobility did not necessarily lead to a homogenization of pharmaceutical presence and practices; space was also left, or created, for a variety of initiatives, and for conceptual, material, and practical cross-fertilizations.[1] Indeed, over time, colonial medicines became harder and harder to define as such, because they were re-appropriated, mimicked, modified, and transformed; their identities and functions were multiplied. Or rather, as I have suggested throughout this book, we should consider as "colonial" not only the products made, brought, and distributed by the colonizers, but, more broadly, *any* medicine that emerged under circumstances of colonial interaction and domination. Thus, colonial medicines were indigenized, Vietnamized, and pluralized by colonial encounters; no longer identifiably "Western," they included products, from local pharmacist-produced specialties to hybrid and neo-traditional medicines, that were both local, in various ways, and modern, and, as I was able to determine, also became quite popular.

Escaping the purview of their initial producers and especially of their official, public distributors – that is, of AMI staff and especially state-qualified (first French, then also Vietnamese) doctors and pharmacists – colonial medicines reveal trajectories that took surprising twists and turns, and which implicated unexpected actors and practices. Due to their growing number and ease of circulation, medicines, as objects of study, shed light on dimensions of colonial medicalization that, until now, have remained hazy, even hidden. They show how the medicalization process was able, at times, to adapt itself, but they especially reveal its limitations, deep rifts, and highly variable reach. These limits are perhaps most eloquently illustrated by the development of an essential medicines outlets network after 1920. In investigating the conditions of accessibility of these pharmaceutical products, it is hard not to be struck by the utter rigidity of the AMI system and of its legislative underpinnings, which seem so ill-adapted to the living conditions, daily lives, means, and expectations of the majority of Vietnamese at the time. This gap, and an inability to bridge it, made even the endeavor to supply the "masses" with quinine, the colonial medicine par excellence, identified as a means to curb the territory's most devastating endemic disease, a source of constant frustration, and failure. Widespread inability, whether for geographic or economic reasons, to gain access to quality care throws into relief just how chronically underfunded and thinly spread the colonial health care system was, especially in rural areas.

This was a system with *at least* two tiers, forcing the majority of the population to seek makeshift solutions, circumvent the law, and resort to

---

[1] Arjun Appadurai, *Modernity At Large: Cultural Dimensions of Globalization* (Minneapolis: University of Minnesota Press, 1996).

medicines that were neither free nor safe, or were ineffective, for lack of alternatives. Most rural residents had no other option but to use the services of therapists who were often poorly trained and sometimes dishonest. Those who happened to have a medicines outlet nearby probably usually found it to be poorly stocked, and, anyhow, they had to pay for even a single a dose of Antipyrin or santonin. Those who were fortunate enough to make it to a fixed consultation site were unlikely to find a pharmacist onsite who was authorized to prepare medicines, even less likely to find a doctor to prescribe these. The poorest, wherever they lived, usually had the fewest choices. Urban residents with modest incomes may have been able to buy, on occasion, one of the cheapest commercial specialties, which might have alleviated incapacitating symptoms but was unlikely to cure a case of syphilis, pneumonia, or trachoma.

This persistent lack of accessibility suggests that modern medicine's insistence on its own superiority, and on the prerogatives and exclusivity of its agents, was ill-suited to the colonial terrains to which it was exported. But that is not all: on top of this predictably arrogant attitude came the more surprising and stubborn therapeutic skepticism of colonial doctors, as well as, by extension, of some biomedically trained Vietnamese doctors. In the tropics, in the era of the rise of bacteriology and of the Pastorian model of war against infectious disease, prevention reigned supreme; this left little or no role for therapeutics. For quite some time, drugs could not be defined as tools of civilization, in that they were not considered to "teach" the modern principles of hygiene and prevention. Furthermore, in (South) East Asia, there were additional obstacles to defining medicines as legitimate and effective tools of medicalization. Remedies, which had an important role in longstanding therapeutic practices, were already familiar to local populations; they were too popular to be "good" and were thus also objects of fierce competition. This perceptible, though usually implicit, biomedical denial of therapeutics was a fundamental error of judgment on how to successfully medicalize the colonies. Yet it also echoed, to some extent, a similarly divergent response to medicines in the metropole, where professional therapeutic skepticism, which was particularly strong within the French medical profession, came up against a popular enthusiasm that made medicines a potentially potent vector of modernization.

Today, the traces of this posture are difficult to discern, for doctors' therapeutic skepticism has, everywhere, given way to a "therapeutic furor," to quote the French philosopher François Dagognet, a volte-face that has not yet been fully elucidated.[2] Yet in some global health

[2] Dagognet, *La raison*, 321.

interventions, particularly in vertical programs targeting a "priority" disease, there still seems to be some ambivalence toward medicines. Preferably, medicines should be a tool of mass prevention, such as vaccines, or curative drugs distributed on a large enough scale to procure a population-level effect (i.e., what is called treatment-as-prevention).[3] At the same time, in view of their risky potential for autonomy, their consumption should, it is emphasized, be closely and medically monitored. Unless these conditions are met, medicines remain largely inaccessible, reserved to the lucky few, and often ill adapted – physically, culturally, financially – to the populations they are destined for.[4]

In Vietnam, high-level public officials seem to view medicines not so much with contempt as with indifference; this translates, in post-Đổi mới health policies, as an underfunding of medicines in the state system and a deregulation of their distribution. These two trends have had a significant impact, and some of the resulting realities are clear reminders of the colonial period: according to the WHO, Ho Chi Minh City's Department of Health granted licenses to 5,800 businesses selling medicines (3,356 pharmacists and more than 300 businesses specialized in "traditional medicines") in just the first half of 2008; yet its pharmacy inspection service disposed of only four qualified pharmacists that year. In the countryside, most Vietnamese continue to resort to the nearest nhà thuốc, shops whose managers are rarely qualified as pharmacists.[5] Despite the variable cost of drugs, their purchase and consumption remains the preferred option in seeking health care, especially given the lack of alternatives for more extensive or better care.[6] In their non-consumption as much as in their consumption, colonial medicines reveal glaring problems of accessibility to public and quality health care in Vietnam under French colonial rule. These problems, to some extent, have persisted beyond independence. Medicines nonetheless capture some of the realities of social change in the colony, and as such remain captivating objects of study. For, as I hope will be obvious by now, they were and are highly versatile, much to health authorities' annoyance. Circulating with ease, they can be ingested and appraised without the need for any mediation or specific expertise. Even injectable products, especially those used as tonics (whether or not these were indicated as

[3] On the concept of treatment-as-prevention, see, in particular, Vinh-Kim Nguyen et al., "Remedicalizing an Epidemic: From HIV Treatment as Prevention to HIV Treatment Is Prevention," *AIDS* 25, 3 (2010): 291–93; Lachenal, *Le médicament*

[4] Kremer, "Pharmaceuticals," 68–69.

[5] Wulffers, "The Role of Pharmaceuticals," 1329.

[6] In 2001, per capita drug spending was US$5.50, up from only US$0.30 in 1990: Daniel Simonet, "Une analyse du marché pharmaceutique vietnamien," *Cahiers d'études et de recherches francophones/Santé*, 11, 3 (2001):155.

such), were traded illicitly from very early on; this was still the case at the time of Vietnam's reunification in 1975, and is still the case today, especially with Western-manufactured products.[7]

Increasingly conspicuous enthusiasm for a growing variety of Western medicines in the interwar years was symptomatic of broader transformations; these arose from changes not only in health care practices but also in ways of thinking, and even in the types of health issues faced, and solutions sought, at both individual and collective levels. Modern therapeutic consumption was the sign of new conceptual reference points, most obviously for understanding health and well-being, but also for dealing with risk, anxiety, and various problems – of modernity, of nutritional deficiency (vitamins), or of sterility (hormones) – and even for making claims to health as a right. These new concepts did not arise ex nihilo, nor did they simply arrive from the West: the success of organ-based therapies, for example, is illustrative of how older therapeutic understandings – in this case, of the permeability between the categories of food and medicine – could take on a new life. Similarly, the quick appropriation of specialties in pill form was in continuity with the familiarity that emerged from contact with convenient pharmaceutical forms imported from neighboring China, long before French colonization. Still, these ways of thinking about health and medicines were strongly shaped by the nature and growth of the market for colonial medicines, whose identity was increasingly defined in terms of mass production, publicity, trademarks, as well as efficacy and practicability.

On the eve of World War II, and the many more years of war to come, medicines were on their way to becoming *commodities* in Vietnam. Foremost among their qualities were scientificity and efficacy. This led to early "deviations," especially because, at that time, the population lacked widespread access to anti-infectious products that were recognized to be safe and effective. I have described not only the strength of illicit drug networks for quinine, 914, and Dagénan, but also the extent to which counterfeiting flourished from the earliest years of colonial rule. Defined broadly as a set of practices of illicit imitation, counterfeiting activities grew increasingly well-structured and sophisticated. Exploiting gaps in accessibility, they specifically targeted landmark products that were well known and highly sought after. It is difficult not to draw a parallel between the sale of false QE beginning in the 1910s – some tablets were apparently so well-manufactured and difficult to trace that they could calmly be sold in AMI outlets – and the more recent circulation of fake Artesunate, a synthetic derivative of artemisinin used

---

[7] Wolffers, "The Role of Pharmaceuticals," 1330.

to treat malaria that is now widely, and rather ingeniously, counterfeited. According to a study published in *The Lancet* in 2001, nearly 30 percent of all tablets on the private market that are labeled "AS" in fact contained no artemisinin at all. Yet they appeared, to the naked eye, to have been duly manufactured by Guilin Pharma, the drug's main Shanghai-based producer. Only an often much lower price aroused suspicion.[8] This was also the case in the 1930s when pharmacy inspectors seized QE tablets.

Both private and illicit networks of medicines mark an indigenization of the medicalization process in colonial Vietnam. They illuminate the role of unexpected, and forgotten, mediators, including agents of traditional health care and other indigenous commercial actors, in these processes, especially in the domestication of the pharmaceutical products introduced by the colonizers. Qualified pharmacists had no monopoly over the capacity to market attractive, modern products that might fulfill local expectations while also mobilizing other labels. Whatever else these practices of therapeutic manipulation and consumption may (or may not) demonstrate, these networks and multiple actors certainly reveal a degree of patient agency among the Vietnamese. They were colonized subjects, but they nevertheless exercised a certain capacity to act, to choose, and therefore to refuse, as well as to appropriate some of the colonizers' conceptual references. This process of appropriation is still under-examined in the field of colonial studies and of global public health, even though it foreshadowed a real conversion to biomedicine, or at least to some of its principles (the toxicity/efficacy calculus, for example), tools, and techniques (such as injections).[9] In this space of relative but paradoxical freedom, new forms of medical pluralism could take root and a new interpretive grid for medicines emerged, characterizing Chinese and Western medicines as hot and effective but toxic, and (re)defining Vietnamese remedies as cold and mild, yet slow-acting and unsuited to treating serious disease – an analytical grid that can still be observed both in Vietnam and among Vietnamese immigrant

[8] Paul Newton et al., "Fake Artesunate in Southeast Asia," *The Lancet* 357, 9272 (2001): 1948–50. Artemisinin is isolated from, and named after, the plant *Artemisia annua* or sweet wormwood. The plant has long grown abundantly in southern China, where it has been used for millennia, as a decoction, to treat fever. The Vietnam War stimulated research on its efficacy in the 1960s, but it was military Chinese researchers who isolated its active substance, artemisinin, in 1972.
[9] The study of the colonial history of medicines also provides an opportunity to see that this biomedical conversion did not necessarily depend on the mobilization of effective means of persuasion or of physical coercion: Dipesh Chakrabarty, *Provincializing Europe. Postcolonial Thought and Historical Difference* (Princeton and Oxford: Princeton University Press, 2007 [2000]), 44.

communities.[10] In parallel, a therapeutic learning process based on biological as well as cultural experiences of medicines unfolded.[11]

We can link this agency back to a more distant East Asian past, and thus make it an echo of the Confucian obligation to educate oneself and manage one's own health. We can also say that the experience of colonialism sustained this tendency, by sparking a creative, modernizing popular press and a dynamic, diversified medicines market, allowing, in the end, for a considerable degree of continuity between pre- and post-colonial periods. It is surely not merely a coincidence that, even after three decades of war, the Vietnamese population has continued to rely heavily on mass media and specialized health publications (manuals, pharmaceutical compendiums, therapeutic mementos, etc.) as key sources of information and ideas on health.[12] Even now, Vietnamese health-seekers' capacity to act continues, very often, to manifest itself, in Vietnam but also in the diaspora, as interactions with pharmacists as advisors and mediators of choice.[13] And despite the strict codification of pharmacists' prerogatives by the Vietnamese state and, before that, by the colonial administration, their professional identities have in fact remained highly fluid and fashioned by lay interpretations. Pharmacists were already playing such roles in the 1930s in Vietnam's cities; so too, probably, were a plethora of traders of medicines, including, of course, merchants of traditional remedies who, as has been emphasized throughout this book, walked a fine legal line, yet were surely on the front lines of medicalization.

In a context of political claims, which, spurred by inequalities – including in access to health care – became increasingly radical from the 1920s and especially the 1930s, the growth of a market for colonial medicines led to a revitalization in the field of traditional medicines. It thus also contributed to the reinvention (we might even say the *invention*) of a Vietnamese medicine, soon to be erected as a scientific and especially as a national medicine – one able to distinguish itself from the Chinese

[10] Marie-Ève Blanc and Laurence Monnais, "Culture, immigration et santé. La consommation de médicaments chez les Vietnamiens de Montréal," *Revue européenne des migrations internationales* 23, 3 (2007): 167.

[11] These can be called "embodied molecules," whose effects are produced by the encounter between a drug, an ingesting body, and the sociocultural context in which its effects are resituated: Margaret Lock and Patricia Kaufert, "Menopause, Local Biologies, and Culture of Aging," *American Journal of Human Biology* 13, 4 (2001): 494–504.

[12] Finer, *Pressing Priorities*, 22–25.

[13] E. Olsson et al., 2002, "Health Professionals' and Consumers' Views of the Role of the Pharmacy Personnel and the Pharmacy Service in Hanoi, Vietnam – A Qualitative Study," *Journal of Clinical Pharmacy and Therapeutics* 27, 4 (2002): 273–80. This study specifies that pharmacists are often perceived by the Vietnamese population as having the capacity to act as doctors.

model and which remained relatively accessible, "close to the people," making it suited to a collaboration with biomedicine in the framework of an integrative health care system. Here, again, colonial history can offer us keys for better understanding a current phenomenon, a "hybrid modernity," that is playing out in postcolonial Vietnam.[14] I cannot overemphasize the extent to which pluralism, whether institutionalized or private (one might even say intimate and embodied), is made up of constructed and rational practices and concepts. Far from monolithic, its determinants and modalities are not only varied and complex, but also intertwined.

Likewise, it becomes quickly impossible to strictly distinguish between that which is (a) modern (drug) and that which is an empirical remedy, that which is Western or Asian, professional or lay, biomedical or alternative, which is natural, industrial, or artisanal, official or officious, local or global. The "new medicines" I have sought to better delineate, those specialties that straddled the boundary between traditional and Western, and which were increasingly well advertised during the interwar period, were, in themselves, signs of an emerging pharmaceutical industry in Vietnam that was hybrid to its core, yet was able to assert itself and to expand. This is an industry that, today, denounces Western attempts to take ownership of the region's biodiversity while, at the same time, competing with these ventures. Reinvigorated by privatization, the Vietnamese pharmaceutical industry offers a panoply of highly diverse products, including traditional remedies targeted at a Western market, as is notably the case of the Hanoi-based company Traphaco, which plays on both labels of traditional medicine and of new (bio)technologies.[15] History and its accidents, tradition, a two-way street between "center" and "periphery," have made Vietnamese pharmaceuticals what they are today – impossible to assign to a fixed classification, much less a Western one.

"Pharmaceutical citizenship" – a notion according to which membership within a social (and biomedical) norm can be granted via access to medicines, especially the "right" medicines such as antidepressants, ARVs, or Artesunate – took on specific meanings over the course of the

---

[14] Anne Raffin, "Postcolonial Vietnam: Hybrid Modernity," *Postcolonial Studies* 11, 3 (2008): 329–44. Raffin specifically mentions the case of medicine and health to demonstrate the construction of a distinctive Vietnamese hybrid modernity that transcends the usual politico-historical watersheds, being anchored in the colonial period and persisting until today.

[15] Nguyễn Phu'o'ng Ngọc, "The Post-Đổi Mới Construction of the Vietnamese Pharmacopoeia: The Case of the Pharmaceutical Company Traphaco," in Monnais, Thompson, and Wahlberg, *Southern Medicine*, 179–201.

decades of colonial rule.[16] This highlights how colonial domination influenced the values associated with being, and especially staying, healthy, but also, perhaps more importantly, how it made an (unfulfilled) promise of civilization, or at least of entry into modernity via processes of medicalization and pharmaceuticalization that would meet the needs of the colonized. Among the urban elite, therapeutic pluralism was key to the emergence of a cosmopolitan medicine amid societal transformations and the rise of a consumer culture. In all of its forms and locations, medical pluralism emerged as a plausible norm, despite colonial intentions and the initial imposition of a hegemonic biomedical model as the only guarantor of modern, effective medicalization. These contrasting patterns and logics of pluralism also reveal new forms of differentiation and social tensions around access to health care – and especially to quality care. These demands predate the still very Western-centric postcolonial pressure for a world that must be healthy at all costs, as well as adherent to biomedical norms, and yet which nevertheless continues to pay little heed to widespread problems, economic or other, of accessibility. This intrusive, even invasive, pressure both marginalizes and demarginalizes; it is nonetheless echoed by a "taste for medicines," for *glocal medicines*, that have become priority tools of therapy and of relief, by conviction as much as by obligation, and that have shaped, and continue to shape, conceptual references to health, science, and modernity.

---

[16] The notion of pharmaceutical citizenship is borrowed from Stefan Ecks, "Pharmaceutical Citizenship: Antidepressant Marketing and the Promise of Demarginalization in India," *Anthropology & Medicine* 12, 3 (2005): 241–42.

Bibliography

Archives

Archives nationales d'outre-mer (ANOM), Aix-en-Provence (France)

Affaires politiques
Agence de la France d'outre-mer Ancien fonds Indochine
Fonds des Amiraux
Fonds de la Direction du contrôle
Fonds de la Résidence supérieure d'Annam
Fonds de la Résidence supérieure du Tonkin (nouveau fonds)
Fonds du Gouvernement général de l'Indochine
Gouvernement général de l'Indochine, Service économique
Nouveau fonds Indochine

Archives scientifiques de l'Institut Pasteur de Paris, Paris (France)

Fonds Camille Lataste
Fonds des Instituts Pasteur d'Indochine
Fonds du laboratoire de chimie thérapeutique
Fonds Paul-Louis Simond

Vietnam National Archives (VNA) (Vietnam)

Centre no.1, Hanoi
Fonds de la Direction locale de la santé du Tonkin
Fonds de la mairie de Hanoi
Fonds de la Résidence de Nam Dinh
Fonds de la Résidence de Phu Tho
Fonds de la Résidence supérieure du Tonkin
Fonds de l'Inspection générale de l'hygiène et de la santé publique

263

Centre no. 2, Ho Chi Minh City
Fonds de la Résidence supérieure d'Annam (now centre no. 4, in Dalat)
Fonds du Gouvernement de la Cochinchine
Tòa đại biểu chính phủ Nam Việt

Serials

Official Bulletins

Journal officiel de l'Indochine française, Saigon, 1889–1951

Published in France

General
Chimie et industrie, Paris, 1918–66
La quinzaine coloniale, Paris, 1897–1914
La revue coloniale, Paris, 1895–1911

Medical and Professional Journals
Annales d'hygiène et de médecine coloniale, Paris, 1898–1915
    Followed by: *Annales de médecine et de pharmacie coloniales*, Paris,
      1920–39
    Then: *Médecine tropicale*, Marseille, 1941–
Archives de médecine navale, Paris, 1864–90
    Followed by: *Archives de médecine navale et coloniale*, Paris, 1890–96
    Then: *Archives de médecine navale*, Paris, 1897–1910
Bulletin de la Société de pathologie exotique, Paris, 1908–
Hygiène sociale, Troyes, 1893–
La presse médicale, Paris, 1893–
Paris médical. La semaine du clinicien, Paris, 1910–51
Revue de médecine et d'hygiène tropicales, Paris, 1904–14

Published in Vietnam

Colonial Serials
Bulletin des amis du vieux Hué, Hué, 1914–44
Bulletin économique de l'Indochine, Saigon then Hanoi then Saigon,
    1898–1945
Bulletin de la Société des études indochinoises, Saigon, 1883–1975
La Cochinchine française. Organe quotidien des intérêts franco-annamites,
    Saigon, 1907–14
La dépêche d'Indochine. Quotidien indépendant, Saigon, 1928–42

Medical and Professional Journals

Archives des Instituts Pasteur d'Indochine, Saigon, 1925–44
Bulletin de l'Amicale des médecins auxiliaires de l'Indochine, Hanoi, 1919–24
Bulletin de la Société médico-chirurgicale de l'Indochine, Hanoi, 1908–37
  Followed by: *La revue médicale française d'Extrême-Orient*, Hanoi, 1938–44
  Then: *L'Extrême-Orient médical*, Hanoi, 1949–53

Newspapers

L'Annam nouveau, Hanoi, 1931–42
Báo đồng pháp. Grand journal quotidien d'information en langue annamite, Hanoi, 1925–32
Công luận báo. L'Opinion, Saigon, 1916–39
Đại Việt tạp chí. Revue indigène de l'Indochine. Organe de propagande de la pensée française, Saigon, 1918–42
L'Écho annamite. Organe de défense des intérêts franco-annamites, Saigon, 1920–44
Lực tỉnh tân văn. Gazette de Cochinchine, Saigon, 1907–44
Phụ nữ tân van. La nouvelle revue de la femme, Saigon, 1929–34
Le progrès annamite, Saigon, 1924–31
La tribune indigène, Saigon, 1917–25
  Followed by: *La tribune indochinoise*, Saigon, 1926–42

Health and Science Magazines

Bao an y báo. Revue de vulgarisation médicale, Hanoi, 1934–38
Khoa học tạp chí. Revue de vulgarisation scientifique, Saigon, 1923–26
Nam trung nhút báo. Le courrier de la Cochinchine, Saigon, 1917–21
Trung Kỳ vệ sinh chỉ nam. Moniteur d'hygiène d'Annam, Hué, 1930–31
Vệ sinh báo. Journal de vulgarisation d'hygiène, Hanoi, 1926–33
Vệ sinh y báo. Revue mensuelle de vulgarisation d'hygiène et de médecine, Tourane, 1928
Y học tân thanh. La nouvelle voix de la médecine, Cholon, 1938–39
Y học thường thức. Revue de vulgarisation d'hygiène et de médecine préventive, Hanoi, 1939

References

Anderson, Benedict. *Imagined Communities. Reflections on the Origins and Spread of Nationalism*. New York and London: Verso, 1983.
Anderson, Warwick. *Colonial Pathologies. American Tropical Medicine, Race, and Hygiene in the Philippines*. Durham and London: Duke University Press, 2006.
Andrews, Bridie. "Tuberculosis and the Assimilation of Germ Theory in China, 1895–1937." *Journal of the History of Medicine and Allied Sciences* 52, 1 (1997): 114–57.

Angier, Henry, Dr. *Guide médical. Formulaire pratique de thérapeutique et de pharmacie à l'usage des postes dépourvus de médecins*, 6th ed. Saigon: Portail, 1940.

Appadurai, Arjun. *Modernity at Large: Cultural Dimensions of Globalization*. Minneapolis: University of Minnesota Press, 1996.

Arnold, David. *Toxic Histories. Poison and Pollution in Modern India*. Cambridge: Cambridge University Press, 2016.

Au, Sokhieng. *Mixed Medicines. Health and Culture in French Colonial Cambodia*. Chicago: Chicago University Press, 2011.

Azema, Jacques. "La définition juridique du médicament." In *La philosophie du remède*, edited by Jean-Claude Beaune, 37–44. Paris: Champ-Vallon, 1993.

Balandier, Georges. "La situation coloniale. Approche théorique." *Cahiers internationaux de sociologie* 12 (1951): 44–79.

Barnes, Linda L. *Needles, Herbs, Gods and Ghosts. China Healing and the West to 1848*. Cambridge: Harvard University Press, 2005.

Barton, Patricia. "Powders, Potions and Tablets: The 'Quinine Fraud' in British India, 1890–1939." In *Drugs and Empires. Essays in Modern Imperialism and Intoxication, c. 1500–c. 1930*, edited by James H. Mills and Patricia Barton, 142–61. Basingstoke: Palgrave McMillan, 2007.

Bates, Donald G. "Why Not Call Modern Medicine 'Alternative'?" *Perspectives in Biology & Medicine* 43, 4 (2000): 514–25.

Baverey-Massat-Bourrat, Séverine. "De la copie au nouveau médicament. Le laboratoire de chimie thérapeutique." *Entreprises & histoire* 36 (2004): 48–63.

Bhattacharya, Nandini. "Between the Bazaar and the Bench: Making of the Drugs Trade in Colonial India, ca. 1900–1930." *Medical History* 90, 1 (2016): 61–91.

Bivins, Roberta. *Alternative Medicine. A History*. Oxford: Oxford University Press, 2007.

Blainey, Geoffrey. *The Tyranny of Distance: How Distance Shaped Australia's History*. Melbourne: Sun Books, 1966.

Blanc, Marie-Ève, and Laurence Monnais. "Culture, immigration et santé. La consommation de médicaments chez les Vietnamiens de Montréal." *Revue européenne des migrations internationales* 23, 3 (2007): 151–76.

Blondeau, Alexandre. *Histoire des laboratoires pharmaceutiques en France et de leurs médicaments*, 3 vol. Paris: Le Cherche-Midi, 1992.

Boissière, Jules. *Dans la forêt*. In *Indochine. Un rêve d'Asie*, edited by Alain Quella-Villégier, 9–19. Paris: Omnibus, 1995. Originally published in *Fumeurs d'opium*. Paris: Flammarion, 1896.

Bonah, Christian, and Anne Rasmussen, ed. *Histoire et médicament aux XIXe et XXe siècles*. Paris: Glyphe, 2005.

Bovet, Daniel. *Une chimie qui guérit*. Paris: Payot, 1988.

Brocheux, Pierre, and Daniel Hémery. *Indochine. La colonisation ambiguë, 1858–1954*. Paris: La Découverte, 2001 [1994].

Burke, Timothy. *Lifebuoy Men, Lux Women. Commodification, Consumption and Cleanliness in Modern Zimbabwe*. London: Leicester University Press, 1996.

Cadière, Léopold. *Croyances et pratiques religieuses des Vietnamiens*. Saigon: École française d'Extrême-Orient (EFEO), 1955.

Cassier, Maurice. "Brevets pharmaceutiques et santé publique en France. Opposition et dispositifs spécifiques d'appropriation des médicaments entre 1791 et 2004." *Entreprise & histoire* 36 (2004): 29–46.

Cayez, Pierre. *Rhône-Poulenc, 1895–1975*. Paris: Armand Colin and Masson, 1988.

Chakrabarty, Dipesh. *Provincializing Europe. Postcolonial Thought and Historical Difference*. Princeton and Oxford: Princeton University Press, 2007 [2000].

Charbonnier, Roger. *Contribution à l'étude de la prophylaxie antivénérienne à Hanoi*. Paris: Jouve & Cie, 1936.

Chauveau, Sophie. "Genèse de la 'sécurité sanitaire': Les produits pharmaceutiques en France aux XIXe et XXe siècles." *Revue d'histoire moderne et contemporaine* 51, 2 (2004): 88–117.

Chauveau, Sophie. *L'invention pharmaceutique: La pharmacie française entre l'état et la société au XXe siècle*. Paris: Sanofi-Synthélabo, 1999.

Chauveau, Sophie. "Marché et publicité des médicaments." In *Histoire et médicament aux XIXe et XXe siècles*, edited by Christian Bonah and Anne Rasmussen, 189–213. Paris: Glyphe, 2005.

Cochran, Sherman G. *Chinese Medicine Men: Consumer Culture in China and Southeast Asia*. Cambridge: Harvard University Press, 2006.

Collin, Johanne, Marcelo Otero, and Laurence Monnais, ed. *Le médicament au cœur de la socialité contemporaine. Regards croisés sur un objet complexe*. Sainte Foy: Presses de l'Université du Québec, 2006.

Conklin, Alice. *A Mission to Civilize: the Republican Idea of Empire in France and West Africa, 1895–1930*. Stanford: Stanford University Press, 1997.

Cook, Harold J. *Matters of Exchange: Commerce, Medicine, and Science in the Dutch Golden Age*. New Haven and London: Yale University Press, 2007.

Craig, David. *Familiar Medicine. Everyday Health Knowledge and Practice in Today's Vietnam*. Honolulu: University of Hawai'i Press, 2002.

Cunningham, Charles E. "Thai 'Injection Doctors': Antibiotic Mediators." *Social Science & Medicine* 4 (1970): 1–24.

Dagognet, François. *La raison et les remèdes*. Paris: Presses universitaires de France, 1964.

Debusman, Robert. "Médicalisation et pluralisme au Cameroun allemand: autorité médicale et stratégies profanes." *Outre-mers. Revue d'histoire* 90, 1 (2003): 225–46.

Digby, Anne. "Self-Medication and the Trade in Medicine within a Multi-Ethnic Context: A Case Study of South Africa from the Mid-Nineteenth to Mid-Twentieth Centuries." *Social History of Medicine* 18, 3 (2005): 439–57.

Dikötter, Frank, Lars Laaman, and Zhou Xun, ed. *Narcotic Culture. A History of Drugs in China*. Chicago: Chicago University Press, 2004.

Drucker, Ernest, Philip G. Alcabes, and Preston A. Marx. "The Injection Century: Massive Unsterile Injections and the Emergence of Human Pathogens." *The Lancet* 358 (2001): 1989–92.

Dunn, Frederick L. "Traditional Asian Medicine and Cosmopolitan Medicine as Adaptive Systems." In *Asian Medical Systems: A Comparative Study*, edited by Charles Leslie, 133–58. Berkeley: University of California Press, 1976.

Duong Dat Van, C. W. Binns, and Truyen Van Le. "Availability of Antibiotics as Over-the-Counter Drugs in Pharmacies: A Threat to Public Health in Vietnam." *Tropical Medicine and International Health* 2, 12 (1997): 1133–39.

Dương Bá Bành. *Histoire de la médecine au Viêt nam*. Hanoi: EFEO, 1947–50.

Dutton, George. "Advertising, Modernity, and Consumer Culture in Colonial Vietnam." In *The Reinvention of Tradition. Modernity and the Middle Class in Urban Vietnam*, edited by Van Nguyen-Marshall, Lisa Drummond Welch, and Danièle Bélanger, 21–42. Singapore: Asian Research Institute, 2012.

Eckart, Wolfgang. "The Colony as Laboratory: German Sleeping Sickness Campaigns in German East Africa and in Togo, 1900–14." *History & Philosophy of Life Sciences* 24 (2002): 69–89.

Ecks, Stefan. "Pharmaceutical Citizenship: Antidepressant Marketing and the Promise of Demarginalization in India." *Anthropology & Medicine*, 12, 3 (2005): 239–54.

Ernst, Waltraud, ed. *Plural Medicine, Tradition and Modernity, 1800–2000*. London and New York, Routledge, 2002.

Etkin, Nina L. "'Side Effects': Cultural Constructions and Reinterpretations of Western Pharmaceuticals." *Medical Anthropology Quarterly* 6 (1994): 99–113.

Exposition coloniale internationale (Paris), Bordes, L. A., Dr., *Le paludisme en Indochine*. Hanoi: IDEO, 1931.

Exposition coloniale internationale (Paris), Gaide, Laurent, and Paul Campunaud. *Le péril vénérien en Indochine*. Hanoi: IDEO, 1930.

Fadlon, Judith. "Meridians, Chakras and Psycho-Neuro-Immunology: The Dematerializing Body and the Domestication of Alternative Medicine." *Body & Society* 10, 4 (2004): 69–86.

Fanon, Frantz. 1959, "Médecine et colonialisme." In *L'an V de la révolution algérienne*, 111–40. Paris: François Maspéro, 1959.

Far Eastern Association for Tropical Medicine (FEATM). *Rapports du Xe Congrès de la FEATM*. Hanoi: IDEO, 1938.

FEATM. *Transactions of the Ninth Congress of the Far Eastern Association for Tropical Medicine Held in Nankin, China*. Nankin: National Health Administration, 1935.

Farquhar, Judith. "For Your Reading Pleasure: Self-Health (*Ziwo baojian*) Information in 1990s Beijing." *Positions. East Asia Cultures Critique* 9, 1 (2001): 105–30.

Faure, Olivier. *Les Français et leur médecine au XIXe siècle*. Paris: Belin, 1993.

Faure, Olivier. "Les officines pharmaceutiques françaises: de la réalité au mythe, fin XIXe-début XXe siècle." *Revue d'histoire moderne et contemporaine*, 43 (1996): 672–85.

Feierman, Steven, and John M. Janzen, ed. *The Social Basis of Health and Illness in Africa*. Berkeley: University of California Press, 1992.

Finer, David. *Pressing Priorities: Consumer Drug Information in the Vietnamese Marketplace*. Stockholm: Karolinska Institutet, Department of Public Health Sciences/ Global Health (IHCAR), 1999.

Flint, Karen E. *Healing Traditions. African Medicine, Cultural Exchange, and Competition in South Africa, 1820–1948*. Athens: Ohio University Press, 2008.

Fox, Nick J., and Katie J. Ward. "Pharma in the Bedroom . . . and the Kitchen . . . The Pharmaceuticalisation of Daily Life." *Sociology of Health & Illness* 30, 6 (2008): 856–68.

Frank, Arthur W. "What's Wrong with Medical Consumerism?" In *Consuming Health, the Commodification of Healthcare*, edited by Sara Henderson and Alan Petersen, 11–30. New York and London: Routledge, 2002.

Frank, Robert, and Gunnar Stollberg. "Conceptualizing Hybridization. On the Diffusion of Asian Medical Knowledge to Germany." *International Sociology* 19, 1 (2004): 79–88.

Gaudillière, Jean-Paul. "Drugs Trajectories." *Studies in the History of Biological and Biomedical Sciences* 36 (2005): 603–11.

Gaudillière, Jean-Paul. "Genesis and Development of a Biomedical Object: Styles of Thoughts, Styles of Work and the History of Sex Steroids." *Studies in History and Philosophy of Science* 35, 3 (2004): 525–43.

Goscha, Christopher. "'Le barbare moderne': Nguyen Van Vinh et la complexité de la odernisation coloniale au Viêt nam." *Outre-mers. Revue d'histoire* 88, 2 (2001): 319–46.

Gouvernement général de l'Indochine, Direction des services économiques. *Répertoire des sociétés anonymes indochinoises.* Hanoi: IDEO, 1944.

Gouvernement général de l'Indochine. *Annuaire statistique de l'Indochine, 1923–1929.* Hanoi: IDEO, 1931.

Gouzien, Paul, Dr. *Manuel franco-tonkinois de conversation spécialement à l'usage des médecins.* Paris: Challamel, 1897.

Greene, Jeremy A. *Generic. The Unbranding of Modern Medicine.* Baltimore: Johns Hopkins University Press, 2014.

Greene, Jeremy A. "Making Medicines Essential: The Emergent Centrality of Pharmaceuticals in Global Health." *BioSocieties* 6 (2011): 10–33.

Greene, Jeremy A., Flurin Condrau, and Elizabeth Siegel Watkins, ed. *Therapeutic Revolution. Pharmaceutical and Social Change in the Twentieth Century.* Chicago: Chicago University Press, 2016.

Guénel, Annick. "The Conference on Rural Hygiene in Bandung, 1937: Towards a New Vision of Health Care?" In *Global Movements, Local Concerns. Medicine and Health in Southeast Asia*, edited by Laurence Monnais and Harold J. Cook, 62–80. Singapore: NUS Press, 2012.

Headrick, Daniel R. *The Tools of Empire. Technology and European Imperialism in the Nineteenth Century.* New York and Oxford: Oxford University Press, 1981.

Hocquard, Charles-Édouard., Dr. *Une campagne au Tonkin*, introduced and edited by Philippe Papin. Paris: Arléa, 1999 [1892].

Hodges, Sarah. *Contraception, Colonialism, and Commerce. Birth Control in South India, 1920–40.* Aldershot: Ashgate, 2008.

Hoffman, John P. "The Historical Shift in the Perception of Opiates: From Medicine to Social Menace." *Journal of Psychoactive Drugs* 22, 1 (1990): 53–62.

Hoi-Eun Kim. "Cure for Empire: The 'Conquer-Russia-Pill,' Pharmaceutical Manufacturers, and the Making of Patriotic Japanese, 1904–45." *Medical History* 57 (2013): 249–68.

Hooker, Claire, and Hans Pols. "Introduction. Health Medicine and the Media." *Health & History* 8, 1 (2006): 1–13.

Howard-Jones, Norman. "A Critical Study of the Origins and Early Development of Hypodermic Medication." *Journal of the History of Medicine* 2, 2 (1947): 201–49.

Jankowiak, William, and Daniel Bradburd, ed. *Drugs, Labor, and Colonial Expansion.* Tucson: University of Arizona Press, 2003.

Kelly, Gail P. "Conflict in the Classroom: A Case Study from Vietnam, 1918–1938." *British Journal of Sociology of Education* 8, 2 (1987): 191–212.

Kremer, Michael. "Pharmaceuticals and the Developing World." *The Journal of Economic Perspectives* 16, 4 (2002): 67–90.

Lachenal, Guillaume. *The Lomidine Files. The Untold Story of a Medical Disaster in Colonial Africa.* Baltimore: Johns Hopkins University Press, 2017.

Lachenal, Guillaume. *Le médicament qui devait sauver l'Afrique. Un scandale pharmaceutique aux colonies.* Paris: La Découverte, 2014.

Larcher, Agathe. "La voie étroite des réformes coloniales et la collaboration franco-Annamite, 1917–1928." *Revue française d'histoire d'outre-mer* 82, 309 (1995): 397–420.

Lean, Eugenia. "The Modern Elixir: Medicine as a Consumer Item in the Early Twentieth-century Chinese Press." *UCLA Historical Journal* 15 (1995): 65–92.

Lears, T. J. Jacskon. "From Salvation to Self-realization: Advertising and the Therapeutic Roots of the Consumer Culture, 1880–1930." In *The Culture of Consumerism. Critical Essays in American History, 1880–1980,* edited by Richard Wightman Fox and T. J. Jackson Lears, 1–38. New York: Pantheon Books, 1983.

Le Failler, Philippe. "Le coût social de l'opium au Vietnam. La problématique des drogues dans le philtre de l'Histoire." *Journal asiatique,* 283, 1 (1995): 239–64.

Le Failler, Philippe. *Monopole et prohibition de l'opium en Indochine. Le pilori des chimères.* Paris: L'Harmattan, 2001.

Lesch, John. "Chemistry and Biomedicine in an Industrial Setting: The Invention of Sulfa Drugs." In *Chemical Sciences in the Modern World,* edited by Seymour H. Mauskopf, 158–215. Philadelphia: University of Pennsylvania Press, 1993.

Lesch, John. *The First Miracle Drugs. How the Sulfa Drugs Transformed Medicine.* New York and Oxford: Oxford University Press, 2007.

Lessard, Micheline. "Organisons-nous! Racial Antagonism and Vietnamese Economic Nationalism in the Early Twentieth Century." *French Colonial History* 8 (2007): 171–201.

Liew Kai Khiun. "Newspapers and the Communication of Medical Sciences in Colonial Malaya, 1840s-1941." *EASTS. East Asian Science, Technology and Society. An International Journal* 3, 2–3 (2009): 209–30.

Link, Perry E. *Mandarin Ducks and Butterflies: Popular Fiction in Early Twentieth-Century Chinese Cities.* Berkeley: University of California Press, 1981.

Lock, Margaret, and Patricia Kaufert. "Menopause, Local Biologies, and Culture of Aging." *American Journal of Human Biology* 13, 4 (2001): 494–504.

Löwy, Ilana. "Biotherapies of Chronic Diseases in the Inter-war Period: From Witte's Peptone to Penicillium Extract." *Studies in the History and Philosophy of Biological and Biomedical Sciences* 36 (2005): 675–95.

Magendie, François. *Formulaire pour la préparation et l'emploi de plusieurs nouveaux médicaments tels la noix vomique, la morphine, etc.* Paris: Méquignon-Marvis, 1822.

Marks, Harry M. *The Progress of Experiment: Science and Therapeutic Reform in the United States, 1900–1990.* Cambridge: Cambridge University Press, 1997.

Marr, David G. "Vietnamese Attitudes Regarding Illness and Healing." In *Death and Disease in Southeast Asia. Explorations in Social, Medical and Demographic History*, edited by Norman G. Owen, 162–87. Singapore: Oxford University Press, 1987.

Marr, David G. *Vietnamese Traditions on Trial, 1925–1945.* Berkeley: University of California Press, 1981.

McHale, Shawn F. *Print and Power. Confucianism, Communism, and Buddhism in the Making of Modern Vietnam.* Honolulu: University of Hawai'i Press, 2004.

Melrose, Dianna. *Bitter Pills: Medicines and the Third World Poor.* Oxford: Oxfam, 1982.

Mills, James H., and Patricia Barton, ed. *Drugs and Empires. Essays in Modern Imperialism and Intoxication, c. 1500–c. 1930.* Basingstoke: Palgrave McMillan, 2000.

Monnais, Laurence. "Colonised and Neurasthenic: From the Appropriation of a Word to the Reality of a Malaise de Civilisation in Urban French Vietnam." *Health & History* 14, 1 (2012): 121–42.

Monnais, Laurence. "Traditional, Complementary, and Perhaps Scientific? Professional Views of Vietnamese Medicine in the Age of Colonialism." In *Southern Medicine for Southern People. Vietnamese Medicine in the Making*, edited by Laurence Monnais, C. Michele Thompson, and Ayo Wahlberg, 61–84. Newcastle Upon Tyne: Cambridge Scholars Publishing, 2012.

Monnais, Laurence. "Le Dr Nguyen Van Luyen et ses confrères. La médecine privée dans le Viêt nam colonial." *Moussons. Recherches en sciences humaines sur l'Asie du Sud-est – Social Science Research on Southeast Asia*, 15 (2010): 75–95.

Monnais, Laurence. "'Modern Medicine' in French Colonial Vietnam. From the Importation of a Model to its Nativisation." In *Development of Modern Medicine in non-European Countries: Historical Perspectives*, edited by Hormoz Ebrahimnejad, 127–59. London and New York: Routledge, The Royal Asiatic Society Book Series, 2009.

Monnais, Laurence. "Leprosy and Lepers in Vietnam: Could Confinement be 'Humanized'?" In *Public Health in Asia and the Pacific. Historical and Comparative Perspectives*, edited by Lewis Milton and Kerrie McPherson, 122–38. London and New York: Routledge, 2008.

Monnais, Laurence. "Les premiers pas inédits d'une professionnelle de santé insolite: La sage-femme vietnamienne dans les années 1900–40." In *Le Vietnam au féminin. Viêt Nam: Women's Realities*, edited by Gisèle Bousquet and Nora Taylor, 67–106. Paris: Les Indes Savantes, 2005.

Monnais, Laurence. "La professionnalisation du 'médecin indochinois' au XXe siècle: des paradoxes d'une médicalisation coloniale." *Actes de la recherche en sciences sociales* 43 (2002): 36–43.

Monnais, Laurence, C. Michele Thompson, and Ayo Wahlberg, ed. *Southern Medicine for Southern People. Vietnamese Medicine in the Making*. Newcastle Upon Tyne: Cambridge Scholars Publishing, 2012.

Monnais, Laurence, and Harold J. Cook, ed. *Global Movements, Local Concerns. Medicine and Health in Southeast Asia*. Singapore: NUS Press, 2012.

Monnais, Laurence, and Noémi Tousignant. "The Values of Versatility: Pharmacists, Plants, and Place in the French (post)Colonial World." *Comparative Studies in Society & History* 58, 2 (2016): 432–62.

Monnais-Rousselot, Laurence. *Médecine et colonisation. L'aventure indochinoise, 1860–1939*. Paris: CNRS Éditions, 1999.

Morin, Henri G. S. *Entretiens sur le paludisme et sa prévention en Indochine*. Hanoi: IDEO, 1935.

Mukharji, Projit. *Doctoring Traditions: Ayurveda, Small Technologies, and Braided Sciences*. Chicago: University of Chicago Press, 2016.

Mukharji, Projit, and David Hardiman, ed. *Medical Marginality in South Asia: Situating Subaltern Therapeutics*. Abingdon: Routledge, 2012.

Neill, Deborah. "Paul Ehrlich's Colonial Connections: Scientific Networks and Sleeping Sickness Drug Therapy Research, 1900–14." *Social History of Medicine* 22, 1 (2009): 61–77.

Neukirch, Jacques. "Comment le Français moyen utilise les médicaments?" *Hommes & commerce* 23 (1954): 63–67.

Newton, Paul, Stéphane Proulx, Michael Green et al. "Fake Artesunate in Southeast Asia." *The Lancet* 357, 9272 (2001): 1948–50.

Nguyễn Phương Ngọc. "The Post-Đổi mới Construction of the Vietnamese Pharmacopoeia: The Case of the Pharmaceutical Company Traphaco." In *Southern Medicine for Southern People. Vietnamese Medicine in the Making*, edited by Laurence Monnais, C. Michele Thompson, and Ayo Wahlberg, 179–201. Newcastle Upon Tyne: Cambridge Scholars Publishing, 2012.

Nguyễn Thi Kim Chuc and Göran Tomson. "Doi moi and Private Pharmacies: A Case Study on Dispensing and Financial Issues in Hanoi, Vietnam." *European Journal of Clinical Pharmacology* 55 (1999): 325–32.

Nguyen Thuy Linh. *Childbirth, Maternity and Medical Pluralism in French Colonial Vietnam, 1880–1945*. Rochester, NY: University of Rochester Press, 2016.

Nguyễn Văn Ký. *La société vietnamienne face à la modernité. Le Tonkin de la fin du XIXe siècle à la seconde guerre mondiale*. Paris: L'Harmattan, 1995.

Nguyen, Vinh-Kim, Nathalie Bajos, Françoise Dubois-Arber et al. "Remedicalizing an Epidemic: From HIV Treatment as Prevention to HIV Treatment is Prevention." *AIDS* 25, 3 (2010): 291–93.

Okumura Junko, Wakai Susumu, and Umenai Takusei. "Drug Utilisation and Self-medication in Rural Communities." *Social Science & Medicine* 54, 12 (2002): 1876–86.

Osseo-Asare, Abena. *Bitter Roots: The Search for Healing Plants in Africa*. Chicago: University of Chicago Press, 2014.

Packard, Randall. *The Making of a Tropical Disease. A Short History of Malaria*. Baltimore: Johns Hopkins University, 2007.

Pairaudeau, Natasha. *Mobile Citizens: French Indians in Indochina 1858–1954.* Copenhagen: NIAS Press, 2016.

Parascandola, John. "Alkaloids to Arsenicals: Systematic Drug Discovery before the First World War." In *The Inside Story of Medicines: A Symposium,* edited by Elaine Stroud and Gregory Higby, 72–92. Madison: American Institute for the History of Pharmacy, 1997.

Parascandola, John. "Chaulmoogra Oil and the Treatment of Leprosy." *Pharmacy in History* 45, 2 (2003): 47–57.

Paucot, Dr. *Notions d'hygiène à l'égard des indigènes.* Paris: Challamel, 1908.

Petryna, Adriana, Andrew Lakoff, and Arthur Kleinman, ed. *Global Pharmaceuticals. Ethics, Markets, Practices.* Durham and London: Duke University Press, 2006.

Peycam, Philippe M. F. *The Birth of Vietnamese Political Journalism: Saigon, 1916–1930.* New York: Columbia University Press, 2012.

Pluchon, Pierre. *Histoire des médecins et des pharmaciens de Marine et des Colonies.* Paris: Privat, 1985.

Pols, Hans, C. Michele Thompson, and John Harley Warner, ed. *Translating the Body. Medical Education in Southeast Asia.* Singapore: NUS Press, 2017.

Porter, Roy. "The Patient's View. Doing Medical History from Below." *Theory & Society* 14, 2 (1985): 175–98.

Pound, Pandora, Nicky Britten, Myfanwy Morgan et al. "Resisting Medicines: A Synthesis of Qualitative Studies of Medicine Taking." *Social Science & Medicine* 61, 1 (2005): 133–55.

Quirke, Viviane. *Collaboration in the Pharmaceutical Industry. Changing Relationships in Britain and France 1935–1965.* London: Routledge, 2007.

Raffin, Anne. "Postcolonial Vietnam: Hybrid Modernity." *Postcolonial Studies* 11, 3 (2008): 329–44.

Rasmussen, Anne. "Les enjeux d'une histoire des formes pharmaceutiques: la galénique, l'officine et l'industrie (XIXe-début XXe siècle)." *Entreprises & histoire* 36 (2004): 17–20.

Reid, Anthony. *Southeast Asia in the Age of Commerce, 1450–1680,* vol. 2, "Expansion and Crisis." New Haven, CT: Yale University Press, 1993.

Riethmiller, Steven. "Ehrlich, Bertheim and Atoxyl: The Origins of Modern Chemotherapy." *Bulletin of the History of Chemistry* 23 (1999): 28–33.

Rosenberg, Charles. *Explaining Epidemics and Other Studies in the History of Medicine.* Cambridge: Cambridge University Press, 1992.

Ross, J. E., and S.M. Tomkins. "The British Reception of Salvarsan." *Journal of the History of Medicine and Allied Sciences* 52, 4 (1997): 398–423.

Ruffat, Michèle. *175 ans d'industrie pharmaceutique française. Histoire de Synthélabo.* Paris: La Découverte, 1996.

Sallet, Albert, Dr. *L'officine sino-annamite. La médecine annamite et la préparation des remèdes.* Paris: Imprimerie nationale, 1931.

Sarraut, Albert. *La mise en valeur des colonies françaises.* Paris: Payot, 1923.

Shapiro, Hugh. "The Puzzle of Spermatorrhea in Republic China." *Positions. East Asia Cultures Critique* 6, 3 (1998): 552–96.

Silverman, Milton, Mia Lydecker, and Philip Randolph Lee. *Bad Medicine: The Prescription Drug Industry in the Third World.* Stanford: Stanford University Press, 1992.

Simonet, Daniel. "Une analyse du marché pharmaceutique vietnamien," *Cahiers d'études et de recherches francophones/Santé* 11, 3 (2001):155–60.

Sivaramakrishnan, Kavita. *Old Potions, New Bottles. Recasting Indigenous Medicine in Colonial Punjab (1850–1945)*. Hyderabad: Orient Longman, 2006.

Société des nations (SDN), Organisation d'hygiène. *Enquête sur les besoins en quinine des pays impaludés et sur l'extension du paludisme dans le monde*. Genève: SDN, 1932.

Tagliacozzo, Eric. *Secret Trades, Porous Borders. Smuggling and States along a Southeast Asian Frontier, 1865–1915*. New Haven, CT: Yale University Press, 2005.

Thompson, C. Michele. *Vietnamese Traditional Medicine: A Social History*. Singapore: NUS Press, 2015.

Thompson, C. Michele. "Medicine, Nationalism, and Revolution in Vietnam: the Roots of a Medical Collaboration to 1945." *EASTM Journal* 21 (2003): 114–48.

Tomes, Nancy. "Merchants of Health: Medicine and Consumer Culture in the United States, 1900–40." *The Journal of American History* 88, 2 (2001): 519–47.

Tousignant, Noémi. *Edges of Exposure: Toxicology and the Problem of Capacity in Postcolonial Senegal*. Durham: Duke University Press, 2018.

Tousignant, Noémi. "Trypanosomes, Toxicity and Resistance: The Politics of Mass Therapy in French Colonial Africa." *Social History of Medicine* 25, 3 (2012): 625–43.

Tsikounas, Myriam. "Quand l'alcool fait sa pub. Les publicités en faveur de l'alcool dans la presse française, de la Loi Roussel à la Loi Evin (1873–1998)." *Le Temps des médias* 1, 2 (2004): 99–114.

Van Der Geest, Sjaak, and Susan Reynolds Whyte. "The Charm of Medicines: Metaphors and Metonyms." *Medical Anthropology Quarterly* 3, 4 (1989): 345–67.

Van Der Geest, Sjaak, and Susan Reynolds Whyte. *The Context of Medicines in Developing Countries. Studies in Pharmaceutical Anthropology*. Dordrecht and Boston: Kluwer Academic Publishers, 1988.

Van Der Geest, Sjaak, Susan Whyte, and Anita Hardon. "The Anthropology of Pharmaceuticals: A Biographical Approach." *Annual Review of Anthropology* 25 (1996): 153–78.

Van Nguyen-Marshall, Lisa Drummond Welch, and Danièle Bélanger, ed. *The Reinvention of Tradition. Modernity and the Middle Class in Urban Vietnam*. Singapore: Asian Research Institute, 2012.

Vaughan, Megan. *Curing Their Ills. Colonial Power and African Illness*. Cambridge: Polity Press, 1992.

Vidal, Louis. *Dictionnaire des spécialités pharmaceutiques*. Paris: Office de vulgarisation scientifique, 1940.

Vorapheth, Kham. *Commerce et colonisation en Indochine, 1860–1945*. Paris: Les Indes savantes, 2004.

Vuckovic, Nancy. "Fast Relief: Buying Time with Medications." *Medical Anthropology Quarterly* 13, 1 (1999): 51–68.

Vũ Trọng Phụng. *Dumb Luck. A Novel*, translated and introduced by Peter Zinoman. Ann Arbor: University of Michigan Press, 2002 [1936].

Vũ Trọng Phụng, *Lục Xì. Prostitution and Venereal Disease in Colonial Hanoi*, translated and introduced by Shaun K. Malarney. Honolulu: University of Hawai'i Press, 2011.

Wahlberg, Ayo. "Bio-politics and the Promotion of Traditional Herbal Medicine in Vietnam." *Health. An Interdisciplinary Journal for the Social Study of Health, Illness and Medicine* 10, 2 (2006): 123–47.

Warner, John Harley. *The Therapeutic Perspective: Medical Practice, Knowledge and Identity in America, 1820–85*. Cambridge: Cambridge University Press, 1986.

Weatherhall, Miles. *In Search of A Cure: A History of Pharmaceutical Discovery*. Oxford: Oxford University Press, 1990.

Weisz, George. "Regulating Specialties in France during the first Half of the Twentieth Century." *Social History of Medicine* 15, 3 (2002): 457–80.

White, Luise. "'They Could Make their Victims Dull': Genders and Genres, Fantasies and Cures in Colonial Southern Uganda." *The American Historical Review* 100, 5 (1995): 1379–1402.

Wilde, Sally. "The Elephants in the Doctor-Patient Relationship: Patients' Clinical Interactions and the Changing Surgical Landscape of the 1890s." *Health & History* 9, 1 (2007): 2–27.

Williamson, Judith. *Decoding Advertisements. Ideology and Meaning in Advertisement*. London: Marion Boyars, 1978.

Wolffers, Ivan. "The Role of Pharmaceuticals in the Privatization Process in Vietnam's Health Care System." *Social Science & Medicine* 41, 9 (1995): 1325–32.

Wong, Wendy Suiyi. "Establishing the Modern Advertising Languages. Patent Medicine Newspaper Advertisements in Hong Kong, 1945–1969." *Journal of Design History* 13, 3 (2000): 213–26.

Woodside, Alexander. "The Development of Social Organizations in Vietnamese Cities in the Late Colonial Period." *Pacific Affairs* 41, 1 (1971): 39–64.

World Bank. *Vietnam Living Standards Surveys (1997–1998)*. Washington, DC: World Bank, 2001.

World Health Organization (WHO). *Promoting Rational Use of Medicines: Core Components – WHO Policy Perspectives on Medicines*, No. 005. Geneva: WHO, September 2002.

WHO. *Traditional Medicine Strategy, 2002–2005*. Geneva: WHO, 2002.

Yang, Timothy. "Selling an Imperial Dream: Japanese Pharmaceuticals, National Power, and the Science of Quinine Self-Sufficiency." *EASTS. East Asian Science, Technology and Society. An International Journal* 6, 1 (2012): 101–25.

Yvon-Trân, Florence. "Artisanat et commerce villageois dans le Viêt nam prémoderne, du XIe au XIXe siècle. Le cas de l'ancienne agglomération villageoise de Phu Ninh (région du Kinh Bac)." *Bulletin de l'École française d'Extrême-Orient* 88 (2001): 217–47.

Zhang, Yuehong E. "Switching between Traditional Chinese Medicine and Viagra: Cosmopolitanism and Medical Pluralism Today." *Medical Anthropology* 26 (2007): 53–96.

Zinoman, Peter. "Introduction." In *Dumb Luck. A Novel*, introduced and translated by Peter Zinoman, 1–30. Ann Arbor: University of Michigan Press, 2002.

Zola, Irving Kenneth. "Structural Constraints in the Doctor-Patient Relationship: The Case of Non-compliance." In *The Relevance of Social Science for Medicine*, edited by Leon Eisenberg and Arthur Kleinman, 241–52. Rordrecht: Reidel, 1981.

Unpublished Work

Baruah, Ved. "Addicts, Peddlers and Reformers: A Social History of Opium in Assam, 1826–1947." PhD dissertation, Cardiff University, 2017.

Guénel, Annick. "Malaria, Colonial Economics, and Migrations in Vietnam." Paper presented at the Fourth Annual Conference of the European Association of Southeast Asian Studies, Paris, France, September 1–4, 2004.

Guénel, Annick. "Malaria Control, Land Occupation, and Scientific Developments in Vietnam in the Twentieth Century." Paper presented at the Fifty-First Annual Meeting of the Association for Asian Studies, Boston, USA, March 11–14, 1999.

Guénel, Annick. "Nationalism and Vietnamese Medicine." Paper presented at the Eleventh International Conference on the History of Science in East Asia, Munich, Germany, August 11–13, 2005.

Jeanselme, Édouard, Dr. "Les principaux facteurs de la morbidité et de la mortalité indochinoise." Paper presented at the Congrès colonial français. Compte-rendu de la section de médecine et d'hygiène coloniale, Paris, France May 29–June 5, 1904.

Mertens, Myriam, "Chemical Compounds in the Congo: Pharmaceuticals and the 'Crossed History' of Public Health in Belgian Africa." PhD dissertation, University of Ghent, 2014.

Villemagne-Renard, Claire. "Les commerçants et les colons Français, Acteurs de la vie économique et politique du Tonkin: Les membres des Chambres de commerce et des Chambres d'agriculture, de leur création aux années Doumer." Paper presented at "Le contact colonial," Université Paris-Sorbonne, November 9–10, 2007.

Index